Operative Dictations in Pediatric Surgery

Dominic J. Papandria
Gail E. Besner • R. Lawrence Moss
Karen A. Diefenbach
Editors

Operative Dictations in Pediatric Surgery

Springer

Editors
Dominic J. Papandria
Department of Surgery
Emory University
Atlanta, GA
USA

Gail E. Besner
Department of Pediatric Surgery
Nationwide Children's Hospital
Columbus, OH
USA

R. Lawrence Moss
Nemours Children's Health System
Jacksonville, FL
USA

Karen A. Diefenbach
Nationwide Children's Hospital
Columbus, OH
USA

ISBN 978-3-030-24211-4 ISBN 978-3-030-24212-1 (eBook)
https://doi.org/10.1007/978-3-030-24212-1

This Springer imprint is published by the registered company Springer Nature Switzerland AG
The registered company address is: Gewerbestrasse 11, 6330 Cham, Switzerland

To Smedley, Kinch, and Chumley – my one love and my two epic sidekicks – you followed where the path led and offered up the best parts of yourselves to add delight to the journey. I am a better man every day despite myself and because of you all.

Dominic J. Papandria

To my mother who instilled in me the desire to become a surgeon-scientist before the term was even invented; to my son, Matthew, and daughter, Nicole, who never fail to amaze me; to my husband, David, who has always supported me; and to the many patients who have entrusted their care to me.

Gail E. Besner

To my greatest teachers: the many children and families for whom I have had the great privilege to care. To the many students and residents who have left me confident that surgery has an exciting future and is in the best of hands. To my wife Kris and my three children Jackson, Krissy, and Ruby who mean more than the world to me.

R. Lawrence Moss

To my parents who gave me the courage to pursue my dream; to my sister, my biggest cheerleader; and to my husband for his love and unfailing support, I would not be here without you.

Karen A. Diefenbach

Preface

In the tradition of the adult text, *Operative Dictations in Pediatric Surgery*, this new volume is designed as a concise guide to the pediatric surgical trainee and practicing surgeon alike. The surgical care of children is inherently multidisciplinary, and we are excited to share this work with our community of surgeons, urologists, gynecologists, head and neck surgeons, and allied health providers. We greatly appreciate the support and enthusiasm on the part of Springer Publishing in coordinating the efforts of our fantastic team of authors to produce this inaugural edition. The book provides summary information across a great variety of surgical and endoscopic procedures, together with template operative dictations to orient learners to the pertinent details and technical variations of the operation. Each chapter also includes procedure-specific indications and risks that are relevant to the consent process.

Our collaborating authors – 81 in all – represent 8 distinct surgical subspecialties and are drawn from 18 institutions throughout North America. We are delighted to offer their collective expertise and perspective to our colleagues and trainees who care for children across the surgical spectrum. In preparing this volume, we have attempted to provide appropriate emphasis on minimally invasive approaches and to portray contemporary practice whenever possible. The result reflects the authors' experiences while still addressing common technical variations to ensure that each chapter is broadly reflective of clinical practice. We do recognize that individual practice is informed by surgeon experience, resource constraints, and other factors, and thus adaptation of the materials included is expected to suit each clinical situation.

As the pediatric surgical community continues to advance the science and technical sophistication of the care of this fragile population, we embrace new challenges and strive to invest in the future of this most rewarding discipline. If we can help to perpetuate the continued success of our peers and the understanding of those who will someday follow in the footsteps, that will be our ultimate satisfaction in this endeavor.

Atlanta, GA, USA — Dominic J. Papandria
Columbus, OH, USA — Gail E. Besner
Jacksonville, FL, USA — R. Lawrence Moss
Columbus, OH, USA — Karen A. Diefenbach

Contents

Contributors

Pablo Aguayo, MD, FACS, FAAP Department of Surgery, Children's Mercy Hospital and Clinics/University of Missouri - Kansas City, Kansas City, MO, USA

Jennifer H. Aldrink, MD Nationwide Children's Hospital, The Ohio State University College of Medicine, Division of Pediatric Surgery, Department of Surgery, Columbus, OH, USA

Seth A. Alpert, MD Nationwide Children's Hospital and The Ohio State University Wexner Medical Center, Section of Urology, Columbus, OH, USA

Jamie E. Anderson, MD University of California, Davis, Department of Pediatric General, Thoracic and Fetal Surgery, Sacramento, CA, USA

Charles J. Aprahamian, MD OSF Children's Hospital of Illinois, Division of Pediatric Surgery, Department of Surgery, Peoria, IL, USA

Nicholas Beecroft, BS The Ohio State University College of Medicine, School of Medicine, Columbus, OH, USA

Gail E. Besner, MD Nationwide Children's Hospital, Department of Pediatric Surgery, Columbus, OH, USA

Kim A. Bjorklund, MD, MEd Nationwide Children's Hospital, Department of Plastic, Reconstructive and Hand Surgery, Columbus, OH, USA

Laura A. Boomer, MD Children's Hospital of Richmond, Virginia Commonwealth University, Department of Pediatric Surgery, Richmond, VA, USA

Christopher K. Breuer, MD Nationwide Children's Hospital, Department of Pediatric Surgery, Columbus, OH, USA

Christina B. Ching, MD Nationwide Children's Hospital, Department of Pediatric Urology, Columbus, OH, USA

Dai H. Chung, MD Children's Medical Center Dallas, Department of Surgery, Dallas, TX, USA

Young Chun, MD Johns Hopkins University, Department of Pediatric Surgery, Baltimore, MD, USA

David Coyle, MD, MB BCh BAO Nationwide Children's Hospital, Division of Pediatric Surgery, Columbus, OH, USA

Katherine Culbreath, BS Johns Hopkins Hospital, Department of Surgery, Baltimore, MD, USA

Daniel G. Dajusta, MD Nationwide Children's Hospital, Department of Pediatric Urology, Columbus, OH, USA

Carlos Andrés de la Torre Ramos, MD University Hospital La Paz, Pediatric Surgery, Madrid, Spain

Katherine J. Deans, MD, MHSc Nationwide Children's Hospital, Department of Pediatric Surgery, Columbus, OH, USA

Karen A. Diefenbach, MD Nationwide Children's Hospital, Department of Pediatric Surgery, Columbus, OH, USA

Joseph R. Esparaz, MD University of Illinois College of Medicine at Peoria; OSF Children's Hospital of Illinois, Department of Surgery, Peoria, IL, USA

Renata B. Fabia, MD Nationwide Children's Hospital, Pediatric General Surgery, Columbus, OH, USA

Jeremy G. Fisher, MD Nationwide Children's Hospital, Department of Pediatric Surgery, Columbus, OH, USA

Jason D. Fraser, MD Department of Surgery, Children's Mercy Hospital and Clinics/University of Missouri - Kansas City, Kansas City, MO, USA

Molly E. Fuchs, MD Nationwide Children's Hospital, Department of Pediatric Urology, Columbus, OH, USA

Laura A. Galganski, MD University of California, Davis, Department of Pediatric General, Thoracic and Fetal Surgery, Sacramento, CA, USA

Margaret E. Gallagher, MD Monroe Carell Jr. Children's Hospital at Vanderbilt, Department of Pediatric Surgery, Nashville, TN, USA

Alejandro V. Garcia, MD Johns Hopkins University, Department of Pediatric Surgery, Baltimore, MD, USA

Seth Goldstein, MD, MPH Ann & Robert H Lurie Children's Hospital of Chicago, Chicago, IL, USA

Dani O. Gonzalez, MD Icahn School of Medicine at Mount Sinai, Department of Surgery, New York, NY, USA

Carolyn Gosztyla, MD Walter Reed National Military Medical Center, Department of General Surgery, Bethesda, MD, USA

Greg Grenier, MD Ohio University/Doctors Hospital, Department of Orthopedic Surgery, Columbus, OH, USA

Devin R. Halleran, MD Nationwide Children's Hospital, Center for Colorectal and Pelvic Reconstruction, Columbus, OH, USA

Richard J. Hendrickson, MD Children's Mercy, University of Missouri -Kansas City, Department of Pediatric Surgery, Kansas City, MO, USA

Geri D. Hewitt, MD Nationwide Children's Hospital, Department of Surgery, Columbus, OH, USA

Justin T. Huntington, MD Nationwide Children's Hospital, Department of Pediatric Surgery, Columbus, OH, USA

Christopher Jaeger, MD The Ohio State University Wexner Medical Center, Department of Urology, Columbus, OH, USA

Eric Jelin, MD Johns Hopkins, Department of Surgery, Bloomberg Children's Center, Baltimore, MD, USA

Morgan Johnson, MS The Ohio State University, College of Medicine, Columbus, OH, USA

David Juang, MD, FACS, FAAP Department of Surgery, Children's Mercy Hospital and Clinics/University of Missouri - Kansas City, Kansas City, MO, USA

Lorraine I. Kelley-Quon, MD, MS Children's Hospital Los Angeles, Division of Pediatric Surgery, Department of Surgery, Keck School of Medicine of University of Southern California, Los Angeles, CA, USA

Brian D. Kenney, MD, MPH Pediatric Intensive Care Unit, Nationwide Children's Hospital, Department of Pediatric Surgery, Columbus, OH, USA

Michaela Kollisch-Singule, MD SUNY Upstate Medical University, Department of General Surgery, Syracuse, NY, USA

Afif Kulaylat, MD Nationwide Children's Hospital, Department of Surgery, Columbus, OH, USA

Mitchell R. Ladd, MD, PhD Johns Hopkins Hospital, Department of General Surgery, Baltimore, MD, USA

Amy E. Lawrence, MD Nationwide Children's Hospital, Department of Pediatric Surgery, Columbus, OH, USA

Marc A. Levitt, MD Nationwide Children's Hospital, Center for Colorectal and Pelvic Reconstruction, Columbus, OH, USA

Harold N. Lovvorn III, MD Monroe Carell Jr. Children's Hospital at Vanderbilt, Department of Pediatric Surgery, Nashville, TN, USA

Sara A. Mansfield, MD, MS The Ohio State University Wexner Medical Center, Department of General Surgery, Columbus, OH, USA

Kate A. McCracken, MD Nationwide Children's Hospital, Department of Pediatric & Adolescent Gynecology, Columbus, OH, USA

Daryl J. McLeod, MD, MPH Nationwide Children's Hospital, Department of Surgery, Section of Urology, Columbus, OH, USA

Marc P. Michalsky, MD Professor of Clinical Surgery and Pediatrics, The Ohio State University College of Medicine, Nationwide Children's Hospital, Department of Pediatric Surgery, Columbus, OH, USA

R. Lawrence Moss, MD Nemours Children's Health System, Jacksonville, FL, USA

Anthony J. Munaco, MD OSF Healthcare Children's Hospital of Illinois, University of Illinois College of Medicine at Peoria, Department of Pediatric Surgery, Peoria, IL, USA

Isam Nasr, MD Johns Hopkins Hospital, Department of Pediatric Surgery, Johns Hopkins Children's Center, Baltimore, MD, USA

Bradley J. Needleman, MD The Edwin H. and E. Christopher Ellison Professor of Surgery, The Ohio State University College of Medicine, Wexner Medical Center, Department of Surgery, Columbus, OH, USA

Benedict C. Nwomeh, MD Nationwide Children's Hospital, Department of Pediatric Surgery, Columbus, OH, USA

James A. O'Neill, MD Vanderbilt University Medical Center, Department of Pediatric Surgery, Vanderbilt Children's Hospital, Nashville, TN, USA

Frances C. Okolo, MD University of Pittsburgh Medical Center, Department of General Surgery, Pittsburgh, PA, USA

Ekene A. Onwuka, MD, MS The Ohio State University Wexner Medical Center, Department of General Surgery, Columbus, OH, USA

Dominic J. Papandria, MD Department of Surgery, Emory University, Atlanta, GA, USA

Courtney Pisano, DO, MS Nationwide Children's Hospital, Department of Pediatric Surgery, Columbus, OH, USA

Howard I. Pryor III, MD Division of Pediatric Surgery, Walter Reed National Military Medical Center, Department of Surgery, Bethesda, MD, USA

Laura Rausch, BS, MA, MD Vanderbilt University Medical Center, Department of General Surgery, Nashville, TN, USA

Rebecca M. Rentea, MD Children's Mercy, University of Missouri -Kansas City, Department of Pediatric Surgery, Kansas City, MO, USA

Daniel Rhee, MD, MPH Johns Hopkins School of Medicine, Department of Surgery, Baltimore, MD, USA

Jamie R. Robinson, MD, MS Vanderbilt University Medical Center, Department of General Surgery, Nashville, TN, USA

William B. Rothstein, MD Virginia Commonwealth University Health System, Department of Surgery, Richmond, VA, USA

Payam Saadai, MD UC Davis Medical Center/Shriners Hospital for Children, Division of Pediatric Surgery, Sacramento, CA, USA

Julie Balch Samora, MD, PhD, MPH Nationwide Childrens Hospital, Department of Orthopaedics, Columbus, OH, USA

Kate Savoie, MD, MS Nationwide Children's Hospital, Department of Pediatric Surgery, Columbus, OH, USA

Stefan Scholz, MD University of Pittsburgh School of Medicine, Children's Hospital of Pittsburgh, Department of Pediatric Surgery, Pittsburgh, PA, USA

Rita D. Shelby, MD Nationwide Children's Hospital, Ohio State University Wexner Medical Center, Department of Pediatric Surgery, Columbus, OH, USA

Astrid R. Soares-Medina, MD, FEBPS Assistant Professor of Clinical Surgery and Pediatrics, Ponce Health Sciences University School of Medicine, Mayagüez Medical Center, Department of Pediatric Surgery, Mayagüez, PR, USA

Justin A. Sobrino Department of Surgery, Children's Mercy Hospital and Clinics/University of Missouri - Kansas City, Kansas City, MO, USA

Shawn D. St. Peter, MD Children's Mercy Hospital, Department of Pediatric Surgery, Kansas City, MO, USA

Jennifer Stanger, MD SUNY Upstate Medical University, Department of Pediatric Surgery, Syracuse, NY, USA

Joseph Adam Sujka, MD Children's Mercy Hospital, Department of Pediatric Surgery, Kansas City, MO, USA

Rajan K. Thakkar, MD Nationwide Children's Hospital, Pediatric General Surgery, Columbus, OH, USA

A. Francois Trappey III, MD University of California, Davis, Department of Pediatric General, Thoracic and Fetal Surgery, Sacramento, CA, USA

Kyle J. Van Arendonk, MD, PhD Children's Hospital of Wisconsin, Department of Surgery, Milwaukee, WI, USA

Melissa Vanover, MD University of California, Davis, Department of Pediatric General, Thoracic and Fetal Surgery, Sacramento, CA, USA

Alejandra Vilanova-Sánchez, MD Hospital La Paz, Department of Pediatric Surgery, Madrid, Spain

Paul K. Waltz, MD University of Pittsburgh Medical Center, Department of General Surgery, Pittsburgh, PA, USA

Lea Wehrli, MD Children's Hospital of Pittsburgh of UPMC, Department of Pediatric Surgery, Pittsburgh, PA, USA

Richard J. Wood, MBChB, FCPS(SA) Nationwide Children's Hospital, Center for Colorectal and Pelvic Reconstruction, Columbus, OH, USA

Andrew Yeh, MD University of Pittsburgh, Department of Surgery, Pittsburgh, PA, USA

Jason Zakko, MD Ohio State University Medical Center/Nationwide Children's Hospital, Department of Pediatric Surgery, Columbus, OH, USA

1 Rigid and Flexible Esophagoscopy for Foreign Body Removal

William B. Rothstein and Laura A. Boomer

Indications and Benefits

- Metallic or radiopaque foreign body confirmed radiographically
- Suspected foreign body by history, or impacted organic material
- Benefits: Direct visualization of the foreign material, confirmation of removal, evaluation of the esophageal mucosa

Risks and Alternatives

- Standard risks (bleeding, infection, need for additional procedures, risks of anesthesia)
- Injury to adjacent structures (teeth, pharynx, esophagus)
- Aspiration
- Perforation or laceration of the pharynx or esophagus
- Alternatives: Long laryngoscope with Magill forceps, fluoroscopically guided balloon, or catheter removal

W. B. Rothstein
Virginia Commonwealth University Health System, Department of Surgery, Richmond, VA, USA

L. A. Boomer (✉)
Children's Hospital of Richmond, Virginia Commonwealth University, Department of Pediatric Surgery, Richmond, VA, USA
e-mail: Laura.boomer@vcuhealth.org

Essential Steps

Rigid Esophagoscopy with Foreign Body Removal

1. Place the patient supine with a shoulder roll to facilitate neck extension similar to endotracheal intubation – the "sniffing position." A tooth guard is recommended to avoid dental injury.
2. Select the largest suitable rigid endoscope.
3. Ensure the camera and light source are appropriately set up prior to beginning the procedure, and that all equipment is the appropriate length for the endoscope.
4. Sit or stand at the patient's head.
5. Retract the tongue and protect the teeth with the non-dominant hand, and carefully guard the endotracheal tube, so as to avoid dislodging the tube during the procedure.
6. Insert scope into oral cavity with the lip of the bevel up. Balance it using the thumb and index finger of non-dominant hand as a fulcrum.
7. Under direct visualization, advance scope along posterior pharyngeal wall.
8. Elevate the cricoid with the tip of the scope and advance into the cervical esophagus.
9. Only advance scope when lumen is visualized.
10. Clear secretions with suction while inspecting for foreign body. Inspect for

D. J. Papandria et al. (eds.), *Operative Dictations in Pediatric Surgery*,
https://doi.org/10.1007/978-3-030-24212-1_1

pathology that may be associated with a retained foreign body (esophageal webs, strictures).
11. Use long grasping forceps to remove foreign body. This can be done piecemeal through the lumen of the scope with soft objects. Large solid objects may be grasped tightly to the end of the scope and removed by retracting the scope and grasper together.
12. After removal, reinsert the endoscope to complete the exam by inspecting the lumen at the site of the foreign body to evaluate for damage, and distal to the foreign body to ensure no further obstruction.

Flexible Esophagoscopy with Foreign Body Removal

1. Place patient in the supine position with the neck extended. (Alternatively, the patient may be placed in lateral decubitus position.)
2. Stand at the head of on the right side of the Table.
3. A bite block facilitates easy passage of the scope.
4. Insert an 8–9-mm flexible endoscope over the tongue and advance along the posterior pharynx under direct visualization. In smaller children, a 6-mm pediatric endoscope may be required; however, the working channels of smaller endoscopes will accommodate a smaller range of instruments.
5. Apply gentle insufflation and pressure against the upper esophageal sphincter to advance into cervical esophagus.
6. Clear secretions with suction to adequately visualize the foreign body.
7. Foreign bodies can be grasped with various snares and graspers through the working port of the scope and removed piecemeal or retracted along with the scope.
8. After removal, reinsert the endoscope to complete the exam by inspecting the lumen at the site of the foreign body to evaluate for damage, and distal to the foreign body to ensure no further obstruction.

Table 1.1 Recommended endoscopy sizes

Age	Rigid	Flexible
Premature infant	4	≤6 mm (pediatric gastroscope)
Term infant (0–3 months)	4–5	≤6 mm (pediatric gastroscope)
3–12 months	5–6	≤6 mm (pediatric gastroscope)
1–2 years	6	6–8 mm
2–5 years	6–7	8 mm (adult gastroscope)
5–10 years	7	8 mm (adult gastroscope)
>10 years	8	8 mm (adult gastroscope)

Note These Variations

- The oral cavity can also be navigated by passing the scope along the floor of the mouth, to the right of the tongue, and following the right pyriformis fossa.
- Recommended endoscopy sizes based on patient size listed in Table 1.1.

Template Operative Dictation (Rigid)

Preoperative Diagnosis Esophageal foreign body

Postoperative Diagnosis Esophageal foreign body

Findings
1. Esophageal foreign body at the level of *cricopharyngeus/mid-esophagus/gastroesophageal junction*
2. No evidence of intraluminal injury
3. Normal cervical esophageal anatomy

Procedure(s) Performed Rigid esophagoscopy with foreign body removal

Anesthesia *General endotracheal anesthesia/ Procedural sedation*

Specimen *Coin/foreign object/none*

Estimated Blood Loss None

Indications This is a/an ___-*day/week/month/year*-old *male/female* with a/an ___-*day/hour/week* history of drooling and dysphagia after a choking event. A suspected esophageal foreign body was confirmed radiographically. *He/she* was deemed to be a suitable candidate for rigid esophagoscopy with removal of foreign body.

Procedure in Detail The patient was placed in supine position and appropriately padded after a smooth induction of general anesthesia. A shoulder roll was placed and the neck gently extended. Timeouts were performed using both pre-induction and pre-incision safety checklists with participation of all present in the operative suite. These confirmed the correct patient, procedure, operative site, and additional critical information prior to the start of the procedure. A size ___ rigid endoscope was introduced to the oral cavity and advanced through the upper esophageal sphincter under direct visualization. The foreign body was visualized at the level of the ___. At this point, an optical long grasping forceps was introduced through the lumen of the endoscope and the foreign body was grasped. The foreign body was retracted against the orifice of the endoscope and the endoscope and foreign body were retracted out through the oral cavity. The endoscope was then reinserted past the level of the previous foreign body and slowly withdrawn. The esophageal mucosa appeared intact and undamaged, with no anatomical abnormalities noted. The endoscope was then removed and the procedure terminated.

Upon completion of the procedure, a debriefing checklist was completed to share information critical to the postoperative care of the patient. The patient tolerated the procedure well, was extubated in the operating room, and was transported to the post-anesthesia care unit in stable condition.

Template Operative Dictation (Flexible)

Preoperative Diagnosis Esophageal foreign body

Postoperative Diagnosis Esophageal foreign body

Findings

1. Esophageal foreign body at the level of *cricopharyngeus/mid-esophagus/gastroesophageal junction*
2. No evidence of intraluminal injury
3. Normal cervical esophageal anatomy

Procedure(s) Performed Flexible esophagoscopy with foreign body removal

Anesthesia *General endotracheal anesthesia/Procedural sedation*

Specimen *Coin/foreign object/none*

Estimated Blood Loss None

Indications This is a/an ___-*day/week/month/year*-old *male/female* with a/an ___-*day/hour/week* history of drooling and dysphagia after a choking event. A suspected esophageal foreign body was confirmed radiographically. *He/she* was deemed to be a suitable candidate for flexible esophagoscopy with removal of foreign body.

Procedure in Detail The patient was placed in *supine position/lateral decubitus position* and appropriately padded after a smooth induction of general anesthesia. Timeouts were performed using both pre-induction and pre-incision safety checklists with participation of all present in the operative suite. These confirmed the correct patient, procedure, operative site, and additional critical information prior to the start of the procedure. A bite block was placed in the mouth. A size ___ flexible endoscope was introduced to the oral cavity and advanced through the upper esophagus, maintaining direct vision of the lumen throughout. The foreign body was visualized at the level of the ___. At this point, a grasping forceps was introduced through the working channel of the endoscope and advanced through until the tip could be visualized. The foreign body was grasped and pulled up against the endoscopy channel. The endoscope and foreign body were retracted out through the oral cavity. The endoscope was then reinserted past the level of the previous foreign body and slowly withdrawn. The esophageal mucosa appeared intact and undamaged, with no anatomical abnormalities noted. The endoscope was then removed and the procedure terminated.

Upon completion of the procedure, a debriefing checklist was completed to share information critical to the postoperative care of the patient. The patient tolerated the procedure well, was extubated in the operating room, and was transported to the post-anesthesia care unit in stable condition.

Flexible Esophagoscopy and Fluoroscopically Guided Dilation

2

William B. Rothstein and Laura A. Boomer

Indications and Benefits

- Symptomatic strictures related to anastomotic strictures (after esophageal atresia repair), caustic ingestion, or other cause
- Benefits: Direct visualization of stricture, confirmation of dilation, evaluation of the esophageal mucosa

Risks and Alternatives

- Standard risks (bleeding, infection, need for additional procedures, risks of anesthesia)
- Injury to adjacent structures (teeth, pharynx, esophagus)
- Aspiration
- Perforation of the pharynx or esophagus
- Alternatives: Enteric feeding tube placement, fluoroscopically guided balloon dilation, esophageal resection

W. B. Rothstein
Virginia Commonwealth University Health System, Department of Surgery, Richmond, VA, USA

L. A. Boomer (✉)
Children's Hospital of Richmond, Virginia Commonwealth University, Department of Pediatric Surgery, Richmond, VA, USA
e-mail: Laura.boomer@vcuhealth.org

Essential Steps

Flexible Esophagoscopy with Balloon Dilation of Stricture

1. Place patient in left lateral decubitus or supine position with neck extended.
2. A bite block facilitates easy passage of the scope.
3. Insert a flexible endoscope over the tongue and advance along the posterior pharynx under direct visualization. For sufficiently tight strictures, a bronchoscope may be necessary.
4. Apply gentle insufflation and pressure against the upper esophageal sphincter to advance into cervical esophagus.
5. Advance to the point of stricture. Carefully inspect the mucosa for signs of perforation. If visual findings are inconsistent with pre-procedure diagnosis, consider tissue sample.
6. A wire can be passed through the stricture under fluoroscopic guidance.
7. Pass the balloon dilator through the scope and over the wire.
8. Real-time fluoroscopy may be used to confirm placement of the balloon across the stricture. Balloon should sit with equal portions above and below the point of stricture.
9. Dilation diameter should be selected based on pre-procedure radiographic findings.

D. J. Papandria et al. (eds.), *Operative Dictations in Pediatric Surgery*,
https://doi.org/10.1007/978-3-030-24212-1_2

10. Fill the balloon dilator with water or contrast and maintain for 30 seconds to 1 minute at each chosen dilator diameter.
11. Watch the balloon fill under fluoroscopy to ensure balloon does not slip above or below stricture, as well as directly with the endoscope.
12. Repeat or serial dilations may be necessary depending on the etiology of the stricture.
13. Remove the balloon dilator and again inspect mucosa for bleeding or perforation.
14. It may be possible to traverse the stricture with the flexible endoscope following dilation.

Note These Variations

- Push dilators or bougies may be used in place of a balloon dilator. After passage of a guidewire through the stricture, the bougie is passed over the wire and guided into the stomach by fluoroscopy. Additionally, some bougies do not have the ability to be passed over a wire. These may be inserted directly into the esophagus, but passage should be visualized with fluoroscopy. This method is associated with a greater risk of bleeding and perforation due to the shear stress of the dilator.

Template Operative Dictation

Preoperative Diagnosis Esophageal stricture

Postoperative Diagnosis Esophageal stricture

Findings
1. ___-cm long, circumferential radial stricture in *cervical esophagus/mid-esophagus/distal esophagus*
2. No evidence of esophageal perforation pre- or post-procedure

Procedure(s) Performed
1. Flexible endoscopy with balloon dilation of esophageal stricture
2. Intraoperative fluoroscopy with surgeon interpretation

Anesthesia *General/procedural sedation*

Specimen {Specimen}

Estimated Blood Loss ___ ml

Indications This is a/an ___ *day/week/month/year*-old *male/female* with a history of *esophageal atresia with tracheoesophageal fistula/caustic ingestion/{other primary cause}*. Patient symptoms were concerning for stricture, which was confirmed by *upper GI study/endoscopy. He/she* was deemed to be a suitable candidate for flexible endoscopy with balloon dilation of esophageal stricture.

Procedure in Detail After a smooth induction of anesthesia, the patient was placed in *left lateral decubitus position/supine position* and appropriately padded. Timeouts were performed using both pre-induction and pre-incision safety checklists with participation of all present in the operative suite. These confirmed the correct patient, procedure, operative site, and additional critical information prior to the start of the procedure. A flexible endoscope was introduced to the oral cavity and advanced through the upper esophageal sphincter under direct visualization. A symmetrical, circumferential stricture was visualized in the ___. At this point, a guidewire was inserted through the accessory port of the endoscope and across the stricture under direct fluoroscopy. A ___-mm balloon dilator was introduced through the accessory port of the endoscope over the wire. A small amount of contrast was introduced into the balloon and placement confirmed by fluoroscopy. Once the balloon dilator was able to be passed through the stricture, and its position confirmed on fluoroscopy, the wire was removed. The balloon was then inflated with contrast for 60 seconds to the designated pressure. The balloon was then completely deflated. A second dilation was performed in a similar fashion with a ___-mm balloon. The balloon was again deflated and then withdrawn. After the procedure, the mucosa was inspected carefully with the endoscope. There was a small amount of bleeding, but no other sign of mucosal damage. Upon completion of the procedure, a debriefing checklist was completed to share information critical to the postoperative care of the patient. The patient tolerated the procedure well, was extubated in the operating room, and was transported to the post-anesthesia care unit in stable condition. A post-procedure chest radiograph was obtained in the recovery room.

3 Repair of Esophageal Atresia with Tracheoesophageal Fistula (Open and MIS Approaches)

Dominic J. Papandria and Karen A. Diefenbach

Indications and Benefits

- Esophageal atresia, with or without tracheo-esophageal fistula
- Benefits: Restoration of esophageal continuity, protection of the airway from aspiration when fistula present

Risks and Alternatives

- Standard risks (bleeding, infection, need for additional procedures, risks of anesthesia)
- Injury to adjacent structures (trachea, esophagus, azygous vein, lung, vagus nerve, recurrent laryngeal nerves)
- Chest wall deformity, scoliosis (associated with open approach)
- Anastomotic leak, anastomotic stricture, or recurrence of fistula
- Alternatives: Temporary occlusion/ligation of fistula

D. J. Papandria
Department of Surgery, Emory University, Atlanta, GA, USA

K. A. Diefenbach (✉)
Nationwide Children's Hospital, Columbus, OH, USA
e-mail: Karen.Diefenbach@nationwidechildrens.org

Essential Steps

Thoracoscopic Repair

1. Rigid bronchoscopy with patient in supine position and occlusion of the fistula with Fogarty catheter
2. Position patient in left lateral decubitus position (left side down) and pad and secure patient to operative table
3. Prep and drape
4. Port placement
5. Identification, isolation, and ligation of the tracheoesophageal fistula
6. Identification and mobilization of the upper esophageal pouch
7. Division of the fistula and resection of the tip of the proximal segment of the esophagus
8. Anastomosis of the proximal and distal esophageal segments
9. Injection of local anesthetic to perform intercostal rib blocks for regional anesthetic effect
10. Placement of thoracic drain near the anastomosis
11. Closure of the remaining incisions

Repair by Thoracotomy

1. Rigid bronchoscopy and placement of Fogarty catheter to occlude the fistula

D. J. Papandria et al. (eds.), *Operative Dictations in Pediatric Surgery*,
https://doi.org/10.1007/978-3-030-24212-1_3

2. Position patient in left lateral decubitus position (left side down) and pad and secure patient to operative table
3. Prep and drape
4. Muscle-sparing thoracotomy incision and placement of retractors
5. Identification, isolation, and ligation of the tracheoesophageal fistula
6. Identification and mobilization of the upper esophageal pouch
7. Division of the fistula and resection of the tip of the proximal segment of the esophagus
8. Anastomosis of the proximal and distal esophageal segments
9. Placement of thoracic drain near the anastomosis
10. Closure of the thoracotomy

Note These Variations

- Bronchoscopy is not performed by all surgeons; it is included as many surgeons do it routinely to evaluate tracheal anatomy, identify the location of the distal fistula, rule out a proximal fistula, evaluate for significant tracheomalacia, and optimally place the endotracheal tube.
- At the time of the bronchoscopy, a Fogarty catheter may be used to occlude the fistula to facilitate ventilation and allow general anesthesia including paralytics to be given prior to entrance into the chest and ligation of the fistula.
- Preoperative echocardiogram is performed on all of these patients to evaluate for congenital cardiac anomalies which are frequently associated with TEF/EA and to evaluate the location of the aortic arch. Some surgeons will change their approach from the right to the left if there is a right-sided aortic arch.

Template Operative Dictation (Thoracoscopic)

Preoperative Diagnosis *Esophageal atresia/ esophageal atresia with tracheoesophageal fistula*

Postoperative Diagnosis Same as preoperative diagnosis

Findings Same as postoperative diagnosis

Procedure(s) Performed Thoracoscopic repair of esophageal atresia *with tracheoesophageal fistula*

Anesthesia General

Specimen None

Drains *None/___FR chest tube/___FR drain*

Implants None

Estimated Blood Loss ___mL

Indications This is a/an ___*-day/week/month/ year*-old *male/female* with esophageal atresia *and tracheoesophageal fistula. He/she* was deemed to be a suitable candidate for thoracoscopic repair of the same.

Procedure in Detail Timeouts were performed using both pre-induction and pre-incision safety checklists with participation of all present in the operative suite. These confirmed the correct patient, procedure, operative site, and additional critical information prior to the start of the procedure. General anesthesia was induced and patient remained spontaneously breathing. *A rigid bronchoscopy was performed which noted normal tracheal anatomy, mild/moderate/severe tracheomalacia, and a tracheoesophageal fistula at approximately ___cm proximal to the carina. A 3/4/5 FR Fogarty catheter was passed through the fistula and the balloon inflated to occlude the fistula. The endotracheal tube was then placed in a midtrachea position.* The patient was placed in left lateral decubitus position and appropriately padded and secured. The right chest and axilla were then prepped and draped in the usual sterile fashion. A ___-mm port was placed in the anterior axillary line at the level of the ___ intercostal space. After verifying the position of the port in the chest, the chest was insufflated to a pressure of *4/6* mmHg. Two additional ports were placed under direct vision, one in the anterior axillary line at the ___ intercostal space under direct vision and one in the posterior axillary line in the ___ intercostal space.

[Choose One:]

If tracheoesophageal fistula: Inspection of the chest revealed the azygous vein and blunt dissection revealed the distal esophagus below the vein. Following the distal esophagus superiorly, the fistula was identified where it inserted on the posterior wall of the membranous trachea. *To facilitate safe ligation of the fistula, the azygous vein was ligated and divided using electrocautery/a bipolar sealing device/endoclips.* The fistula was then ligated using *a ___-0 Vicryl suture ligature/ an endoclip.* The fistula was divided and the distal portion of the esophagus was mobilized to minimize tension on the anastomosis.

If pure atresia: {Continue dictation}

Inspection of the chest near the esophageal hiatus revealed a short distal segment of distal esophagus. This was mobilized circumferentially using blunt dissection being careful to avoid injury to any vagal fibers. A bipolar sealing device was used for hemostasis.

{Continue dictation}

Dissection was then performed to expose and mobilize the proximal esophageal pouch using blunt dissection and bipolar sealing device for hemostasis. Gentle pressure on the orogastric tube facilitated this process. Care was taken to dissect closely along the esophagus to avoid injury to the membranous trachea and the recurrent laryngeal nerves. Any vagal fibers were preserved when possible.

Once both the proximal and distal segments of the esophagus were mobilized, the end of the proximal esophageal segment was *excised/ incised* to expose the mucosa. The anastomosis was then performed using interrupted ___-0 Vicryl/PDS suture starting at the far corner of the posterior wall of the anastomosis and completing the back wall. The OG tube was then passed under direct vision into the distal esophagus and the anterior wall of the anastomosis was then completed starting from the farthest corner. A total of ___ sutures were placed. The transanastomotic tube was *removed/passed into the stomach and secured by anesthesia.*

Intercostal rib blocks were performed under direct visualization using ___% Marcaine with epinephrine. A ___FR chest tube/ ___ drain was placed adjacent to the anastomosis and secured as it exited the chest at the inferior, anterior incision using ___-0 Silk/Neurolon/Nylon suture.

The remaining ports were removed and the incisions closed at the level of the fascia using a ___-0 Vicryl suture and a ___-0 Monocryl suture. Dressings were applied to the incisions *and the drain site.*

Upon completion of the procedure, a debriefing checklist was completed to share information critical to the postoperative care of the patient. The patient tolerated the procedure well. *He/she remained intubated and was transported to the NICU* unit in stable condition thereafter.

Template Operative Dictation (Open)

Preoperative Diagnosis *Esophageal atresia/ Esophageal atresia with tracheoesophageal fistula.*

Postoperative Diagnosis Same as preoperative diagnosis

Findings Same as postoperative diagnosis

Procedure(s) Performed Repair of esophageal atresia *with tracheoesophageal fistula*

Anesthesia General

Specimen None

Drains *None/___FR chest tube/___FR drain*

Implants None

Estimated Blood Loss ___ mL

Indications This is a/an ___*-day/week/month/ year*-old *male/female* with esophageal atresia *and tracheoesophageal fistula.* He/she was deemed to be a suitable candidate for repair of the same by thoracotomy.

Procedure: in Detail Timeouts were performed using both pre-induction and pre-incision safety checklists with participation of all present in the operative suite. These confirmed the correct patient, procedure, operative site, and additional critical information prior to the start of the procedure. General anesthesia was induced and patient remained spontaneously breathing. *A rigid bronchoscopy was performed which noted normal tracheal anatomy, mild/moderate/severe tracheomalacia, and a tracheoesophageal fistula at approximately ___cm proximal to the carina. A 3/4/5 FR Fogarty catheter was passed through the fistula and the balloon inflated to occlude the fistula. The endotracheal tube was then placed in a mid-trachea position.* The patient was placed in left lateral decubitus position and appropriately padded and secured. The right chest and axilla were then prepped and draped in the usual sterile fashion. A muscle-sparing incision was made at the level of the fourth intercostal space extending from the anterior axillary line posteriorly for a length of ___ cm. The latissimus dorsi muscle was mobilized and retracted without dividing and the serratus anterior muscle was mobilized from its posterior insertion to expose the ribs and intercostal muscles. The chest was entered at the fourth intercostal space just superior to the fifth rib. *Care was taken to preserve the parietal pleura.* The Finochietto retractor was used to spread the ribs. Blunt dissection was used to separate the parietal pleura from the chest wall posteriorly until the distal esophagus was identified.

[Choose One:]

If tracheoesophageal fistula: Following the distal esophagus superiorly, the fistula was identified where it inserted on the posterior wall of the membranous trachea. *To facilitate safe ligation of the fistula, the azygous vein was ligated and divided using electrocautery/suture ligation.* The fistula was then ligated and divided using *a ___-0 Vicryl suture ligature/interrupted ___-0 ___ sutures*. The distal portion of the esophagus was mobilized to minimize tension on the anastomosis.

If pure atresia: The distal esophagus was mobilized circumferentially to minimize tension on the anastomosis using blunt dissection being careful to avoid injury to any vagal fibers. A bipolar sealing device was used for hemostasis.

{Continue dictation}

Dissection was then performed to expose and mobilize the proximal esophageal pouch using blunt dissection and bipolar sealing device for hemostasis. Gentle pressure on the orogastric tube facilitated this process. Care was taken to dissect closely along the esophagus to avoid injury to the membranous trachea and the recurrent laryngeal nerves. Any vagal fibers were preserved when possible.

Once both the proximal and distal segments of the esophagus were mobilized, the end of the proximal esophageal segment was *excised/incised* to expose the mucosa. The anastomosis was then performed using interrupted ___-0 Vicryl/PDS suture starting at the far corner of the posterior wall of the anastomosis and completing the back wall. The OG tube was then passed under direct vision into the distal esophagus and the anterior wall of the anastomosis was then completed starting from the farthest corner. A total of ___ sutures were placed. The transanastomotic tube was *removed/passed into the stomach and secured by anesthesia.*

A ___FR chest tube/ ___ drain was placed adjacent to the anastomosis and secured as it exited the chest at the anterior and inferior to the incision using ___-0 Silk/Neurolon/Nylon suture.

The incision was closed in layers. Interrupted ___-0 Vicryl sutures were used to approximate the ribs being careful to not obliterate the intercostal space. The serratus anterior muscle was reapproximated to its posterior insertion using interrupted ___-0 Vicryl sutures. The subcutaneous tissue was closed using a running ___-0 Vicryl suture and the skin was closed using a running ___-0 Monocryl suture. Dressings were applied to the incisions *and the drain site.*

Upon completion of the procedure, a debriefing checklist was completed to share information critical to the postoperative care of the patient. The patient tolerated the procedure well. *He/she remained intubated and was transported to the NICU* unit in stable condition thereafter.

Esophageal Replacement

4

Michaela Kollisch-Singule and Jennifer Stanger

Indications and Benefits

- Esophageal stricture (from caustic injury, reflux esophagitis, anastomotic scarring after esophageal atresia repair, achalasia)
- Congenital esophageal stenosis (if not amenable to resection with end-to-end anastomosis)
- Long-gap esophageal atresia
- Benefits: Continuity of gastrointestinal tract to optimize enteral nutrition

Risks and Alternatives

- Standard risks (bleeding, infection, need for additional procedures, risks of anesthesia)
- Injury to adjacent structures (azygous vein, vagus nerve, posterior membranous trachea)
- Vascular insufficiency with necrosis
- Anastomotic stricture/leak/ulcer
- Delayed gastric emptying, disordered peristalsis, ulcers
- Long term: Dilation and dysmotility of the conduit
- Alternatives: Serial dilations of strictures, delayed repair of atresia/stenosis, gastric/jejunal feeding tubes for enteral nutrition

Essential Steps

1. Abdominal incision
2. Mobilization of esophagus
3. Mediastinal dissection of esophagus
4. Neck dissection of esophagus
5. ***If {Colon interposition}***
   (a) Division of gastrocolic ligament
   (b) Mobilization of ascending and descending colon
   (c) Conduit assessment for perfusion
   (d) Ligation of left branch of the middle colic artery and the marginal artery (with preservation of the ascending branch of the left colic artery)
   (e) Transection of transverse colon
   (f) Mobilization of colon up mediastinum
   (g) Division of descending colon
   (h) Transection of stomach distal to gastroesophageal junction
   (i) Withdrawal of esophagogastric specimen from mediastinum through neck
   (j) Creation of colono-gastric anastomosis
   (k) Creation of colo-colonic anastomosis

M. Kollisch-Singule (✉)
SUNY Upstate Medical University, Department of General Surgery, Syracuse, NY, USA
e-mail: KolliscM@upstate.edu

J. Stanger
SUNY Upstate Medical Unversity, Department of Pediatric Surgery, Syracuse, NY, USA

D. J. Papandria et al. (eds.), *Operative Dictations in Pediatric Surgery*,
https://doi.org/10.1007/978-3-030-24212-1_4

6. *If {Gastric tube}*
   (a) Gastrohepatic ligament divided down to pylorus
   (b) Mobilization of greater curvature of stomach
   (c) Ligation of left gastric artery
   (d) {Pyloroplasty}
   (e) Creation of gastric tube with sequential staple loads
   (f) Withdrawal of esophagogastric specimen from mediastinum through neck
7. Transection of cervical esophagus
8. Anastomosis between cervical esophagus and colon/gastric conduit
9. Penrose drain into neck
10. {Jejunostomy feeding tube}
11. Closure

Note These Variations

- Open, laparoscopic, robotic approach
- Conduit choice: Colonic interposition, gastric tube, gastric transposition, jejunal substitution
- Stapled/handsewn anastomoses
- Suture choices
- Placement of jejunostomy feeding tube

Template Operative Dictation (Open)

Preoperative Diagnosis Esophageal *stricture/stenosis/atresia*

Postoperative Diagnosis Same as preoperative diagnosis

Findings Same as postoperative diagnosis

Procedure(s) Performed Esophageal replacement

Anesthesia *General*

Specimen *Esophagus/esophagogastrectomy*

Drains Penrose in neck

Implants None

Estimated Blood Loss ___ mL

Indications This is a/an ___*-day/week/month/year*-old *male/female* with esophageal *stricture/stenosis/atresia*, which was causing *dysphagia/odynophagia/inability to maintain oral nutrition. He/she* was deemed to be a suitable candidate for esophageal replacement with a *colon transposition/gastric tube.*

Procedure in Detail Following satisfactory induction of anesthesia, the patient was placed in a supine position and appropriately padded. {A Foley catheter and nasogastric tube were placed.} Timeouts were performed using both pre-induction and pre-incision safety checklists with participation of all present in the operative suite. These confirmed the correct patient, procedure, operative site, and additional critical information prior to the start of the procedure. The abdomen and left neck were then prepped and draped in the usual sterile fashion. Prophylactic antibiotics were given.

An *upper midline/transverse/subcostal* incision was made into the abdomen and the peritoneal cavity entered. The pars flaccida was incised and dissected to the right crus of the diaphragm. The crural dissection was continued by coming across the anterior arch of the diaphragm. The left crus was similarly dissected as much as possible, which required ligation of the short gastric arteries, until the anterior aspect of the gastroesophageal junction was visualized. The esophagus was retracted laterally to expose the decussation of the crural fibers, and a retroesophageal window was developed until the esophagus was circumferentially mobilized. The esophageal hiatus was widened by incising it anteriorly. The phrenic vein was ligated in order to adequately expose the mediastinum.

The mediastinum was entered and the loose areolar tissue was bluntly dissected around the distal esophagus separating it from the surrounding mediastinal attachments and mobilization carried proximally toward the neck.

Attention was turned to the left neck. Just anterior to the sternocleidomastoid muscle and extending to just above the sternum, a small neck incision was made and carried down along the medial aspect of the sternocleidomastoid muscle. The omohyoid and sternohyoid muscles were divided. The dissection was carried deeper until the vertebral bodies were palpable posteriorly. The esophagus was bluntly dissected free of the posterior membranous trachea anteriorly, and from the vertebral bodies posteriorly. The cervical esophagus was encircled with a/an __-inch Penrose drain and retracted gently caudally allowing for blunt dissection inferiorly toward the previous mediastinal dissection from the transhiatal approach.

[Choose one:]

If {colon interposition}: {The patient preoperatively received a colonic *mechanical/antibiotic* prep.} The gastrocolic ligament was incised, separating the transverse colon from the greater curvature of the stomach. The splenic and hepatic flexures were taken down. In a lateral-to-medial approach, the mobilization of the left colon was continued from the splenic flexure down the white line of Toldt, mobilizing the descending colon off the retroperitoneum to the level of the sigmoid colon. In a similar fashion, the ascending colon was mobilized to the level of the cecum dissecting down from the hepatic flexure sweeping the colon off the hepatorenal fossa and retroperitoneum, while protecting the ureter, duodenum, and kidney. The colon was grasped and elevated to identify the tenting of the mesentery to indicate the regions of the middle and left colic vascular pedicles. {Transillumination was used to identify the arteries.} The peritoneum was incised on either side of these vessels in order to isolate them. {The length of colon required for the conduit was estimated by measuring the distance from the angle of the mandible to the xiphoid process.} The conduit was assessed for adequate perfusion and viability by placing small bulldog clamps on the arteries to be ligated and reassessing for graft viability. After several minutes, the bowel appeared *healthy/dusky* {and flow was confirmed with fluorescein dye injection/mesenteric Doppler flow/inspected for venous congestion}. After demonstrating adequate perfusion, the left branch of the middle colic artery was ligated at its origin and the marginal artery was ligated. The remaining mesentery between the right colic artery and the right branch of the middle colic artery was divided, being cautious to leave the ascending branch of the left colic artery and arcades intact. Using the previously noted required length for guidance, the transverse colon was divided and brought up through the mediastinum and through the cervical neck incision in an isoperistaltic fashion, verifying that there were no twists in the mesentery. The distal colon was divided, verifying adequate conduit length to reach the stomach. An anastomosis was fashioned with a *handsewn/stapled* anastomosis to re-establish continuity of the colon. The stomach was stapled just distal to the gastroesophageal junction. A colono-gastric anastomosis was created with a *handsewn anastomosis/linear cutting staples* verifying no redundancy of the colon within the mediastinum.

If {gastric tube}: The division of the gastrohepatic ligament was continued along the lesser curvature of the stomach to the duodenum, exposing the lesser sac. {No accessory/replaced left hepatic artery was noted.} Attention was then directed to mobilizing the greater curvature of the stomach. The gastrocolic ligament was divided while the right gastroepiploic artery and arcade were carefully preserved. Retrogastric adhesions to the retroperitoneum and pancreas were taken down. Once the lesser sac was completely mobilized, the left gastric pedicle was ligated with a _________ before completely freeing the stomach. {A pyloroplasty was performed.} The nasogastric tube was withdrawn. The gastric conduit was created in an *isoperistaltic/retroperistaltic fashion* over a _____ French chest tube, using a stapler along the greater curvature of the stomach. The left gastroepiploic arcade was identified and preserved throughout this process. Sequential staple loads were used until adequate length of the tube was obtained to reach the cervical incision. {The suture line was oversewn with ___ suture.} The gastric conduit was withdrawn into the cervical neck wound and visualized directly from the abdomen to verify that the staple line remained lateral and the specimen did not twist.

The cervical esophagus was transected sharply and the esophagus and *colon/gastric* conduit were lifted out of the mediastinum via the neck incision. The *colon/gastric* conduit was opened and a heel stitch secured between the cervical esophagus and *gastric/colonic* conduit. A *cutting stapler/handsewn anastomosis* was used to create a *side-to-side/end-to-end* anastomosis between the cervical esophagus and the conduit. The remaining defect was then closed with *interrupted __ sutures/TA stapler* and a nasogastric tube was then passed distally into the neo-esophagus. After completing the anastomosis, the conduit was grasped and pulled down into the abdomen until the cervical anastomosis seated down into the neck, ensuring a straight conduit. Hemostasis was verified. The nasogastric tube was secured at __cm at the level of the nares. {A jejunostomy feeding tube was placed.}

The abdomen was irrigated and hemostasis verified. The abdominal fascia was closed with __ suture. The wound was irrigated and closed with ___. A Penrose drain was placed in the cervical neck incision and secured. The neck incision was closed with interrupted _ suture and the skin was reapproximated with __ and dressed.

Upon completion of the procedure, a debriefing checklist was completed to share information critical to the postoperative care of the patient. The patient tolerated the procedure well, *was extubated in the operating room*, and was transported to the post-anesthesia care unit in stable condition thereafter.

5 Esophagomyotomy (Open and MIS Approaches)

Kate Savoie and Karen A. Diefenbach

Indications and Benefits

- Esophageal achalasia not responding to medical management

Risk and Alternatives

- Risks: Bleeding, infection, trocar placement injuries, pneumothorax/capnothorax, vagal injury, full-thickness injury to the esophagus, splenic injury, incomplete myotomy
- Alternatives: Weight loss, medical management of reflux disease, lifestyle modifications, magnetic gastroesophageal junction rink (e.g., LINX® device, Ethicon US, LLC, Shoreview, MN, USA)

Essential Steps

1. Upper midline incision or trocars placed
2. Exposure of the esophageal hiatus
3. Division of the anterior phrenoesophageal ligaments
4. Myotomy dividing longitudinal and circular muscles
5. Divide short gastric vessels if performing fundoplication
6. Identify anterior vagus
7. Mediastinal dissection for esophageal exposure
8. Crural reapproximation
9. Crural mesh reinforcement
10. Fundoplication (Dor/Toupet)
11. Abdominal wall closure *OR* port removal and fascial closure

Notes These Variations

- A fundoplication case be performed and should be based on preoperative discussion with patient/family regarding long-term risk of GERD.
- Some surgeons elect to not place mesh at the hiatus.

Template Operative Dictation

Preoperative Diagnosis *Esophageal achalasia*

Postoperative Diagnosis Same as preoperative diagnosis

Findings Same as postoperative diagnosis

Anesthesia General

K. Savoie
Nationwide Children's Hospital, Department of Pediatric Surgery, Columbus, OH, USA

K. A. Diefenbach (✉)
Nationwide Children's Hospital, Columbus, OH, USA
e-mail: Karen.Diefenbach@nationwidechildrens.org

D. J. Papandria et al. (eds.), *Operative Dictations in Pediatric Surgery*,
https://doi.org/10.1007/978-3-030-24212-1_5

Specimen Hernia sac

Drains {Drains}

Implants {Implants}

Estimated Blood Loss ____ mL

Indications This is *a/an* ___-*year*-old *male/female* with __________. A preoperative diagnostic evaluation including *an esophagram and manometry* confirmed the diagnosis of esophageal achalasia. *He/she* was deemed to be a suitable candidate for an *open/minimally invasive* esophagomyotomy (Heller myotomy) and presents for this procedure.

Procedure in Detail Following satisfactory induction of anesthesia, the patient was placed in a lithotomy position and appropriately padded. Timeouts were performed using both pre-induction and pre-incision safety checklists with participation of all present in the operative suite. These confirmed the correct patient, procedure, operative site, and additional critical information prior to the start of the procedure.

[Choose One:]

If open technique was performed: An upper midline incision was made and carried down to the fascia with electrocautery. The linea alba was incised to reveal the peritoneum. This was grasped and divided sharply with Metzenbaum scissors.

If minimally invasive technique was performed: A/an ___-mm *transumbilical/infraumbilical* incision was made and a Veress needle/___-mm port placed through this incision into the peritoneal cavity. Once intraperitoneal placement was confirmed, the abdomen was insufflated to a pressure of ___ mmHg. Two additional 5-mm ports were placed in the right and left upper quadrants triangulated to the esophageal hiatus. Retraction of the left lobe of the liver to expose the esophageal hiatus was achieved via a *falciform retraction stitch/Nathanson retractor placed in a subxiphoid location/a laparoscopic liver retractor placed in the right upper quadrant lateral to the previously placed port.* Finally, a 5-mm assistant port was placed in the left upper quadrant lateral to the working port. The patient was then placed into reversed Trendelenburg.

{Continue dictation}

The short gastric vessels were sequentially divided with *suture ligation/a vessel sealer*. The esophagus was then dissected free of the left crus. The esophagus was dissected circumferentially being careful to preserve the anterior and posterior branches of the vagus nerve and the left gastric artery. The right crus was identified and the esophagus mobilized from this structure.

The phrenoesophageal was carefully divided. A Penrose was then placed around the esophagus and gentle caudal retraction applied. A careful mediastinal dissection was then carried out to elongate the intraabdominal portion of the esophagus. The anterior vagus nerve was identified and a location chosen to start the myotomy. The longitudinal and circular muscles were divided down to the level of the submucosa and the myotomy extended a minimum of 4 cm above the GE junction on the anterior wall of the esophagus and at least 2 cm below the GE junction onto the anterior wall of the stomach.

Endoscopy was used to evaluate the myotomy and confirm that the mucosa was intact once the myotomy was completed. The esophagus was then retracted anteriorly and the right and left crus reapproximated with ___-0 *Vicryl/Monocryl/Prolene/PDS* in an interrupted fashion.

[Choose One:]

If a Dor fundoplication was performed: The cardia of the stomach was then grasped and sufficient dissection of the short gastric vessels confirmed. A Dor fundoplication was performed using interrupted ___-0 Ethibond sutures. The fundus was secured on the left side with a suture from the apex of the left crus to the cut edge of the myotomy. A second suture was placed 2 cm inferiorly in the same fashion. Third and fourth sutures were used to secure the fundus to the opposite edge of the myotomy and the right crus.

If a Toupet fundoplication was performed: The cardia of the stomach was then grasped and sufficient dissection of the short gastric vessels confirmed. The cardia was then passed posterior to the esophagus and a "shoeshine" maneuver performed. The left side of the fundus was then secured to the edge of the esophageal myotomy and the left crus with ___-0 Ethibond in an interrupted fashion. The right side was similarly secured to the edge of the myotomy and the right crus.

The abdomen was inspected and hemostasis confirmed.

If open technique was performed: The fascia was then closed with a __-0 Vicryl/Prolene/PDS in an interrupted/running/figure-of-eight fashion.

If minimally invasive technique was performed: The liver retractor was carefully removed under direct visualization. The ports were removed and the fascia at the umbilical incision was closed using a ___-0 *Vicryl/Prolene/PDS* suture. *The fascia at the remaining incisions was closed using a ___-0 ___suture.*

{Continue dictation}

All counts were correct at the end of the case and the attending of record was present and scrubbed for *all/key* portions of the case.

Upon completion of the procedure, a debriefing checklist was completed to share information critical to the postoperative care of the patient. The patient tolerated the procedure well, *was extubated in the operating room*, and was transported to the post-anesthesia care unit in stable condition.

6 Esophagogastric Fundoplication (Open and MIS Approaches)

Dani O. Gonzalez and Payam Saadai

Indications and Benefits

- Gastroesophageal reflux with severe esophagitis
- Failure of medical management of reflux
- Respiratory symptoms (recurrent pneumonia, aspiration, dyspnea, apneic episodes, choking)
- Esophageal stricture
- Feeding intolerance
- Failure to thrive
- Laryngospasm leading to severe cyanotic or apneic events
- Hiatal or paraesophageal hernia
- Benefits: Can facilitate enteral autonomy in patients with feeding intolerance and aids in the prevention of morbidity in infants with reflux

D. O. Gonzalez
Icahn School of Medicine at Mount Sinai, Department of Surgery, New York, NY, USA

P. Saadai (✉)
UC Davis Medical Center/Shriners Hospital for Children, Division of Pediatric Surgery, Sacramento, CA, USA
e-mail: psaadai@ucdavis.edu

Risks and Alternatives

- Standard risks (bleeding, infection, need for additional procedures, risks of anesthesia)
- Injury to adjacent structures (esophagus, spleen, vagus nerves, aorta)
- Pneumothorax
- Tight or narrow fundoplication
- Failed or slipped fundoplication
- Dysphagia
- Alternatives: gastrojejunostomy feeding tube, medical management

Essential Steps

1. Position the patient in the supine or low lithotomy position at the foot of the bed.
2. Place a nasogastric or orogastric tube.
3. Use a liver retractor to elevate the left lobe of the liver to expose the esophageal hiatus.
4. Ligate the short gastric arteries to mobilize gastric fundus.
5. Open gastrohepatic ligament at the pars flaccida.
6. Identify and preserve both vagus nerves throughout the procedure.
7. Develop a circumferential plane between the esophagus and diaphragmatic crura.
8. If present, reduce hiatal hernia and repair crural defect.

D. J. Papandria et al. (eds.), *Operative Dictations in Pediatric Surgery*,
https://doi.org/10.1007/978-3-030-24212-1_6

9. Grasp fundus and pass it posterior to the esophagus.
10. Create a short floppy wrap by placing interrupted sutures over the gastric tube or bougie.
11. If desired, place gastropexy sutures to prevent migration into the mediastinum.

Note These Variations

- A variety of liver or abdominal retractors may be used for exposure.
- Some surgeons prefer limited crural dissection and minimal division of the short gastric vessels.
- The crura may not be reapproximated if there is no defect.
- Gastropexy sutures may be added to secure the fundus to the diaphragm.
- 3-mm or 5-mm ports and instruments may be used depending on the size of the child.

Template Operative Dictation (Open)

Preoperative Diagnosis *Refractory gastroesophageal reflux/feeding intolerance/paraesophageal hernia/hiatal hernia*

Postoperative Diagnosis Same as preoperative diagnosis

Findings See operative note

Procedure(s) Performed Esophagogastric fundoplication

Anesthesia General

Specimen None

Drains None

Implants None

Estimated Blood Loss ___ mL

Indications This is a/an ___*-day/week/month/year*-old *male/female* with *severe reflux esophagitis/feeding intolerance/failure to thrive/paraesophageal hernia/hiatal hernia.* Medical management had failed and he/she was deemed to be a suitable candidate for esophagogastric fundoplication.

Procedure in Detail Following satisfactory induction of anesthesia, the patient was placed in supine and appropriately padded. Timeouts were performed using both pre-induction and pre-incision safety checklists with participation of all present in the operative suite. These confirmed the correct patient, procedure, operative site, and additional critical information prior to the start of the procedure. The abdomen was then prepped and draped in the usual sterile fashion.

A *nasogastric/orogastric* tube was placed to decompress the stomach. A *midline upper abdominal/left subcostal* skin incision was made. The subcutaneous tissues were carefully dissected. The abdomen was inspected. A liver retractor was placed to elevate the left lobe of the liver anterosuperiorly and expose the esophageal hiatus. *The left triangular ligament of the liver was taken down for additional exposure.* Using electrocautery, the short gastric vessels were carefully ligated in order to mobilize gastric fundus and free it from its attachments to the spleen. The stomach was then retracted caudally to provide downward traction on the phrenoesophageal ligament. The gastrohepatic ligament was opened at the pars flaccida. A plane was dissected between the right and left diaphragmatic crura and the esophagus in order to develop a circumferential plane. Both the anterior and posterior vagus nerves were carefully identified and preserved throughout the procedure. *A vessel loop/Penrose drain was placed around the esophagus incorporating the posterior vagus nerve.* The distal esophagus was mobilized to allow for sufficient intra-abdominal length. *A small/large hiatal hernia was present and the contents were reduced.* __ interrupted nonabsorbable sutures were placed posteriorly to reapproximate the right and left crura.

The fundus was grasped and folded posterior to the esophagus. A "shoeshine" maneuver was performed to ensure adequate mobility of the fundus. *The nasogastric/orogastric tube was exchanged for a ___ French bougie.* A 360-degree fundoplication was created with ___ interrupted nonabsorbable sutures to create a ___-cm long fundoplication, incorporating the anterior wall of the esophagus on the two superior sutures. The wrap was noted to be floppy without any evidence of tension on the fundus or the sutures. *The nasogastric tube/orogastric tube/bougie was removed. The fundoplication was tacked to the diaphragmatic crus using ___ interrupted nonabsorbable sutures to prevent the wrap from migrating into the mediastinum.*

The abdomen was then inspected and hemostasis was ensured. The liver retractor was removed. The fascia was closed with *running/interrupted* ___ suture. The skin incision was closed with absorbable suture in layers and a dressing was applied.

Upon completion of the procedure, a debriefing checklist was completed to share information critical to the postoperative care of the patient. The patient tolerated the procedure well, *was extubated in the operating room*, and was transported to the post-anesthesia care unit in stable condition.

Template Operative Dictation (Laparoscopic)

Preoperative Diagnosis *Refractory gastroesophageal reflux/feeding intolerance/paraesophageal hernia/hiatal hernia*

Postoperative Diagnosis Same as preoperative diagnosis

Findings See operative note

Procedure(s) Performed Laparoscopic esophagogastric fundoplication

Anesthesia General

Specimen None

Drains None

Implants None

Estimated Blood Loss ___ mL

Indications This is a/an ___*-day/week/month/year*-old *male/female* with *severe reflux esophagitis/feeding intolerance/failure to thrive/paraesophageal hernia/hiatal hernia.* Medical management had failed and he/she was deemed to be a suitable candidate for laparoscopic esophagogastric fundoplication.

Procedure in Detail Following satisfactory induction of anesthesia, the patient was placed in *supine/low lithotomy* position at the foot of the table and appropriately padded. Timeouts were performed using both pre-induction and pre-incision safety checklists with participation of all present in the operative suite. These confirmed the correct patient, procedure, operative site, and additional critical information prior to the start of the procedure. The abdomen was then prepped and draped in the usual sterile fashion.

A *nasogastric/orogastric* tube was placed to decompress the stomach. A skin incision was made *at/above* the umbilicus for placement of a 5-mm port. The abdomen was insufflated and a 5-mm, 30-degree laparoscopic was placed. There were no noted injuries from initial port placement. Three additional 5-mm ports were placed, including two operating ports in the right and left upper quadrants along the mid-clavicular lines, and a retracting port in the left mid-abdomen.

{If Nathanson liver retractor used} In the midline of the epigastrium, a skin incision was made for a Nathanson liver retractor. The liver retractor was placed to elevate the left lobe of the liver and expose the esophageal hiatus.

{If flexible liver retractor used} In the right anterior axillary line, a skin incision was made for a snake liver retractor. The liver retractor was placed to elevate the left lobe of the liver and expose the esophageal hiatus.

The short gastric vessels were carefully divided *using a vessel sealing device/hook electrocautery* to mobilize gastric fundus. The stomach was then retracted caudally to provide downward traction on the phrenoesophageal ligament. The gastrohepatic ligament was then opened at the pars flaccida. A plane was dissected between the right and left diaphragmatic crura and the esophagus in order to develop a circumferential plane. Both the anterior and posterior vagus nerves were carefully identified and preserved throughout the procedure. *A vessel loop/Penrose drain was placed around the esophagus incorporating the posterior vagus nerve.* The distal esophagus was mobilized to allow for sufficient intra-abdominal length. *A small/large hiatal hernia was present and the contents were reduced.* ___ interrupted nonabsorbable sutures were placed posteriorly to reapproximate the right and left crura.

The fundus was grasped and folded posterior to the esophagus. A "shoeshine" maneuver was performed to ensure adequate mobility of the fundus. *The nasogastric/orogastric tube was exchanged for a ___ French bougie.* A 360-degree fundoplication was created with ___ interrupted non-absorbable sutures to create a/an __-cm long fundoplication, incorporating the anterior wall of the esophagus on the two superior sutures. The wrap was noted to be floppy without any evidence of tension on the fundus or the sutures. *The nasogastric tube/orogastric tube/bougie was removed. The fundoplication was tacked to the diaphragmatic crus using ___ interrupted non-absorbable sutures to prevent the wrap from migrating into the mediastinum.*

The abdomen was then inspected and hemostasis was ensured. The liver retractor was removed under vision. The ports were removed and the abdomen desufflated. The umbilical fascial defect was closed with interrupted absorbable sutures. Skin incisions were closed with absorbable sutures and a dressing was applied.

Upon completion of the procedure, a debriefing checklist was completed to share information critical to the postoperative care of the patient. The patient tolerated the procedure well, *was extubated in the operating room*, and was transported to the post-anesthesia care unit in stable condition.

Hiatal and Paraesophageal Hernia (Open and MIS Approaches)

7

Kate Savoie and Karen A. Diefenbach

Indications and Benefits

- Hiatal hernia not responding to medical management
- Hiatal hernias in patients not wanting long-term medical management
- Type II–IV paraesophageal hernias

Risk and Alternatives

- Risks: Bleeding, infection, trocar placement injuries, pneumothorax/capnothorax, vagal injury, full-thickness injury to the esophagus, splenic injury, incomplete myotomy
- Alternatives: Weight loss, medical management of reflux disease, lifestyle modifications, magnetic gastroesophageal junction rink (e.g., LINX® device, Ethicon US, LLC, Shoreview, MN, USA)

Essential Steps

1. Upper midline incision or ports placed
2. Exposure of the esophageal hiatus
3. Anterior phrenoesophageal ligaments divided
4. Divide short gastric vessels
5. Identify anterior and posterior vagus branches
6. Mediastinal dissection for esophageal exposure and lengthening
7. Crural reapproximation
8. Crural mesh reinforcement
9. Fundoplication (Nissen/Toupet)
10. Abdominal wall closure or port removal and fascial closure

Notes These Variations

- A fundoplication case be performed and should be based on preoperative reflux symptoms.
- Some surgeons elect to not place mesh at the hiatus.

Template Operative Dictation

Preoperative Diagnosis *Hiatal hernia/Type II paraesophageal hernia/Type III paraesophageal hernia/Type IV paraesophageal hernia*

Postoperative Diagnosis Same as preoperative diagnosis

Findings Same as postoperative diagnosis

Anesthesia General

K. Savoie
Nationwide Children's Hospital, Department of Pediatric Surgery, Columbus, OH, USA

K. A. Diefenbach (✉)
Nationwide Children's Hospital, Columbus, OH, USA
e-mail: Karen.Diefenbach@nationwidechildrens.org

D. J. Papandria et al. (eds.), *Operative Dictations in Pediatric Surgery*,
https://doi.org/10.1007/978-3-030-24212-1_7

Specimen Hernia sac

Drains {Drains}

Implants {Implants}

Estimated Blood Loss ____ mL

Indications This is *a/an* ___*-month/year*-old *male/female* with a *hiatal/paraesophageal* hernia. A preoperative diagnostic evaluation of *esophagogastroduodenoscopy/barium swallow* confirmed the diagnosis. *He/she* was deemed to be a suitable candidate for an *open/minimally invasive hiatal/paraesophageal* hernia repair.

Procedure in Detail Following satisfactory induction of anesthesia, the patient was placed in a lithotomy position and appropriately padded. Timeouts were performed using both pre-induction and pre-incision safety checklists with participation of all present in the operative suite. These confirmed the correct patient, procedure, operative site, and additional critical information prior to the start of the procedure.

[Choose One:]
If open technique was performed: An upper midline incision was made and carried down to the fascia with electrocautery. The linea alba was incised to reveal the peritoneum. This was grasped and divided sharply with Metzenbaum scissors.

If minimally invasive technique was performed: A/an ___-mm *transumbilical/infraumbilical* incision was made and a veress needle/___-mm port placed through this incision into the peritoneal cavity. Once intraperitoneal placement was confirmed, the abdomen was insufflated to a pressure of ___ mmHg. Two additional 5-mm ports were placed in the right and left upper quadrants triangulated to the esophageal hiatus. Retraction of the left lobe of the liver to expose the esophageal hiatus was achieved via a *falciform retraction stitch/Nathanson retractor placed in a subxiphoid location/a laparoscopic liver retractor placed in the right upper quadrant lateral to the previously placed port.* Finally, a 5-mm assistant port was placed in the left upper quadrant lateral to the working port. The patient was then placed into reversed Trendelenburg.

{Continue dictation}

The contents of the hernia sac were then reduced into the abdomen using gentle traction to avoid injury. The short gastric vessels were sequentially divided with *suture ligation/a vessel sealer*. The esophagus was then dissected free of the left crus. The esophagus was dissected circumferentially being careful to preserve the anterior and posterior branches of the vagus nerve and the left gastric artery. The right crus was identified and the esophagus mobilized from this structure. *The hernia sac was then incised circumferentially from the margins of the hiatus/completely excised.* Care was taken to avoid entry into the pleural space.

A penrose was then placed around the esophagus and gentle caudal retraction applied. A careful mediastinal dissection was then carried out to elongate the intraabdominal portion of the esophagus.

The esophagus was then retracted anteriorly and the right and left crus reapproximated with ___-0 *vicryl/monocryl/prolene/PDS* in an interrupted fashion. A piece of synthetic mesh was then fashion for the hiatus and placed overlying the crural repair. This was secured in place with *surgical glue/sutures*.

[Choose One:]
If a Nissen fundoplication was performed: *A ___ FR bougie was then placed into the stomach.* The cardia of the stomach was then grasped and sufficient dissection of the short gastric vessels confirmed. The cardia was then passed posterior to the esophagus and a "shoeshine" maneuver performed. The edges of the cardia were approximated around the distal esophagus and secured to each other and the underlying esophagus with ___-0 *vicryl/prolene/PDS/Ethibond* sutures in an interrupted fashion. This was repeated twice in order to form a 2-cm wrap. The bougie was then removed.

If a Toupet fundoplication was performed: The cardia of the stomach was then passed posterior to the esophagus and a "shoeshine" maneuver performed. The left side of the fundus was then secured to the esophagus with ___-0 *vicryl/prolene/PDS/Ethibond* in an interrupted fashion. The right side was similarly secured to the anterolateral aspect of the esophagus and to the right crus.

The abdomen was inspected and hemostasis confirmed.

If open technique was performed: The fascia was then closed with a __-0 vicryl/prolene/PDS in an interrupted/running/figure-of-eight fashion.

If minimally invasive technique was performed: The liver retractor was carefully removed under direct visualization. The ports were removed and the fascia at the umbilical incision was closed using a ___-0 *vicryl/prolene/PDS* suture. *The fascia at the remaining incisions was closed using a ___-0 ___suture.*

{Continue dictation}

All counts were correct at the end of the case and the attending of record was present and scrubbed for *all/key* portions of the case.

Upon completion of the procedure, a debriefing checklist was completed to share information critical to the postoperative care of the patient. The patient tolerated the procedure well, *was extubated in the operating room*, and was transported to the post-anesthesia care unit in stable condition.

Esophagogastroduodenoscopy and Percutaneous Endoscopic Gastrostomy

8

Justin T. Huntington and Karen A. Diefenbach

Indications and Benefits

- Anatomic evaluation of the upper gastrointestinal tract
- Pathologic sampling of the upper gastrointestinal tract, including malignancy
- Diagnosis of esophagitis (Barrett's), gastritis, duodenitis, ulcer disease, gastroesophageal reflux disease, achalasia
- Evaluation for non-cardiac chest and epigastric pain
- Therapeutic interventions such as removal of foreign body, dilatation for stricture, control of upper gastrointestinal bleeding, and stent placement
- Benefits: Relatively non-invasive, allows for visualization and pathologic sampling, can be diagnostic and therapeutic

Risks and Alternatives

- Standard risks (bleeding, infection, need for additional procedures, risks of sedation/anesthesia)
- Injury to adjacent structures (teeth, mouth, oropharynx, esophagus, stomach, small intestine)
- Procedure-specific risks: Upper gastrointestinal perforation
- Alternatives: Cross-sectional imaging or upper gastrointestinal series can be used for diagnostics but not therapeutics

Essential Steps

1. Visualization of the entire upper gastrointestinal tract including esophagus, stomach, and duodenum
2. Retroflexion of the endoscope to evaluate the gastroesophageal junction and any evidence of hiatal hernia
3. Adequate biopsy samples of any pathologic findings

Note These Variations

- Additional procedures including possible percutaneous endoscopic gastrostomy placement when indicated

Template Operative Dictation

Preoperative Diagnosis Gastritis/esophagitis/gastroesophageal reflux disease/peptic ulcer disease

J. T. Huntington
Nationwide Children's Hospital, Department of Pediatric Surgery, Columbus, OH, USA

K. A. Diefenbach (✉)
Nationwide Children's Hospital, Columbus, OH, USA
e-mail: Karen.Diefenbach@nationwidechildrens.org

D. J. Papandria et al. (eds.), *Operative Dictations in Pediatric Surgery*,
https://doi.org/10.1007/978-3-030-24212-1_8

Postoperative Diagnosis Same as preoperative diagnosis

Findings *Normal anatomy and mucosal appearance/esophagitis/gastritis/duodenitis/ulceration/bleeding noted at ___*

Procedure(s) Performed

1. Esophagogastroduodenoscopy *with/without* biopsy
2. *Percutaneous endoscopic gastrostomy tube placement*

Anesthesia *Procedural sedation/general anesthesia*

Specimens *Snare/forceps biopsies taken at ____*

Drains None

Implants None

Estimated Blood Loss *None/minimal/___ mL*

Indications This is a/an __*-day/week/month/year*-old *male/female* who presents to the operative/endoscopy suite for diagnostic upper endoscopy with possible intervention and biopsy due to concern for *bleeding/abdominal pain* evaluation.

Procedure in Detail Following satisfactory induction of anesthesia/sedation, the patient was placed in a supine position and padded appropriately *and a bite block was placed.* A timeout was performed using both pre-induction and pre-incision safety checklists with participation of all present in the operative/endoscopy suite. These confirmed the correct patient, procedure, operative site, and additional critical information prior to the start of the procedure. All endoscopy equipment was checked for proper function and setup prior to the beginning of the procedure. No prep or preoperative antibiotics were required.

The endoscope was then placed in the oral cavity and passed to the oropharynx. Under visualization and with the use of insufflation, the upper esophagus was identified and intubated. The endoscope was then passed distally into the stomach, ensuring that the lumen was visualized and no undue resistance was met. The stomach was grossly visualized and then retroflexion was used to carefully inspect the cardia of the stomach and to ensure no evidence of hiatal hernia. The endoscope was then straightened and passed to the pylorus and then into the proximal duodenum. Inspection of the duodenum identified *no evidence/evidence* of duodenitis and showed *no evidence/evidence* of gastric outlet obstruction. The endoscope was then slowly withdrawn to inspect the proximal duodenum and then the entire stomach. Aspiration of gastric contents *was/was not* required to assist with visualization of the stomach mucosa. There were not any masses, extrinsic compression, gastritis, or ulcerations visualized. The stomach was then suctioned to remove excess air and the endoscope withdrawn to the level of the gastroesophageal junction. The Z-line/gastroesophageal junction appeared *normal/abnormal. No/__* biopsies were performed *at the following sites: ____*. The endoscope was then slowly withdrawn along the entire course of the esophagus to ensure no esophagitis and no evidence of iatrogenic injury. The endoscope was then withdrawn from the oropharynx and mouth.

[Choose One:]

No gastrostomy placement: The procedure was then terminated and insufflated air aspirated prior to removal of the endoscope.

Percutaneous endoscopic gastrostomy: Upon completion of a complete esophagogastroduodenoscopy being sure to exclude gastric outlet obstruction, an area in the left upper quadrant of the abdomen was prepped and draped in a sterile fashion. The stomach was fully insufflated and distended. The greater curvature was identified endoscopically and palpation of the abdomen was noted to correlate with an acceptable location in the mid to distal stomach to place a gastrostomy tube. Care was taken to select a location one to two finger breadths below the rib cage for placement. One-to-one palpation was noted at the chosen site and transillumination was achieved at this site. Having completed the above measures, the patient was felt to be a suitable percutaneous endoscopic gastrostomy candidate and the kit was opened. The abdomen was then prepped and draped in a normal sterile fashion. Local anesthetic was instilled at the chosen site and then a finder needle was used to confirm position. The needle was inserted slowly and continuous aspiration was performed. There was no aspiration of air until the needle was seen endoscopically. The larger needle was then attached to a syringe and inserted into the same location using the same trajectory. Continuous aspiration was again used and no aspiration noted until the tip of the needle was seen within the stomach. The guidewire was then inserted through the needle. An endoscopic snare was placed around the needle prior to deploying the guidewire. Adequate guidewire length was passed into the lumen of the stomach and grasped with the snare. The needle was then backed out over the wire. A stab incision with an 11-blade scalpel was used on the skin around the wire. The entire endoscope was removed while continuing to hold the guidewire with the snare. The guidewire was then looped around a 16 French PEG tube and snugged to the loop in the guidewire. Lubrication was placed around the PEG tube. The guidewire and PEG were then pulled from the abdominal side of the patient until snug in the stomach. The location of the PEG at the skin level was noted. Repeat upper endoscopy showed the internal bumper to be in a good position, not causing outlet obstruction, and with no signs of bleeding. The stomach was completely aspirated. The endoscope was slowly withdrawn and the esophageal mucosa was examined to ensure no iatrogenic injury. The external bumper was then applied and placed snug but not tight at the skin level and a dressing applied *with antibiotic ointment*. The occlusion clamp was then placed on the PEG tube, which was cut to an appropriate length. The connector housing was then fitted to the end of the tube and attached to a drainage bag.

Upon completion of the procedure, a debriefing checklist was completed to share information critical to the postoperative care of the patient. The patient tolerated the procedure well, *was extubated in the operating room*, and was transported to the post-anesthesia care unit in stable condition thereafter.

9 Gastrostomy Placement (Open and Laparoscopic Approach)

Justin T. Huntington and Karen A. Diefenbach

Indications and Benefits

- Malnutrition, failure to thrive, decreased oral intake, feeding intolerance, oral aversion, need for long-term enteral access
- Dysphagia/aspiration, neurologic impairment
- Esophageal atresia, intestinal discontinuity, gastric decompression
- Benefits: Provides long-term enteral access for nutritional support, ease of administration of enteric medications, more comfortable and durable as compared to nasoenteric feeding access

Risks and Alternatives

- Standard risks (bleeding, infection, need for additional procedures, risks of sedation/anesthesia)
- Injury to adjacent structures (intra-abdominal organs)
- Leakage around gastrostomy tube, dislodgment of the gastrostomy tube (early postoperatively can lead to leakage into the peritoneal cavity, later can lead to buried bumper syndrome, or complete externalization of the tube), tube malfunction (including clogging, cracks in the tubing, breaks in the balloon leading to the tube falling out of the patient requiring replacement), distal displacement or distal initial placement leading to gastric outlet obstruction.
- Alternatives: long-term nasoenteric feeding access

J. T. Huntington
Nationwide Children's Hospital, Department of Pediatric Surgery, Columbus, OH, USA
e-mail: Justin.Huntington2@nationwidechildrens.org

K. A. Diefenbach (✉)
Nationwide Children's Hospital, Columbus, OH, USA
e-mail: Karen.Diefenbach@nationwidechildrens.org

Essential Steps

1. Appropriate position of the gastrostomy on the abdominal wall to decrease future complications
2. Confirmation of intra-luminal placement of the enterostomy tube
3. Securing the stomach to the abdominal wall (Stamm technique)
4. Snugging the external bumper but not overtightening
5. Securing the tube externally with a suture, dressing to buttress the tube, or in combination
6. Careful management postoperatively to include avoidance of torqueing the tube, avoidance of overtightening the external bumper, and local wound care to avoid excess moisture on the skin leading to skin breakdown and wound issues

D. J. Papandria et al. (eds.), *Operative Dictations in Pediatric Surgery*,
https://doi.org/10.1007/978-3-030-24212-1_9

Note These Variations

- Use of endoscopy to perform laparoscopic-assisted PEG placement or confirmation of intraluminal location of enterostomy balloon (see Chap. 10).

Template Operative Dictation (Open)

Preoperative Diagnosis Need for long-term enteral access due to ___

Postoperative Diagnosis Same as preoperative diagnosis

Findings *Stomach amenable to gastrostomy tube placement*

Procedure(s) Performed *Laparoscopic/open* gastrostomy placement

Anesthesia *General anesthesia*

Specimens none

Drains none

Implants gastrostomy (__ French, __ cm, *tube/button* type, *secured at __ cm*)

Estimated Blood Loss *none/minimal/___ mL.*

Indications This is a __ *day-/week-/month-/year-*old *male/female* who presents to the operative suite for placement of gastrostomy tube due to feeding difficulty secondary to ___.

Procedure in Detail Following satisfactory induction of general anesthesia, the patient was placed in a supine position and padded appropriately. A timeout was performed using both pre-induction and pre-incision safety checklists with participation of all present in the operative suite. These confirmed the correct patient, procedure, operative site, and additional critical information prior to the start of the procedure. The abdomen was prepped and draped in a normal sterile fashion and appropriate preoperative antibiotics were administered prior to incision.

[Choose One:]
Laparoscopic gastrostomy tube placement: The subcostal margin on the left was identified and a line was drawn one fingerbreadth below this to mark an appropriate position for a feeding tube prior to insufflation. A location approximately 1–2 cm to the left of midline along this line was deemed an appropriate position for the gastrostomy tube and marked. An umbilical incision was then created and dissection carried down to the level of the umbilical stalk and fascia. This was grasped and elevated. An incision was carried out on the fascia and while lifting with a clamp on the umbilical stalk, a Veress needle was inserted into the abdomen and a saline drop test was reassuring for intraperitoneal placement. The abdomen was insufflated to a pressure of *12* mm Hg. A 5 mm port was then inserted at this umbilical site. The abdomen was inspected and ensured that no injury occurred from initial port placement.

The stomach was visualized and appeared adequate for gastrostomy tube placement. A small finder needle was used at the previously marked location and was clamped at the skin level immediately upon being visualized at the level of the peritoneum. This length was then measured and 4 mm added to this measurement (typical thickness of the stomach) to determine the length of the low-profile gastrostomy button tube. Under direct visualization, a 5 mm port was placed at the previously marked location for the gastrostomy tube. A bowel grasper was used through the left upper quadrant port to grasp the stomach along the greater curvature of the stomach approximately two-thirds of the way from the gastroesophageal junction to the pylorus. This area of the stomach reached the port site and was grasped firmly. The abdomen was desufflated and the left upper quadrant port was removed while maintaining the grasper on the stomach. The stomach was carefully externalized through the port site and a 2-0 stay suture was placed as a stay suture and a snap was placed on the suture. The grasper was then removed from the field. A 3-0 absorbable braided purse-string suture was placed widely on the stomach and directed inferiorly from the stay suture to allow sufficient room for the gastrostomy site. This was placed to a straight snap. Two Stamm sutures were placed, one lateral and one medial. *3-0* absorbable braided sutures were used for this and they were placed from fascia to stomach (outside the purse-string) and then back to fascia. They were placed to curve snaps and placed to the corresponding side of the patient.

The abdomen was then insufflated and the laparoscope was inserted and the area of the stomach to be used for the gastrostomy was visualized. A needle was placed into the stomach within the purse-string and just below the stay suture. Aspiration of air or gastric contents was achieved and then a flexible guidewire placed through the needle. This appeared to be within the stomach on laparoscopy. The needle was backed off of the guidewire and then a Seldinger technique was used with a series of well-lubricated dilators passing easily into the stomach under direct visualization. Once dilated to a size *16* French dilator, the *14* French low-profile gastrostomy button was then passed over the guidewire and passed easily into the stomach. The balloon was inflated with sterile water to *5* mL and appeared to be within the stomach. The guidewire was removed and the appropriate tubing connected to the gastrostomy tube and a large syringe was used to inject *30–60* mL of air into the stomach. This visually inflated the stomach and aspiration decompressed the stomach.

Having completed all confirmatory testing of intra-gastric location, the stay suture was removed and then the purse-string suture was tied followed by the Stamm sutures. These were then trimmed short and the abdomen was desufflated. The fascia at the umbilical port site was closed with *3-0* braided absorbable suture and the skin closed with *deep dermal 5-0 braided* absorbable suture and sterile dressing applied. The gastrostomy tube was then secured with a dressing and left to a gravity bag.

Open gastrostomy tube placement: The subcostal margin on the left was identified and a line was drawn one fingerbreadth below this to mark an appropriate position for a feeding tube prior to insufflation. A location approximately 1–2 cm to the left of midline along this line was deemed an appropriate position for the gastrostomy tube and marked. A small upper midline/upper transverse laparotomy was performed. The abdomen was entered safely and the stomach identified. A location two-thirds of the way from the gastroesophageal junction to the pylorus along the greater curvature was identified as a suitable location for gastrostomy tube placement, and it was ensured that this would reach the abdominal wall at the previously marked location without tension. A 3-0 silk purse-string was placed at this location on the stomach wall. The previously marked location for gastrostomy tube was incised and the abdomen was bluntly entered with a hemostat while protecting the viscera with a malleable retractor. A hemostat from inside the abdomen was snapped to the transabdominal hemostat and passed through the abdominal wall. A 14 French gastrostomy tube was grasped and pulled through the abdominal wall. The balloon was checked for patency by instilling sterile water in the balloon port and then desufflated. Within the purse-string suture, a full thickness gastrotomy was created with cautery and gastric contents were encountered. The gastrostomy tube was inserted into the stomach and the purse-string was tied down. The balloon was inflated with 5 cc of sterile water and was felt to be within the stomach and patent. Two Lembert sutures were placed on either side of the tube with 3-0 silk, taking care to avoid the balloon. Four 3-0 silk Stamm sutures were placed from the abdominal wall to the seromuscular portion of the stomach outside of the purse-string suture, beginning with the lateral suture, which was snapped with an identifying hemostat. These sutures were then tied down beginning with the lateral suture. These sutures were trimmed and again the balloon was confirmed to be intact and the gastrostomy tube was instilled with air and then aspirated to confirm appropriate functionality. The skin level on the tube was noted and the tube was secured to the skin with 3-0 nylon suture. The fascia was closed with running 3-0 braided absorbable suture, and then the skin was closed with running subcuticular 5-0 braided absorbable suture and sterile dressings applied. The external bumper was placed snuggly but not tight. The gastrostomy tube was then secured with a dressing and left to a gravity bag.

Laparoscopic-assisted percutaneous endoscopic gastrostomy (PEG) tube placement: The subcostal margin on the left was identified, and a line was drawn one fingerbreadth below this to mark an appropriate position for a feeding tube prior to insufflation. A location approximately 1–2 cm to the left of midline along this line was deemed an appropriate position for the gastrostomy tube and marked. An umbilical incision was then created and dissection carried down to the level of the umbilical stalk and fascia. This was grasped and elevated. An incision was carried out on the fascia and while lifting with a clamp on the umbilical stalk, a Veress needle was inserted into the abdomen and a saline drop test was reassuring for intraperitoneal placement. The abdomen was insufflated to a pressure of 12 mm Hg. A 5 mm port was then inserted at this umbilical site. The abdomen was inspected and ensured that no injury occurred from initial port placement.

Attention was then turned to performing a complete esophagogastroduodenoscopy being sure to exclude gastric outlet obstruction. The stomach was fully insufflated and distended. The greater curvature was identified endoscopically and the area of light transillumination was seen from the endoscope by laparoscopy. The previously marked area on the abdominal wall was within a reasonable distance to pass a needle from this site into the stomach near the greater curvature of the stomach away from the pylorus. The needle was visualized entering the stomach by the endoscope. An endoscopic snare was placed around the needle prior to deploying the guidewire. Adequate guidewire length was passed into the lumen of the stomach and grasped with the snare. The needle was then backed out over the wire. A stab incision with an 11-blade scalpel was used on the skin around the wire. The entire endoscope was removed while continuing to hold the guidewire with the snare. The guidewire was then looped around a 16 French PEG tube and snugged to the loop in the guidewire. Lubrication was placed around the PEG tube. The guidewire and PEG were then pulled from the abdominal side of the patient until snug in the stomach. The location of the PEG at the skin level was noted. Repeat upper endoscopy showed the internal bumper to be in a good position, not causing outlet obstruction, and with no signs of bleeding. The stomach was completely aspirated. The endoscope was slowly withdrawn and the esophageal mucosa was examined to ensure no iatrogenic injury. The external bumper was then applied and placed snug but not tight at the skin level and a dressing applied. The PEG tube was cut to an appropriate length and attached to a drainage bag. The umbilical stalk and fascia were closed with 2-0 absorbable braided suture, and the skin at the umbilicus was closed with a deep dermal 4-0 absorbable braided suture and a sterile dressing applied on top of this.

Upon completion of the procedure, a debriefing checklist was completed to share information critical to the postoperative care of the patient. The patient tolerated the procedure well, *was extubated in the operating room*, and was transported to the post-anesthesia care unit in stable condition thereafter.

10 Pyloromyotomy (Open and Laparoscopic Approach)

Justin T. Huntington and Karen A. Diefenbach

Indications and Benefits

- Hypertrophic pyloric stenosis (ultrasound findings of 4 mm thickness or greater, 14 mm channel length or greater, some variation is found at differing institutions, can also be diagnosed by upper gastrointestinal series)
- Benefits: Provides surgical correction results in resolution of this problem, there can be postoperative gastric atony that requires patience from the surgeon and family for resolution

Risks and Alternatives

- Standard risks (bleeding, infection, need for additional procedures, risks of sedation/anesthesia)
- Injury to adjacent structures (duodenum, stomach)
- Duodenal injury, full thickness injury at the pylorus requiring repair and additional myotomy, incomplete myotomy, delayed gastric emptying
- Alternatives: in very poor surgical candidates, patients can be maintained with orogastric decompression and transpyloric feeding or TPN while allowing time for this problem to resolve

Essential Steps

1. Correct dehydration and electrolyte derangements prior to surgical intervention.
2. Ensure adequate myotomy (typically by demonstration of independent movement of superior and inferior margins).
3. Ensure no full-thickness injury.

Note These Variations

- Use of air insufflation via a preoperatively placed nasogastric tube to test for leakage/full-thickness injury at myotomy site.
- Open procedure may be performed via supraumbilical curvilinear skin incision and midline fascial division superiorly at the linea alba.
- Full-thickness injury during myotomy: primary repair of the full-thickness injury with interrupted sutures and then rotate pylorus to perform the pyloromyotomy on a different aspect of the pylorus. Omental patch can be used on top of the perforation. The OG catheter can be left in place and postoperative upper gastrointestinal series completed to ensure no active leaking from the repair.

J. T. Huntington
Nationwide Children's Hospital, Department of Pediatric Surgery, Columbus, OH, USA

K. A. Diefenbach (✉)
Nationwide Children's Hospital, Columbus, OH, USA
e-mail: Karen.Diefenbach@nationwidechildrens.org

D. J. Papandria et al. (eds.), *Operative Dictations in Pediatric Surgery*,
https://doi.org/10.1007/978-3-030-24212-1_10

Template Operative Dictation (Laparoscopic)

Preoperative Diagnosis Hypertrophic pyloric stenosis

Postoperative Diagnosis Same as preoperative diagnosis

Findings consistent with postoperative diagnosis

Procedure(s) Performed Laparoscopic pyloromyotomy

Anesthesia *General anesthesia*

Specimens none

Drains none

Implants none

Estimated Blood Loss *none/minimal*

Indications This is a __ *day/week* old *male/female* who presents to the operative suite for pyloromyotomy due to preoperative findings of hypertrophic pyloric stenosis. The patient was admitted preoperatively and resuscitated with intravenous fluids and correction of electrolyte derangements was confirmed by laboratory results.

Procedure in Detail Following satisfactory induction of anesthesia/sedation, the patient was placed in a supine position and padded appropriately. A timeout was performed using both pre-induction and pre-incision safety checklists with participation of all present in the operative suite. These confirmed the correct patient, procedure, operative site, and additional critical information prior to the start of the procedure. *Appropriate perioperative antibiotics were administered.*

The patient was placed transversely on the OR table in a supine position with head slightly up and a monitor placed across from the operating surgeon. An OG catheter was placed and kept to low intermittent wall suction. The abdomen was prepped and draped in a normal sterile fashion. Local anesthetic was instilled around the umbilicus, and then the umbilicus was grasped and the base of the appendix was bluntly opened with a curved hemostat. The instrument was noted to be intraperitoneal by showing mobility in all directions. A 3 mm port was then placed and insufflation to 10 mmHg was achieved. A laparoscope was inserted. This showed the stomach to be decompressed with the OG catheter and the pylorus appeared thickened.

Under direct visualization, local anesthetic was instilled in the right upper quadrant just below the level of the liver near the mid-clavicular line. This was followed by an 11 blade being used to create a stab incision under direct visualization until the peritoneum was penetrated. A duodenal grasper was then placed through this incision site under direct visualization. Local anesthetic was then instilled under direct visualization in the left upper quadrant above and just to the patient's left of the pylorus. This was followed by an 11 blade being used to create a stab incision under direct visualization until the peritoneum was penetrated. A long-tip insulated Bovie electrocautery device was then placed through this incision site under direct visualization. The cautery was set to 0 and coagulation set to 10. The duodenal grasper was used to gently grasp the proximal duodenum and to roll the pylorus into the field of view.

The cautery pencil was used to palpate the proximal and distal extent of the hypertrophic muscle and then was used with coagulation to mark deliberately the area to be used for pyloromyotomy while avoiding vessels and being sure to not dissect too proximally or distally. A second pass was used to score the entire line. The tip of the Bovie was then used to bluntly dissect at the center of the scored line and bluntly dissect through the hypertrophic muscle. This was rotated 360 degrees. The cautery was then exchanged for a blunt, hockey-tip style pyloric spreader. This was engaged in the center of the dissection line and once within the muscle was spread slowly under direct visualization. The mucosa was seen bulging below this and was intact. The pyloric spreader was then used proximally and distally until the muscle splayed out. The graspers were then used to ensure independent movement of the upper and lower aspects of the muscle.

If air insufflation leak test performed: the anesthesiologist then instilled air through the OG tube until the stomach was distended while the duodenum was occluded. There was no bubbling visualized nor any bilious fluid seen. The duodenal occlusion was released and air was seen going through the pylorus and filling the duodenum. The stomach was then aspirated of all air and the orogastric tube removed.

The instruments were removed under visualization and there were no signs of bleeding. The abdomen was desufflated and the umbilical stalk was closed with 3-0 absorbable braided suture. Skin was closed with 5-0 absorbable braided suture and surgical glue was placed on top of this in multiple layers.

Upon completion of the procedure, a debriefing checklist was completed to share information critical to the postoperative care of the patient. The patient tolerated the procedure well, *was extubated in the operating room*, and was transported to the postanesthesia care unit in stable condition thereafter.

Template Operative Dictation (Open)

Preoperative Diagnosis Hypertrophic pyloric stenosis

Postoperative Diagnosis Same as preoperative diagnosis

Findings consistent with postoperative diagnosis

Procedure(s) Performed Open pyloromyotomy

Anesthesia *General anesthesia*

Specimens none

Drains none

Implants none

Estimated Blood Loss *none/minimal*

Indications This is a __ *day/week* old *male/female* who presents to the operative suite for pyloromyotomy due to preoperative findings of hypertrophic pyloric stenosis. The patient was admitted preoperatively and resuscitated with intravenous fluids and correction of electrolyte derangements was confirmed by laboratory results.

Procedure in Detail The patient was placed on the OR table in a supine position. An OG catheter was placed and kept to low intermittent wall suction. The abdomen was prepped and draped in a normal sterile fashion. A small transverse incision was created just to the right of midline at the level of the edge of the liver. The anterior rectus sheath, rectus muscle, and posterior rectus sheath were divided and the abdomen was entered safely. The stomach and pylorus were identified and the pylorus was externalized and the pylorus did appear thickened, consistent with the diagnosis of hypertrophic pyloric stenosis. The proximal and distal extents of the pyloric stenosis were identified. Bovie electrocautery was used to create a longitudinal mark along the pyloric stenosis and the muscle was superficially divided. A blunt pyloric spreader was then used and inserted into the muscle and slow traction was used to divide the muscle down to the level of bulging mucosa. The proximal and distal extents were spread similarly until the muscle splayed out and the upper and lower portion showed independent movement. Air was then given via the orogastric tube. This caused distention of the stomach and pylorus. There was no bubbling or bilious drainage seen. Hemostasis was satisfactory. The stomach was aspirated of all air and the pylorus delivered back into the abdomen. The fascia was closed in two layers with 3-0 absorbable braided suture, and the skin was closed with running subcuticular 5-0 absorbable braided suture followed by a sterile dressing.

If air insufflation leak test performed: the anesthesiologist then instilled air through the OG tube until the stomach was distended while the duodenum was occluded. There was no bubbling visualized nor any bilious fluid seen. The duodenal occlusion was released and air was seen going through the pylorus and filling the duodenum. The stomach was then aspirated of all air and the orogastric tube removed.

Upon completion of the procedure, a debriefing checklist was completed to share information critical to the postoperative care of the patient. The patient tolerated the procedure well, *was extubated in the operating room*, and was transported to the postanesthesia care unit in stable condition thereafter.

11 Exploratory Laparotomy for Complications of Peptic Ulcer Disease

Justin T. Huntington and Karen A. Diefenbach

Indications and Benefits

- Perforation secondary to peptic ulcer disease
- Bleeding peptic ulcers despite maximum medically stable or in the severely hemodynamically unstable bleeding peptic ulcer patient
- Stricture due to peptic ulcer disease
- Failure of medical management to clear peptic ulcer disease or unable to rule out underlying malignancy
- Benefits: Tissue diagnosis, definitive surgical management

Risks and Alternatives

- Standard risks (bleeding, infection, need for additional procedures, risks of sedation/anesthesia)
- Injury to adjacent structures (esophagus, stomach, duodenum, bile/pancreatic ducts)
- Procedure-specific risks: Ongoing bleeding, anastomotic leak/stricture, ongoing peptic ulcer disease, post-vagotomy syndromes, marginal ulcers
- Alternatives: Endoscopic therapies, angioembolization, medical therapies with acid suppression

Essential Steps

1. Stop bleeding for peptic ulcer disease with active bleeding.
2. Source control and repair for perforated ulcer.
3. Biopsy or resect gastric ulcerations to rule out underlying malignancy.
4. *Helicobacter pylori* testing (serum or biopsy).

Note These Variations

- Significant variability depending on presentation, underlying issue, surgeon preferences.
- In the event of an antrectomy, a Billroth I (described here), Billroth II, or Roux-en-Y reconstruction may be performed depending on patient factors and surgeon preference.

Template Operative Dictation (Open)

Preoperative Diagnosis Peptic ulcer disease refractory to medical management, complicated by *bleeding/perforation/obstruction*

J. T. Huntington
Nationwide Children's Hospital, Department of Pediatric Surgery, Columbus, OH, USA

K. A. Diefenbach (✉)
Nationwide Children's Hospital, Columbus, OH, USA
e-mail: Karen.Diefenbach@nationwidechildrens.org

D. J. Papandria et al. (eds.), *Operative Dictations in Pediatric Surgery*,
https://doi.org/10.1007/978-3-030-24212-1_11

Postoperative Diagnosis Same as preoperative diagnosis

Findings Peptic ulcer disease, *with ___ perforation/obstruction/hemorrhage*

Procedure(s) Performed

1. Exploratory laparotomy
2. *Repair of duodenal perforation/oversewing of bleeding peptic ulcer*
3. *Truncal/selective vagotomy and pyloroplasty*
4. *Subtotal gastrectomy*

Anesthesia General anesthesia

Specimens None/partial gastrectomy/biopsy for malignancy and/or *H. Pylori*

Drains *None/__ French Jackson Pratt*

Implants None

Estimated Blood Loss *__ mL*

Indications This is a/an *__-day/week/month/year*-old *male/female* who presents to the operative suite for __ due to concern for peptic ulcer disease with *refractory bleeding/perforation/obstruction/concern for malignancy.*

Procedure in Detail Following satisfactory induction of anesthesia/sedation, the patient was placed in a supine position and padded appropriately. A timeout was performed using both pre-induction and pre-incision safety checklists with participation of all present in the operative/endoscopy suite. These confirmed the correct patient, procedure, operative site, and additional critical information prior to the start of the procedure. Appropriate perioperative antibiotics were administered.

[Choose One:]

If perforated duodenal ulcer (primary repair): The stomach and duodenum were inspected and a perforation was noted along the second portion of the duodenum with ___ contamination that was addressed with irrigation until effluent was clear. The remainder of the stomach, small bowel, and colon showed no other abnormalities. The NG tube was palpated within the stomach and was in a good position. The edges of the bowel were healthy and therefore were primarily repaired with interrupted 3-0 Vicryl in a single-layer closure. A pedicle of omentum was then used to cover this repair in a modified Graham patch. Three 2-0 Silk sutures were used to take bites on each side of the repair and the tongue of omentum passed under these sutures and then tied to approximate but not crush the tissue.

If perforated duodenal ulcer (Graham patch): The stomach and duodenum were inspected. There was noted to be perforation along the second portion of the duodenum. The abdomen was irrigated thoroughly until effluent was clear. The remainder of the stomach, small bowel, and colon showed no other abnormalities. The NG tube was palpated within the stomach and was in a good position. The edges of the bowel were *ischemic/irregular/attenuated* and therefore primary closure was not attempted. A pedicle of omentum was then used to cover this repair as a Graham patch. 2-0 silk sutures were used to take seromuscular bites circumferentially about the defect and the tongue of omentum was transfixed within the defect in the duodenal wall. The sutures were then tied to approximate but not crush the tissue.

If perforated duodenal ulcer (jejunal buttress repair): The stomach and duodenum were inspected. There was noted to be perforation along the second portion of the duodenum. The abdomen was irrigated thoroughly until effluent was clear. The remainder of the stomach, small bowel, and colon showed no other abnormalities. The NG tube was palpated within the stomach and was in a good position. The edges of the bowel were *ischemic/irregular/attenuated* and therefore primary closure was not attempted. As there was insufficient omentum to effect a Graham patch, a loop of jejunum was identified __ cm from the ligament of Treitz, which was mobilized to the level of the perforation via an *antecolic/retrocolic* route. Interrupted 2-0 silk sutures were used to take seromuscular bites of the duodenal wall and jejunal buttress circumferentially about the defect in an only repair. The sutures were then tied to approximate but not crush the tissue.

If bleeding peptic ulcer: A Kocher maneuver was performed to achieve better visualization of the duodenum. Preoperative workup showed the bleeding ulcer to be in the proximal duodenum (or specify location). A longitudinal duodenotomy was then performed. The ulcer was identified on the posterior wall of the duodenum and direct digital pressure was used to control bleeding. This was then replaced with a sponge stick which controlled bleeding. 3-0 silk sutures were used to control the bleeding in a three-point ligation technique. These sutures were placed superior, inferior, and toward the patient's left side to control all branches of the bleeding vessel. Care was taken to identify the ampulla and avoid injury to the common bile duct. *The duodenotomy was then extended along the stomach parallel to the greater curvature and the gastric lumen further explored in search of a gastric nidus of bleeding. The incision was continued through the pylorus and a Heineke-Mikulicz/Finney pyloroplasty was performed to close the distal extent of the gastrotomy and duodenotomy, which was located at the ___.* The area was irrigated and observed. There was no additional bleeding present. The duodenum was then closed transversely with full-thickness interrupted 3-0 Vicryl sutures and then 3-0 interrupted silk Lembert sutures were placed over this.

If perforated gastric ulcer or mass: The area of the stomach with the perforation/mass was identified. The remainder of the abdomen was inspected and showed no other evidence of masses or metastatic disease.

If stapled resection: A wedge resection using a series of linear stapler cutter (using *purple/green/black* loads) *with/without* staple reinforcement. *The staple line was then oversewn with 2-0/3-0/4-0 silk/Vicryl in interrupted Lembert sutures/with a running seromuscular suture.*

If handsewn reconstruction: The affected portion of the stomach was excised with coagulating monopolar current and the resulting defect closed in *a single layer/two layers* with interrupted ___-0 silk/Vicryl sutures. *The location of the resection necessitated division of right/left gastric/gastroepiploic vessels with the LigaSure vessel sealer/clamps and ___-0 silk ties.*

Upper endoscopy was completed to ensure no additional ulcers or masses and a water leak test was used to ensure no leak of the wedge resection area and the staple line was inspected for any bleeding. The resection did not create any areas of stenosis by upper endoscopy or by external visualization of the stomach.

If vagotomy performed: The most proximal stomach was then identified and the pars flaccida was incised. The proximal stomach was dissected free from surrounding structures to the level of the right crus taking care to avoid any accessory left hepatic artery. Once this was completed, the left side of the stomach was mobilized from surrounding structures to expose the left crus. The retroesophageal space was dissected free at the gastroesophageal junction and a Penrose drain was placed at this level and inferior traction was used. The left (anterior) vagus was identified traveling along the anterior esophagus quite adherent to the esophagus. A 1-cm section was removed between clips and sent for frozen pathology. The right (posterior) vagus was identified posterior to the esophagus slightly away from the esophagus. It was resected in the same manner and sent for frozen pathology. Subsequent pathologic examination showed nerve tissue for both specimens.

[Choose One or None:]

If pyloroplasty: A longitudinal incision was then placed along the anterior aspect of the pylorus with coagulating current. This was subsequently closed transversely with interrupted *___-0 silk* sutures to fashion a *Heineke-Mikulicz pyloroplasty.*

If antrectomy: The anterior and posterior branches of the vagus nerve were identified and a truncal vagotomy performed with a segment of each nerve sent for pathologic examination. A full Kocher maneuver was performed. An energy device was used to ligate the right gastroepiploic vessels, the vessels along the greater curvature of the stomach, the right gastric vessels, and the distal gastrohepatic ligament. The posterior stomach was then dissected free from surrounding structures. A stapler (with or without staple reinforcement) was used to divide the stomach at the level of healthy tissue and near the level of the angularis. A distal resection was carried out distal to the pylorus on the proximal duodenum through healthy tissue with a stapling device, taking care to avoid the common bile duct and pancreas. The specimen was sent for permanent pathology (unless any concern for malignancy in which case it would be sent for frozen pathology). The duodenum was able to be brought to the greater curvature of the stomach to perform a Billroth I reconstruction. This was performed by opening the staple line on the duodenum and the same length of staple line on the inferior staple line of the stomach (on the side of the greater curvature). The posterior duodenum and posterior stomach were approximated by taking seromuscular bites with interrupted 3-0 silk sutures to approximate the entire posterior anastomosis. A 3-0 running Vicryl suture was then used to take full-thickness bites beginning in the mid-posterior wall and two separate sutures (one run inferior and one superior). At the inferior and superior aspects of the anastomosis, a Connell-type suture technique was used to avoid anastomotic stenosis and then these sutures were run on the anterior aspect of the anastomosis and tied to one another. The entire remainder of the anastomosis not previously approximated with silk suture was oversewn with interrupted 3-0 silk Lambert sutures to cover the running anastomosis. The fascia was then closed with interrupted 2-0 Vicryl and then skin closed loosely with 5–0 deep dermal sutures and a sterile dressing applied.

A closed suction drain was then placed next to the identified lesion. The fascia was then closed with interrupted 2-0 Vicryl and then skin closed loosely with 5-0 deep dermal sutures and a sterile dressing applied.

Upon completion of the procedure, a debriefing checklist was completed to share information critical to the postoperative care of the patient. The patient tolerated the procedure well, *was extubated in the operating room*, and was transported to the post-anesthesia care unit in stable condition thereafter.

Placement of Gastric Electrical Stimulator

12

Dominic J. Papandria and Karen A. Diefenbach

Indications and Benefits

- Gastroparesis
- Gastrointestinal dysmotility
- Benefits: improvement in gastric emptying

Risks and Alternatives

- Standard risks (bleeding, infection, need for additional procedures, risks of anesthesia)
- Injury to adjacent structures (stomach, colon, liver)
- Dislodgement or displacement of gastric electrical stimulation leads
- Non-therapeutic procedure with persistence of preoperative symptoms, discomfort related to stimulation
- Need for additional procedures or surgery, specifically conversion of temporary stimulation to placement of permanent stimulator, replacement of generator and battery
- Alternatives: Continued medical management of impaired gastric emptying

Essential Steps

Endoscopic

1. Lead preparation
2. Esophagogastroscopy
3. Nasogastric passage of temporary leads
4. Securement of leads to gastric mucosa using endoscopic clips
5. Connection of leads and initial programming of stimulator generator
6. Securement of extracorporeal lead

Laparoscopic

1. Abdominal access and diagnostic laparoscopy
2. Intramural securement of leads at the gastric antrum, with or without simultaneous endoscopic visualization
3. Connection of leads and initial programming of stimulator generator
4. Formation of subcutaneous pocket and placement of stimulator generator
5. Closure of incisions

D. J. Papandria
Department of Surgery, Emory University,
Atlanta, GA, USA

K. A. Diefenbach (✉)
Nationwide Children's Hospital,
Columbus, OH, USA
e-mail: Karen.Diefenbach@nationwidechildrens.org

D. J. Papandria et al. (eds.), *Operative Dictations in Pediatric Surgery*,
https://doi.org/10.1007/978-3-030-24212-1_12

Open

1. Laparotomy
2. Intramural securement of leads at the gastric antrum, with or without simultaneous endoscopic visualization
3. Connection of leads and initial programming of stimulator generator
4. Formation of subcutaneous pocket and placement of stimulator generator
5. Closure of incisions

Note These Variations

- Intraoperative endoscopy can be used to confirm intramural placement of permanent leads and avoid violation of the gastric mucosa as leads are advanced.
- Dictation reflects placement of an Enterra II (Medtronic, Minneapolis, MN), but other approved gastric neurostimulator products can be utilized.
- The presence of a gastrostomy, gastrojejunostomy, or diverting enterostomy requires careful exclusion of these sites from the operative field as well as possible adjustment to port placement and generator siting to avoid contamination of the implanted device.
- Generator replacement for battery failure is typically performed locally, without the need to obtain intraperitoneal access or adjust lead placement/positioning.

Template Operative Dictation (Endoscopic)

Preoperative Diagnosis Impaired gastric emptying

Postoperative Diagnosis Same as preoperative diagnosis

Findings Same as postoperative diagnosis

Procedure(s) Performed
1. Upper endoscopy
2. Temporary Placement of gastric electrical stimulator with nasogastric leads

Anesthesia *General/procedural sedation*

Specimen None

Drains None

Implants
1. ____ gastric neurostimulator generator, Serial number: ____
2. ____ neurostimulator multi-polar lead, Serial number: ____

Estimated Blood Loss None

Indications This is a/an ___-*year*-old *male/female* with impaired gastric emptying secondary to ____. He/she was evaluated and deemed to be a suitable candidate for temporary placement of gastric electrical stimulator to assess potential benefit prior to placement of an implanted device.

Procedure in Detail Following satisfactory induction of *anesthesia/sedation*, the patient was placed in supine position and appropriately padded. Timeouts were performed using both pre-induction and pre-incision safety checklists with participation of all present in the operative suite. These confirmed the correct patient, procedure, operative site, and additional critical information prior to the start of the procedure. *The patient was then fitted with a bite block.*

A flexible gastroscope was introduced per oris, traversing the pharynx and esophagus under endoscopic vision to access the stomach. All visualized structures were unremarkable *with the exception of* ___. A site for stimulator lead placement was identified along the anterior greater curve and the temporary lead was introduced per the *left/right* naris and advanced blindly/under endoscopic vision until the electrode tip reached the site of interest.

[Choose One:]

If securing with ties and clips: The multi-channel stimulator lead was then prepared for insertion by fashioning loops in a 2-0 silk tie and tying this to the distal end of the lead. Care was taken not to obstruct the contact electrodes present in the distal lead housing. The lead was then secured using the endoscopic clip applier, affixing the silk loops to the gastric mucosa *at four points*.

If securing with clips alone: The mucosa was then imbricated over the tip of the lead using the endoscopic clip applier, completely covering the electrodes.

The lead placement was then inspected and found to be satisfactory. The lead terminals were then connected to the generator and interrogated using designated equipment provided by the manufacturer, verifying impedance (___ Ohm) and current within goal range. The generator was then programmed with the following settings:

Voltage: ___ V
Pulse window: ___ ms
Time on: ___ sec
Time off: ___ sec
Frequency: ___ Hz

Insufflated gas was then aspirated, endoscopy terminated, and the endoscope removed. Upon completion of the procedure, a debriefing checklist was completed to share information critical to the postoperative care of the patient. The patient tolerated the procedure well, *was extubated in the operating room*, and was transported to the post-anesthesia care unit in stable condition thereafter.

Template Operative Dictation (Open)

Preoperative Diagnosis Impaired gastric emptying

Postoperative Diagnosis Same as preoperative diagnosis

Findings Same as postoperative diagnosis

Procedure(s) Performed

1. Placement of gastric electrical stimulator (*left/right*-sided)
2. *Upper endoscopy*

Anesthesia *General/procedural sedation*

Specimen None

Drains None

Implants

1. ____ gastric neurostimulator generator, Serial number: ____
2. ____ neurostimulator leads, Serial numbers: ____, ____

Estimated Blood Loss None

Indications This is a/an ___-*year*-old *male/female* with impaired gastric emptying secondary to ____. He/she was evaluated and deemed to be a suitable candidate for open placement of gastric electrical stimulator *by clinical criteria/following trial of a temporary stimulator.*

Procedure in Detail Following satisfactory induction of anesthesia, the patient was placed in supine position and appropriately padded. Timeouts were performed using both pre-induction and pre-incision safety checklists with participation of all present in the operative suite. These confirmed the correct patient, procedure, operative site, and additional critical information prior to the start of the procedure. The abdomen was then prepped and draped in the usual sterile fashion *and an Ioban impermeable drape was applied.* A site for subcutaneous placement of the stimulator generator was identified and marked in the *left lower quadrant.*

A/an ___-mm *midline/left paramedian* incision was placed and carried down to the level of the fascia using electrocautery laparotomy. This was then divided using electrocautery, proceeding to the peritoneum. This was placed on anterior traction and sharply incised, then opened along the whole of the incision using cautery. A cursory inspection of the intraperitoneal contents revealed no traumatic sequelae of abdominal access.

[Choose One:]

If using intraoperative endoscopy: *The patient was fitted with a bite block* and simultaneous flexible endoscopy was then performed. A flexible gastroscope was introduced per oris, traversing the pharynx and esophagus under endoscopic vision to access the stomach. All visualized structures were unremarkable *with the exception of* ___. The site for stimulator lead placement was confirmed and maintained under endoscopic surveillance. The gastric mucosa was observed endoscopically during lead placement and this was not violated. Insufflated gas was then aspirated and the endoscope removed on completion of lead placement.

The guide suture was placed longitudinally within the gastric wall using a needle driver. Gentle traction was then applied to the suture to draw the attached electrode into proper position. This was repeated to place the second lead. The leads were then transfixed to the stomach by placing interrupted *0 Ethibond* first bilaterally through the silicone retention flange on each lead, then taking seromuscular bites of the adjacent antrum. Silicone retention discs were then introduced per the port and the guide sutures were passed through the center of each. Both discs were then secured to the stomach with bilateral interrupted *0 Ethibond* sutures in similar fashion to the flange. Finally, each lead's retention suture was fixed at the level of the disc using the medium clip applier. The exposed segments of the guide sutures were then transected and the needles removed from the peritoneum.

A 6-cm transverse incision was placed at the previously identified site for generator placement in the *left lower quadrant*. This was carried down through the skin and subcutaneous tissues to the level of the fascia using electrocautery. The extraperitoneal segments of the leads were then tunneled to this wound bed. The pocket for the stimulator was developed using a combination of blunt dissection and electrocautery along the anterior fascia *inferior*. On completion, this accommodated the implant without tension of the overlying skin.

The laparotomy incision was then closed in layers, starting with interrupted *0 Vicryl* for the fascia leaving a 3-mm defect for the traversing leads. This was followed by closure of the deep dermal layer with interrupted *4-0 Vicryl* and skin closure with *5-0 Monocryl* in continuous subcuticular fashion.

The device to be implanted was then connected to the leads and interrogated and then disabled using designated equipment provided by the manufacturer, verifying impedance (___ Ohm) and current within goal range. The generator was then programmed with the following settings:

Voltage: ___ V
Pulse window: ___ ms
Time on: ___ sec
Time off: ___ sec
Frequency: ___ Hz

The device was then deactivated to permit the use of monopolar cautery and placed within the subcutaneous pocket. Redundant lead wiring was coiled and placed behind the generator within the pocket. The wound was then closed in layers, using interrupted *3-0 Vicryl* for Scarpa's fascia, interrupted deep dermal *4-0 Vicryl* sutures, and skin closure with *5-0 Monocryl* in continuous subcuticular fashion. All incisions were then dressed with surgical skin adhesive. The device was re-interrogated and activated following confirmation of acceptable lead impedance.

Upon completion of the procedure, a debriefing checklist was completed to share information critical to the postoperative care of the patient. The patient tolerated the procedure well, was extubated in the operating room, and was transported to the post-anesthesia care unit in stable condition thereafter.

Template Operative Dictation (Laparoscopic)

Preoperative Diagnosis Impaired gastric emptying

Postoperative Diagnosis Same as preoperative diagnosis

Findings Same as postoperative diagnosis

Procedure(s) Performed
1. Diagnostic laparoscopy
2. Laparoscopic Placement of gastric electrical stimulator (*left/right*-sided)
3. *Upper endoscopy*

Anesthesia General

Specimen None

Drains None

Implants
1. ____ gastric neurostimulator generator, Serial number: ____
2. ____ neurostimulator leads, Serial numbers: ____, ____

Estimated Blood Loss ___ mL

Indications This is a/an ___-*year*-old *male/female* with impaired gastric emptying secondary to ____. He/she was evaluated and deemed to be a suitable candidate for laparoscopic placement of gastric electrical stimulator *by clinical criteria/following trial of a temporary stimulator.*

Procedure in Detail Following satisfactory induction of anesthesia, the patient was placed in supine position and appropriately padded. Timeouts were performed using both pre-induction and pre-incision safety checklists with participation of all present in the operative suite. These confirmed the correct patient, procedure, operative site, and additional critical information prior to the start of the procedure. The abdomen was then prepped and draped in the usual sterile fashion *and an Ioban impermeable drape was applied.* A site for subcutaneous placement of the stimulator generator was identified and marked in the *left lower quadrant.*

A 5-mm umbilical incision was placed and carried down to the level of the fascia using blunt dissection. The abdomen was entered, followed by placement of a 5-mm trocar. The abdomen was then insufflated to a pressure of *15* mmHg and the laparoscope was introduced into the peritoneal cavity. A cursory survey of the abdominal contents revealed no traumatic sequelae of abdominal access. Local anesthetic infiltration and stab incisions were then placed at two additional trocar sites: a 5-mm port was placed in the *left upper quadrant* and a 10–12 mm port in *left lower quadrant* under laparoscopic vision. The incision for the latter port was placed at the previously marked generator site; this was extended transversely by 5 cm and carried down to the level of the fascia with electrocautery. The fascia was divided with electrocautery and the abdomen entered bluntly with a hemostat. This was replaced with a Veress needle within a dilating sheath, which was then used to insufflate the abdomen to a pressure of 12 mmHg, and this was well tolerated. The needle was removed and a 5-mm radially dilating port was placed per the sheath and a 5-mm laparoscope introduced into the abdomen. A cursory laparoscopic examination of the intra-abdominal contents revealed no traumatic sequelae of abdominal access. Local anesthetic infiltration and stab incisions were then placed, followed by placement of 5-mm radially dilating ports in the *left lower quadrant* and *left upper quadrant.* Finally, the umbilical port was replaced with a 10–12 mm radially dilating port and all port placements were performed under laparoscopic vision.

The two stimulator leads were then introduced per *the left lower quadrant* port and positioned to lie without tension on the stomach at favorable sites on the anterior gastric wall.

[Choose One:]

If using intraoperative endoscopy: *The patient was fitted with a bite block* and simultaneous flexible endoscopy was then performed. A flexible gastroscope was introduced per oris, traversing the pharynx and esophagus under endoscopic vision to access the stomach. All visualized structures were unremarkable *with the exception of* ___. The site for stimulator lead placement was confirmed and maintained under endoscopic surveillance. The gastric mucosa was observed endoscopically during lead placement and this was not violated. Insufflated gas was then aspirated and the endoscope removed.

The guide suture was placed longitudinally within the gastric wall using a laparoscopic needle driver. Gentle traction was then applied to the suture to draw the attached electrode into proper position. This was repeated to place the second lead. The leads were then transfixed to the stomach by placing interrupted *0 Ethibond* first bilaterally through the silicone retention flange on each lead, then taking seromuscular bites of the adjacent antrum. Silicone retention discs were then introduced per the port and the guide sutures were passed through the center of each. Both discs were then secured to the stomach with bilateral interrupted *0 Ethibond* sutures in similar fashion to the flange. Finally, each lead's retention suture was fixed at the level of the disc using the 5-mm clip applier. The exposed segments of the guide sutures were then transected and the needles removed from the peritoneum. The extraperitoneal segments of the leads were then delivered through the *left lower quadrant* port, which was then removed.

The remaining port was then removed under laparoscopic vision and site was noted to be hemostatic. Following desufflation of the abdomen, the 5-mm sites were closed at the fascia using interrupted *3-0 Vicryl* and 10–12 mm site using *2-0 Vicryl* in similar fashion, securing the leads. The pocket for the stimulator was developed using a combination of blunt dissection and electrocautery just superficial to the anterior fascia *inferior* to the incision in the *left lower quadrant*. On completion, this accommodated the implant without tension of the overlying skin.

The device to be implanted was then connected to the leads and interrogated and then disabled using designated equipment provided by the manufacturer, verifying impedance (___ Ohm) and current within goal range. The generator was then programmed with the following settings:

Voltage: ___ V
Pulse window: ___ ms
Time on: ___ sec
Time off: ___ sec
Frequency: ___ Hz

The device was then deactivated to permit the use of monopolar cautery and placed within the subcutaneous pocket. Redundant lead wiring was coiled and placed behind the generator within the pocket. The wound was then closed in layers, using interrupted *3-0 Vicryl* for Scarpa's fascia, interrupted deep dermal *4-0 Vicryl* sutures, and skin closure with *5-0 Monocryl* in continuous subcuticular fashion. Skin at the port sites was then closed in a similar fashion. All incisions were then dressed with surgical skin adhesive. The device was re-interrogated and activated following confirmation of acceptable lead impedance.

Upon completion of the procedure, a debriefing checklist was completed to share information critical to the postoperative care of the patient. The patient tolerated the procedure well, was extubated in the operating room, and was transported to the post-anesthesia care unit in stable condition thereafter.

Removal of Bezoars and Other Ingested Foreign Bodies (Open and MIS Approaches)

13

Frances C. Okolo and Stefan Scholz

Indications and Benefits

- Large gastric bezoars
- Failure of medical management or endoscopy
- Benefits: *If laparoscopic*—smaller incision size, less pain, faster recovery time, and better cosmesis; *if open*—shorter operative time and decreased costs

Risks and Alternatives

- Standard risks: Bleeding, infection, need for additional procedures, and risks of anesthesia
- Injury to adjacent structures (liver, spleen)
- Gastric perforation and ileus

Essential Steps

1. ***If laparoscopic***: Create pneumoperitoneum via Hasson open technique, place infraumbilical port, and insert 30 degree camera. Inspect for iatrogenic injuries and insert additional ports.
2. ***If open***: Upper midline abdominal incision or left transverse abdominal/subcostal incision.
3. Place patient in moderate reverse Trendelenburg position.
4. Lyse adhesions (if present).
5. ***If open***: Grasp the stomach and perform a gastrotomy on the anterior wall from the mid antrum to the body of the stomach.
6. ***If laparoscopic***: Place transabdominal traction sutures and insert 12-mm trocar into the stomach in a sheath technique, use endoscope as intragastric camera.
7. Aspirate stomach contents.
8. Mobilize the bezoar and extract the bezoar (preferably in one piece).
9. Inspect stomach for any remnant fragments and extract if found.
10. Repair the gastrotomy by suture or with stapler.
11. Explore abdominal cavity for debris.
12. Irrigate abdominal cavity.
13. Close incisions: ***If laparoscopic***—remove ports, deflate abdomen, and close port sites. ***If open***—close fascia and skin.

F. C. Okolo
University of Pittsburgh Medical Center, Department of General Surgery, Pittsburgh, PA, USA

S. Scholz (✉)
University of Pittsburgh School of Medicine, Children's Hospital of Pittsburgh, Department of Pediatric Surgery, Pittsburgh, PA, USA
e-mail: stefan.scholz@chp.edu

D. J. Papandria et al. (eds.), *Operative Dictations in Pediatric Surgery*,
https://doi.org/10.1007/978-3-030-24212-1_13

Note These Variations

- Various trocar sizes, positioning of additional ports.
- ***If laparoscopic:*** A 15-mm port may be inserted into the gastric lumen to facilitate retrieval of large bezoar in pieces; a ballooned trocar may be used as an alternative to the sheath trocar.
- The endoscope can be used as an intragastric camera during laparoscopic retrieval.
- An additional port may be placed for liver retraction.
- ***If open:*** Stay sutures may be applied to the stomach at the site of gastrotomy.
- The stomach may be sutured to the fascia circumferentially to prevent spillage of contaminated gastric content into abdominal cavity. An appropriately sized wound protector may be placed into the gastric lumen to prevent spillage and maximize exposure.
- ***If laparoscopic surgery***: One of the port incisions may need to be extended for en bloc removal versus piecemeal removal through port site with a claw grabber ("mother-in-law").
- Gastrotomy repair: One- or two-layer closure with absorbable sutures or stapler.
- Fascia closure*:* ***If laparoscopic surgery***—open versus laparoscopic suture passer for 12 mm/15 mm port site. ***If open surgery***—repair is performed with nonabsorbable suture in a continuous fashion.

Template Operative Dictation (Open)

Preoperative Diagnosis Giant gastric bezoar not amenable to endoscopic retrieval

Postoperative Diagnosis Same as preoperative diagnosis

Findings Same as postoperative diagnosis

Procedure(s) Performed Exploratory laparotomy, removal of gastric bezoar

Anesthesia General

Specimen Gastric foreign body

Estimated Blood Loss ___ mL

Indications This is a/an ___-day/week/month/year-old *male/female* with history of ___ who presented with progressive abdominal pain and palpable abdominal mass. Abdominal CT scan with contrast revealed a large intraluminal gastric mass suggestive of a/an ___. He/she was deemed to be a suitable candidate for open gastric bezoar removal.

Procedure in Detail Following satisfactory induction of anesthesia, the patient was placed in supine position and appropriately padded. Time-outs were performed using both preinduction and preincision safety checklists with participation of all present in the operative suite. These confirmed the correct patient, procedure, operative site, and additional critical information prior to the start of the procedure. The abdomen was then prepped and draped in the usual sterile fashion.

A 5-cm *vertical upper midline/transverse left upper quadrant* skin incision was performed and carried down to the fascia using electrocautery. The peritoneum was identified and incised to enter the abdominal cavity. *A wound protector was placed and a wound retractor was applied for additional exposure.* The table was then placed in reverse Trendelenburg position. *A small amount of thin adhesions were identified and lysed using Metzenbaum scissors under direct visualization.* The stomach was identified, noted to be distended secondary to the palpable giant bezoar. The anterior wall of the stomach was grasped with Allis tissue forceps. *Two stay sutures were then placed, one on the body of the stomach and one at the mid antrum.* A 4-cm gastrotomy was then performed from the mid antrum to the body using a harmonic scalpel with immediate visualization of the bezoar. Fluid was evacuated from the stomach. *The gastrotomy opening was then sutured to the fascia in all four quadrants and the wound protector was placed into the lumen of the stomach.*

[Choose One:]
If bezoar unable to be removed in one piece: *Attempt to extract the bezoar in one piece was unsuccessful. The bezoar was thus fragmented using clamps and removed piecemeal.*

If bezoar removable in one piece: *The bezoar was successfully extracted in one piece using clamps.*

The proximal and distal stomach were digitized to identify and extract any remnants. The specimen was then sent to pathology. The gastrotomy was then closed *with a stapler after both edges were aligned in two layers with a continuous 2-0 vicryl suture.* The abdomen was copiously irrigated with 1 L warm NS followed by fascial closure with running 2-0 PDS suture after hemostasis was confirmed. The skin was closed with a running 4-0 monocryl suture.

Upon completion of the procedure, a debriefing checklist was completed to share information critical to the postoperative care of the patient. The patient tolerated the procedure well, *was extubated in the operating room,* and was transported to the postanesthesia care unit in stable condition thereafter.

Template Operative Dictation (Laparoscopic)

Preoperative Diagnosis Large bezoar, not amendable to endoscopic retrieval

Postoperative Diagnosis Same as preoperative diagnosis

Findings Same as postoperative diagnosis

Procedure(s) Performed Laparoscopic removal of large bezoar under endoscopic control

Anesthesia General

Specimen Gastric bezoar

Estimated Blood Loss ___

Indications This is a/an __-day/week/month/year-old male/female with history of ___ who presented with progressive abdominal pain and palpable abdominal mass. Abdominal CT scan with contrast revealed a large intraluminal gastric mass suggestive of a/an ___. He/she was deemed to be a suitable candidate for laparoscopic gastric bezoar removal.

Procedure in Detail Following satisfactory induction of anesthesia, the patient was placed in supine position and appropriately padded. Time-outs were performed using both preinduction and preincision safety checklists with participation of all present in the operative suite. These confirmed the correct patient, procedure, operative site, and additional critical information prior to the start of the procedure. The abdomen was then prepped and draped in the usual sterile fashion.

A skin incision was made at the umbilicus and carried down to the fascia using electrocautery. The peritoneum was incised and entry into the peritoneal cavity was confirmed. Two stay sutures were placed through the fascia and a 5-mm trocar was inserted through the fascial opening into the peritoneal cavity and secured with the stay sutures. Carbon dioxide insufflation was performed with intra-abdominal pressure set to 12–15 mmHg. Once pneumoperitoneum was achieved and stable patient hemodynamics were confirmed, a 5-mm, 30 degree laparoscope was inserted and the abdomen was inspected for any injuries. The stomach was identified and a 5-mm trocar was placed in the left upper abdomen. The stomach was identified and noted to be distended secondary to the bezoar. An upper endoscope was placed into the stomach and the stomach mildly inflated. The stomach was grasped through the 5-mm trocar and pulled to the abdominal wall. Two transabdominal stay sutures were then placed on the anterior surface of the stomach. Under direct vision with the laparoscope and the endoscope, a Veress needle and a sheath were placed into the stomach using the transabdominal sutures for retraction. A *12-mm/15-mm sheath trocar/ballooned trocar* was then placed into the lumen of the stomach between the stay sutures.

[Choose One:]

If bezoar cannot be removed through the 12-mm/15-mm port in pieces: Two additional laparoscopic ports were placed into the abdomen and a larger gastrotomy was performed with the harmonic scalpel. The gastric contents were suctioned to avoid spillage. Two additional gastric retraction sutures were placed at the edge of the gastrotomy. The bezoar was then removed from the stomach and placed into an endocatch bag. The endocatch bag was then retrieved through the extended 12-mm/15-mm port site and inspected to ensure it was intact.

If bezoar can be removed through the 12-mm/15-mm port in pieces: Using the endoscope as an intragastric camera, we then extracted the large bezoar piecemeal with the Claw Grasper through the 12-mm/15-mm left upper quadrant port.

The bezoar was then sent to pathology as a specimen in pieces. The stomach was then inspected for any residue and remaining remnants were removed, and then irrigated and closed with a laparoscopic staple device. The abdomen was copiously irrigated with warm NS and hemostasis was ensured. The intra-abdominal CO_2 was evacuated and ports were removed under direct visualization. Fascial closure was performed with vicryl suture and the skin was closed with a running 4-0 monocryl suture.

Upon completion of the procedure, a debriefing checklist was completed to share information critical to the postoperative care of the patient. The patient tolerated the procedure well, *was extubated in the operating room*, and was transported to the postanesthesia care unit in stable condition thereafter.

14 Sugiura Procedure (Esophagogastric Devascularization)

Andrew Yeh and Stefan Scholz

vIndications

- Bleeding esophageal varices in patients refractory to medical treatment that are:
  - Not candidates for portosystemic shunts or liver transplantation
  - Relatively well-preserved liver function (Child–Pugh class A or B)

Risks and Alternatives

- Standard risks (bleeding, infection, need for additional procedures, and risks of anesthesia)
- Injury to adjacent structures (lungs, portal vein, pancreas)
- Esophageal stricture
- Rebleeding due to remaining varices
- Portal vein thrombosis
- Esophageal fistula or leak

A. Yeh
University of Pittsburgh, Department of Surgery, Pittsburgh, PA, USA

S. Scholz (✉)
University of Pittsburgh School of Medicine, Children's Hospital of Pittsburgh, Department of Pediatric Surgery, Pittsburgh, PA, USA
e-mail: stefan.scholz@chp.edu

Essential Steps

1. Selective right lung ventilation is required.
2. Make a left lateral thoracotomy incision.
3. Isolate the distal half of the distal esophagus circumferentially.
4. Ligate and divide all perforating veins in the distal esophagus.
5. Transect the distal esophagus at the hiatus while leaving the posterior muscle layer intact.
6. Perform esophageal reanastomosis.
7. Close chest and transition to abdominal portion of the procedure.
8. Perform a splenectomy.
9. Devascularize the abdominal esophagus, the cardia of the stomach, and the greater and lesser curvature of the stomach.

Thoracic Portion

1. Selective right lung ventilation is required.
2. Place patient in the right lateral decubitus position with appropriate padding.
3. Make left lateral thoracotomy incision in the sixth or seventh intercostal space.
4. Incise the inferior mediastinal pleura longitudinally anterior to the descending aorta to access the esophagus. The dilated adventitial venous plexus of the esophagus

D. J. Papandria et al. (eds.), *Operative Dictations in Pediatric Surgery*,
https://doi.org/10.1007/978-3-030-24212-1_14

should be visualized. This plexus communicates with submucosal varices via large perforators.
5. Isolate the distal half of the esophagus circumferentially using careful blunt dissection.
6. Encircle esophagus with tape to allow for easy manipulation.
7. Visualize dilated perforating veins surrounding the esophagus that feed into the submucosa of the esophagus.
8. Ligate and divide all perforating veins along approximately 10–15 cm of distal esophagus. The inferior pulmonary vein serves as the superior border and the inferior border is the preperitoneal fat. There may be as many as 50 perforating vessels. Leaving any collateral veins will increase the risk of rebleeding.
9. If a nasogastric tube has been placed, retract it proximal to the planned transection point.
10. Clamp the esophagus distal and proximal to the desired transection point using noncrushing and nonslipping bowel clamps. Transection should occur at the level of the hiatus.
11. Divide the anterior muscle layer at the desired transection point with a scalpel.
12. Encircle the submucosa of the esophagus with tape.
13. Divide the submucosa and mucosa, but leave the posterior muscle layer intact. This prevents twisting and stricture formation after reanastomosis.
14. Reanastomose the mucosal layer using nonabsorbable 5-0 suture.
15. Prior to reanastomosis of the anterior mucosal layer, carefully advance nasogastric tube distal to the anastomosis.
16. Complete the anastomosis of the mucosal layer.
17. Close the anterior muscle layer using absorbable 4-0 suture.
18. Close the chest in the standard fashion. Leave a minimum of one chest tube.

Abdominal Portion

19. Make a left subcostal or upper midline abdominal incision.
20. Perform a splenectomy. This will allow for better exposure for the paraesophagogastric devascularization.
21. Divide the splenic ligaments (splenorenal, splenocolic, splenophrenic, and gastrosplenic) to completely mobilize the spleen.
22. Divide the short gastric vessels. Stay close to the stomach to avoid injuring the gastroepiploic vessels.
23. Doubly ligate and divide the main splenic artery and vein and remove the spleen. Be careful not to injure the pancreas.
24. Devascularize the abdominal esophagus, the cardia of the stomach, and the greater and lesser curvatures of the stomach. The length of devascularization should be approximately 7 cm from the gastric cardia. Ensure that the left gastric vessels are left intact. Division of the posterior vagus nerve is necessary. The esophagus and cardia should be completely mobilized.
25. Abdominal incision is closed in the standard fashion.

Note These Variations

- The original Sugiura procedure was a two-step procedure where the thoracic and abdominal portions were separated by 4–6 weeks. The procedure is now performed as a single procedure.
- The original Sugiura procedure included division of the anterior vagus nerve. If this is done, a gastric emptying procedure (i.e., pyloroplasty) is necessary.
- Feeding jejunostomy tube can be placed for postoperative feeding.
- A modified Sugiura procedure is performed entirely using an abdominal incision. No thoracic incision is necessary. The abdominal portion begins similarly to the original

Sugiura procedure. A splenectomy is performed. Devascularization and mobilization of the distal esophagus and proximal stomach are completed. Once the distal esophagus is mobilized, a Penrose drain is used to encircle the esophagus for traction. The esophageal hiatus is opened and the thoracic esophageal dissection is completed of approximately 10 cm. Care should be taken to divide only transverse veins. Once this is completed, the esophageal transection is performed. An anterior gastrotomy is made to introduce an EEA stapler. The stapler is opened and introduced 2 cm superior to the esophagogastric junction. A 0 suture is passed behind the esophagus and used to tie down the esophagus to the opened stapler. The stapler is then closed and fired. The anastomosis can be inspected through the gastrotomy. The gastrotomy is closed in two layers and a Nissen fundoplication is performed to prevent reflux.

Template Operative Dictation

Preoperative Diagnosis Life-threatening bleeding esophageal varices refractory to medical therapy

Postoperative Diagnosis Same as preoperative diagnosis

Findings Large esophageal varices

Procedure(s) Performed Sugiura procedure or esophagogastric devascularization and transection

Anesthesia General

Specimen None

Drains None

Implants None

Estimated Blood Loss ___ mL

Indications This is a/an ___-day/week/month/year-old male/female with life-threatening bleeding esophageal varices refractory to medical therapy. He/she was deemed to be a suitable candidate for Sugiura procedure or esophagogastric devascularization and transection.

Procedure in Detail Following satisfactory induction of anesthesia including the placement of a double lumen endotracheal tube and nasogastric tube, the patient was placed in the right lateral decubitus position and appropriately padded. Time-outs were performed using both preinduction and preincision safety checklists with participation of all present in the operative suite. These confirmed the correct patient, procedure, operative site, and additional critical information prior to the start of the procedure. The left chest was then prepped and draped in the usual sterile fashion. A left lateral thoracotomy incision was made in the sixth intercostal space. Care was taken to establish hemostasis using electrocautery and to avoid injury to the intercostal neurovascular bundle. Upon entering the chest, anesthesia proceeded with selective right lung ventilation.

The distal esophagus was exposed by incising the inferior mediastinal pleura and mobilized using blunt circumferential dissection with special care not to injure the adventitial venous plexus. Perforating veins from the adventitial venous plexus were carefully dissected, ligated, and divided for a length of 15 cm starting from the preperitoneal fat. The nasogastric tube was then retracted proximally and the esophagus was clamped proximally and distally to the transection point. The anterior esophageal muscle layer was then transected using a scalpel at the level of the hiatus and the submucosal layer was circumferentially and bluntly dissected away from the posterior esophageal muscle layer. Varices encountered during transection were ligated. The mucosal layer of the esophagus was then reanastomosed in an interrupted fashion using 5-0 nonabsorbable suture. The anterior muscle layer was then reapproximated in an interrupted fashion using 4-0 absorbable suture. The nasogastric tube was carefully advanced to pass the anastomosis into the stomach. A careful evaluation for hemostasis was made. A chest tube was then placed in the left chest cavity and the thoracotomy incision was closed layer by layer in the standard fashion.

The patient was then repositioned to be supine and double lung ventilation was reinitiated. The abdomen was then prepped and draped in the usual sterile fashion. A left subcostal incision was made. Care was taken to establish hemostasis using electrocautery. The abdomen was explored for aberrant anatomy or pathology for which none was found. The spleen was then mobilized by dividing its ligamentous attachments using a vessel sealing device. The splenic artery and vein were identified and doubly ligated using 0 silk suture proximally and distally and then divided. The spleen was then removed. Care was taken not to injure the tail of the pancreas.

Devascularization of the abdominal esophagus and the proximal stomach was then completed. The short gastric vessels were divided with a vessel sealing device close to the stomach taking care not to injure the gastroepiploic vessels. The left gastric vessels and the anterior vagus nerve were identified and left intact. During the devascularization of the distal esophagus, the posterior vagus nerve was identified and divided. A careful evaluation for hemostasis was made. The abdominal incision was then closed layer by layer in the standard fashion.

Upon completion of the procedure, a debriefing checklist was completed to share information critical to the postoperative care of the patient. The patient tolerated the procedure well, *was extubated in the operating room*, and was transported to the postanesthesia care unit in stable condition thereafter.

15 Laparoscopic Sleeve Gastrectomy

Astrid R. Soares-Medina, Marc P. Michalsky, and Bradley J. Needleman

Indications and Benefits

- BMI ≥35 kg/m^2 or 120% of the 95th percentile with clinically significant comorbid conditions such as obstructive sleep apnea (apnea–hypopnea index >5), type 2 diabetes, idiopathic intracranial hypertension, nonalcoholic steatohepatitis, Blount's disease, slipped capital femoral epiphysis, gastroesophageal reflux disease, or hypertension.
- BMI ≥40 kg/m^2 or 140% of the 95th percentile (whichever is lower).
- Benefits: To reduce excess body weight and remit associated comorbid diseases in the adolescent population.

A multidisciplinary team must also consider whether the patient and family have the ability and motivation to adhere to the recommended treatments pre- and postoperatively, including consistent use of micronutrient supplements.

Contraindications for Adolescent MBS Include

- A medically correctable cause of obesity.
- An ongoing substance abuse problem (within the preceding year).
- A medical, psychiatric, psychosocial, or cognitive condition that prevents adherence to postoperative dietary and medication regimens.
- Current or planned pregnancy within 12–18 months of the procedure.

Risks and Alternatives

- Standard risks: Bleeding, infection, need for additional procedures, and risks of anesthesia
- Injury to adjacent structures (spleen, liver, pancreas, stomach)
- Staple line leak
- Fistula, stenosis, twisting
- GERD
- Alternatives: Roux-en-Y gastric bypass

A. R. Soares-Medina (✉)
Assistant Professor of Clinical Surgery and Pediatrics, Ponce Health Sciences University School of Medicine, Mayagüez Medical Center, Department of Pediatric Surgery, Mayagüez, PR, USA

M. P. Michalsky
Professor of Clinical Surgery and Pediatrics, The Ohio State University College of Medicine, Nationwide Children's Hospital, Department of Pediatric Surgery, Columbus, OH, USA

B. J. Needleman
The Edwin H. and E. Christopher Ellison Professor of Surgery, The Ohio State University College of Medicine, Wexner Medical Center, Department of Surgery, Columbus, OH, USA

D. J. Papandria et al. (eds.), *Operative Dictations in Pediatric Surgery*,
https://doi.org/10.1007/978-3-030-24212-1_15

Essential Steps

1. Supine position:
   (a) Patient should be secured to the operating table using appropriate belt and a large foot board to insure safe intraoperative repositioning.
   (b) Antiembolic stockings and intermittent compression devices are employed to prevent venous thromboembolism.
   (c) A naso/orogastric tube for gastric decompression should be placed.
2. Stab Veress needle in the left upper quadrant and induce pneumoperitoneum.
3. Insert a 5-mm laparoscopic optical port in the left upper quadrant at the midclavicular line.
4. Inspect abdomen to confirm lack of iatrogenic injury from Veress insertion.
5. Place additional ports: A 5-mm supraumbilical port site (around 12–15 cm below the xiphoid process), a 15-mm right upper quadrant port site, and a 5-mm right and 5-mm left subcostal port sites.
6. Through a stab incision in the subxiphoid space, insert a liver retractor (i.e., Nathanson liver retractor) in order to expose the gastroesophageal junction.
7. Position the patient in a reverse Trendelenburg position, and the table slightly tilted right side down.
8. Measure a 6-cm distance proximal to the pylorus and divide the small branches of the gastroepiploic arcade with a preferred energy device in order to enter the lesser sac.
9. Using a preferred energy device, dissect along the greater curvature of the stomach up to the angle of His. Care should be taken to avoid thermal injury near the gastroesophageal junction.
10. Once the hiatus is reached, lift the stomach up to expose its posterior aspect, and free all lesser sac attachments of the stomach while exposing the left diaphragmatic crus.
11. Inspect the hiatus for hiatal hernia, *and if necessary, repair it using a nonabsorbable braided suture.*
12. Instruct anesthesia to remove all *oro/naso*gastric tubes except the endotracheal tube and then to slowly pass a blunt-tipped bougie (i.e., typically 36–40 French; per individual surgeon preference) into the stomach. The surgeon can guide it along the lesser curvature of the stomach under laparoscopic vision.
13. Create the gastric sleeve using an endostapling device (staple height and possible buttress material according to individual surgeon preference) dividing from 6 cm proximal to the pylorus along the bougie toward the angle of His. Care should be taken to avoid acute angulation along the resulting "sleeve" with close attention paid to avoid narrowing at the angularis. Inspect the stapler line to confirm hemostasis and the integrity of the staple lines.
14. Intraoperative flexible endoscopy should be performed in order to inspect the intraluminal portion of the staple line (i.e., for disruption or hemorrhage) and to carry out a leak test under direct vision.
15. Remove the 15-mm port and place a wound protector under direct vision. Bring the stomach out through this incision.
16. Close the 15-mm incision at the facial level using a fascial suture device.
17. Remove all port sites under direct vision and release pneumoperitoneum.
18. Close skin incisions using a 4-0 braided absorbable suture.

Note These Variations

- Initial access via Veress needle technique versus optical trocar technique versus direct fascial cutdown technique.
- Various bariatric trocar types and sizes are available.
- 15-mm trocar can be placed in the RUQ or periumbilical.
- Staple line may be enhanced with surgeon's choice of buttress material or oversewn.
- 10 mm versus 5 mm and 0 versus 30° laparoscope (angled scope allows for better visualization of the angle of His).

- Removal of stomach remnant through the 15-mm incision using a wound protector or laparoscopic bag retrieval system.
- Various liver retractors options.
- Drain placement (usually not indicated).
- Fascia closure at large trocar sites, open versus laparoscopic with suture passer.

Template Operative Dictation (Laparoscopic)

Preoperative Diagnosis Severe obesity (BMI ___ kg/m^2) with *major/minor* comorbid disease

Postoperative Diagnosis Same as preoperative diagnosis

Findings Same as postoperative diagnosis

Procedure(s) Performed Laparoscopic vertical sleeve gastrectomy (VSG)

Anesthesia General

Specimen Excised stomach

Drains None

Implants None

Estimated Blood Loss Minimal

Indications This is a/an__-year-old *male/female* with severe obesity (BMI ___ kg/m^2) and *type 2 diabetes/glucose intolerance, pseudotumor cerebri, severe nonalcoholic steatohepatitis, mild/moderate/severe obstructive sleep apnea, hypertension, dyslipidemia, impaired weight-related quality of life. He/she* was deemed to be a suitable candidate for laparoscopic vertical sleeve gastrectomy (VSG).

Procedure in Detail Following satisfactory induction of anesthesia, the patient was placed in supine position and appropriately padded and secured. Time-outs were performed using both preinduction and preincision safety checklists with participation of all present in the operative suite. These confirmed the correct patient, procedure, operative site, and additional critical information prior to the start of the procedure. The abdomen was then prepped and draped in the usual sterile fashion.

[Choose One:]
If Veress needle: *A skin incision was made and the Veress needle inserted in the left upper quadrant. Proper position was confirmed by aspiration and saline meniscus test and then a 0 degree camera was used to insert a 5-mm optical trocar safely in the left upper quadrant.*

If optical trocar: *A skin incision in the left upper quadrant was made and the optical trocar was used to enter the abdomen safely under direct laparoscopic visualization using a 5-mm 0 degree camera.*

The patient's abdomen was insufflated to a pressure limit of ___ mmHg at a flow of ___ L/min of carbon dioxide. Once the abdomen was insufflated, the camera was used to confirm lack of iatrogenic injury from *Veress/optical* trocar insertion. The patient tolerated insufflation well. The remaining ports were placed under direct vision. This included a 5-mm supraumbilical port site, a 15-mm right upper quadrant port site, and two 5-mm right and left subcostal port sites. On inspection of the patient's intra-abdominal cavity, normal anatomy was observed. A Nathanson liver retractor was placed in the subxiphoid region to allow retraction of the liver in a cephalad position. Once all trocars were in satisfactory position, the patient was placed in a reverse Trendelenburg position, and the table slightly tilted right side down.

The procedure was initiated by measuring a 6-cm distance proximal to the pylorus using a premeasured piece of umbilical tape. At this position, the small branches of the gastroepiploic arcade were divided and the lesser sac entered. The dissection was continued proximally along the greater curvature of the stomach using a preferred energy device, dividing the short gastric vessels, with care taken to avoid injury to the spleen. Once the hiatus was reached, the stomach was lifted up to expose its posterior aspect and the lesser sac attachments of the stomach were divided taking care to avoid injury to the pancreas, splenic vessels, *and/or* the left gastric artery. The dissection was inspected and found to be hemostatic.

At this point, anesthesia was instructed to remove all *oro/naso*gastric tubes except the endotracheal tube, and then to pass a 36-French bougie which was placed properly into the stomach and guided along the lesser curvature of the stomach under laparoscopic vision. Once in place, an endostapling device was used to divide the stomach along the bougie. ___ staple loads were used in order to form the gastric sleeve by continuing this division along the bougie up to the angle of His. The staple line was inspected and noted to be intact. No obvious bleeding was observed. The bougie was removed under direct vision. The 15-mm port was removed and a wound protector was placed under direct vision and the gastric remnant was removed through this incision. Then the 15-mm port was inserted back through the same incision. At this point, the table was placed in neutral position and the gastric sleeve was submerged in warm sterile saline and an endoscope was inserted through the mouth into the esophagus and down through the sleeve. No leak was noted with insufflation. The staple line was noted to be intact and hemostatic intraluminally. The endoscope was then removed *and absorbable hemostatic powder was sprayed in the staple line*. The 15-mm incision was closed at the fascial level with a fascial closure device using 0 braided absorbable suture. All port sites were removed under direct vision. The Nathanson liver retractor was also removed under direct vision. Pneumoperitoneum was released. The skin was closed using ___-0 braided absorbable suture. All incisions were locally anesthetized and sterile dressings were applied.

Upon completion of the procedure, a debriefing checklist was completed to share information critical to the postoperative care of the patient. The patient tolerated the procedure well, *was extubated in the operating room*, and was transported to the postanesthesia care unit in stable condition thereafter.

16 Laparoscopic Roux-En-Y Gastric Bypass

Astrid R. Soares-Medina, Marc P. Michalsky, and Bradley J. Needleman

Indications and Benefits

- BMI ≥35 kg/m² or 120% of the 95th percentile with clinically significant comorbid conditions such as obstructive sleep apnea (apnea–hypopnea index >5), type 2 diabetes, idiopathic intracranial hypertension, nonalcoholic steatohepatitis, Blount's disease, slipped capital femoral epiphysis, gastroesophageal reflux disease, or hypertension.
- BMI ≥40 kg/m² or 140% of the 95th percentile (whichever is lower).
- Benefits: To reduce excess body weight and reverse associated comorbid diseases in the adolescent population.

A multidisciplinary team must also consider whether the patient and family have the ability and motivation to adhere to the recommended treatments pre- and postoperatively, including consistent use of micronutrient supplements.

The principles of gastric bypass include the creation of an approximately 30-ml proximal gastric pouch based on the lesser curve of the stomach, a 75–150-cm Roux limb anastomosed to the gastric pouch with an approximately 12-mm stoma, a more than 30 cm biliopancreatic limb, and long common channel.

Contraindications for adolescent MBS include:

- A medically correctable cause of obesity
- An ongoing substance abuse problem (within the preceding year)
- A medical, psychiatric, psychosocial, or cognitive condition that prevents adherence to postoperative dietary and medication regimens
- Current or planned pregnancy within 12–18 months of the procedure

Risks and Alternatives

- Standard risks: Bleeding, infection, need for additional procedures, and risks of anesthesia
- Injury to adjacent structures (spleen, liver, pancreas, stomach)
- Anastomotic stenosis and/or hemorrhage at the gastrojejunostomy
- Proximal anastomotic leaks or staple-line disruptions

A. R. Soares-Medina (✉)
Assistant Professor of Clinical Surgery and Pediatrics, Ponce Health Sciences University School of Medicine, Mayagüez Medical Center, Department of Pediatric Surgery, Mayagüez, PR, USA

M. P. Michalsky
Professor of Clinical Surgery and Pediatrics, The Ohio State University College of Medicine, Nationwide Children's Hospital, Department of Pediatric Surgery, Columbus, OH, USA

B. J. Needleman
The Edwin H. and E. Christopher Ellison Professor of Surgery, The Ohio State University College of Medicine, Wexner Medical Center, Department of Surgery, Columbus, OH, USA

D. J. Papandria et al. (eds.), *Operative Dictations in Pediatric Surgery*, https://doi.org/10.1007/978-3-030-24212-1_16

- Internal hernias
- Gallstone formation
- Marginal ulcers
- Thromboembolic events
- Gastrogastric fistula
- "Candy cane" redundant Roux syndrome
- Nutritional/vitamin deficiencies
- Bacterial overgrowth syndromes
- *Alternatives*: Laparoscopic sleeve gastrectomy

Essential Steps

Position and Trocars Placement

1. *Supine position or lithotomy ("French") position in steep reverse Trendelenburg.* Patient should be secured to the table. Antiembolic stockings and intermittent compression devices are employed to prevent venous thromboembolism. A *naso/oro*gastric tube for gastric decompression should be placed.
2. Stab Veress needle in the left upper quadrant and induce pneumoperitoneum.
3. Insert a 5-mm laparoscopic optical trocar in the left upper quadrant, subcostal at the midclavicular line. Additional trocars include: a 5-mm port in the left lateral position, a 12-mm port in the midline (around 12–15 cm below the xiphoid process) for the camera, a 15-mm port at the midclavicular line in the right side of the abdomen, and an additional 5-mm right lateral port.
4. Inspect abdomen to confirm lack of iatrogenic injury from Veress insertion.

Creation of the Biliopancreatic Limb (Jejunojejunostomy)

1. Retract the omentum cephalad over the transverse colon to identify the ligament of Treitz.
2. Trace the small bowel distally. Divide the small bowel at approximately 40–100 cm from the ligament Treitz using the endoscopic stapler device ensuring that the distal small bowel can easily reach up to the level of the upper stomach.
3. Divide the distal mesentery using *the endoscopic staplers or preferred energy device.*
4. Suture a Penrose drain (or similar) on the distal small bowel (Roux limb) for later identification.
5. Run the distal bowel approximately 75–150 cm distally (based on surgeon's criteria).
6. At this point create a side-to-side functional jejunojejunal anastomosis.

[Choose One:]

If stapled anastomosis: *Make small enterotomies along the proximal limb of the small bowel previously divided and the jejunum. Create a side-to-side stapled anastomosis using a linear cutter endostaplers. Close the enterotomy transversely, approximating the edges and then firing an endostapler across the enterotomy.*

If sutured anastomosis: *Fix both limbs with interrupted seromuscular stitches, then create small enterotomies and suture the posterior side of the anastomosis (single or two layers and in an interrupted or continuous fashion). Then suture the anterior anastomosis in the same manner using an absorbable suture.*

7. Close the mesenteric defect using a running nonabsorbable suture.

Creation of the Gastric Pouch

1. Place a Nathanson liver retractor in the subxiphoid region through an additional 5-mm port site incision in order to retract the left lobe of the liver superiorly.
2. Open the lesser omentum to identify the lesser curvature of the stomach and enter the lesser sac (this can be divided with a stapler or window can be created along the lesser curve of stomach preserving the vagus and vascular structures).

3. Open the distal stomach with preferred energy device to pass the anvil of the EEA stapler through the gastrostomy into the upper part of the stomach. This can be done by measuring the distance from the gastroesophageal junction (approximately 5 cm) or below the first vein.
4. Bring out the anvil of the EEA on the anterior surface of the upper gastric pouch remnant.
5. Create the proximal pouch by dividing the stomach using endostaplers in order to create an approximately 30-ml gastric pouch.
6. Close the distal stomach enterotomy using endostaplers.

Gastrojejunostomy

1. Divide the greater omentum using a preferred energy device in anticipation of an antecolic and antegastric orientation of the Roux limb.
2. Identify the distal limb of the small bowel previously divided (demarcated with a previously placed Penrose drain) and bring it up to the level of the gastric pouch.
3. Open the claw of the distal small bowel with advance cutting device.
4. Introduce the EEA stapler through the abdominal wall and advance it into the small bowel.
5. Open the EEA stapler in order to have the bar of the EEA exiting through the side wall of the small bowel.
6. Attach the anvil to the EEA stapler. Screw down and fire the EEA stapler.
7. Remove the EEA stapler from the abdominal cavity and open it to identify two complete donuts.
8. Close off the end of the small bowel with an endostapler.

Upper Endoscopy, Leak Test, and Closure

1. Perform intraoperative endoscopy to perform a leak test under direct vision and evaluate for bleeding, pouch, and stoma size.
2. Close the 15- and 12-mm ports incisions at the fascial level using a fascial suture device.
3. Remove all port sites under direct vision and release pneumoperitoneum.
4. Close skin incisions using a ___-0 braided absorbable suture.

Note These Variations

- Initial access via Veress needle technique versus optical trocar technique.
- Various bariatric trocar types and sizes are available.
- 10 mm versus 5 mm and 0 versus 30° laparoscope.
- Various liver retractors options.
- Drain placement (usually not indicated).
- Fascia closure at large trocar sites, open versus laparoscopic with suture passer.
- The Roux limb can also be passed retrocolic and/or retrogastric, especially if it is felt there will be too much tension on the anastomosis.
- Attention must be directed to avoid kinking or twisting the Roux limb or inadvertently performing the notorious Roux-en-O by not properly identifying each limb prior to the jejunojejunostomy anastomosis.
- Divide the omentum using an advanced bipolar cutting device to decrease the tension of the gastrojejunostomy anastomosis.
- Silk sutures can be placed medially and laterally at the gastrojejunostomy for reinforcement.
- Different variations for the gastrojejunostomy exist: handsewn, linear stapler, or EEA anastomosis.
- Different EEA sizes exist and the anvil can be passed transgastric as described or transoral via a nasogastric tube.
- The Petersen's defect, the space between the Roux limb and the transverse mesocolon can be closed with interrupted sutures or purse-string sutures to help prevent herniation in this space.

- Transversus abdominis plane blocks (TAP blocks) can be performed by the surgeon laparoscopically at the beginning or end of the case or by anesthesia with ultrasound guidance.

Template Operative Dictation (Laparoscopic)

Preoperative Diagnosis Severe obesity (BMI ___ kg/m^2) with *major/minor* comorbid disease

Postoperative Diagnosis Same as preoperative diagnosis

Findings Same as postoperative diagnosis

Procedure(s) Performed Laparoscopic Roux-en-Y gastric bypass

Anesthesia General

Specimen None

Drains None

Implants None

Estimated Blood Loss Minimal

Indications This is a/an __-year-old *male/female* with severe obesity (BMI ___ kg/m^2) and *type 2 diabetes/glucose intolerance, pseudotumor cerebri, severe nonalcoholic steatohepatitis, mild/moderate/severe obstructive sleep apnea, hypertension, dyslipidemia, impaired weight-related quality of life. He/she* was deemed to be a suitable candidate for laparoscopic Roux-en-Y gastric bypass.

Procedure in Detail Following satisfactory induction of anesthesia, the patient was placed in supine position and appropriately padded and secured. Time-outs were performed using both preinduction and preincision safety checklists with participation of all present in the operative suite. These confirmed the correct patient, procedure, operative site, and additional critical information prior to the start of the procedure. The abdomen was then prepped and draped in the usual sterile fashion.

[Choose One:]

If Veress needle: *A skin incision was made and the Veress needle inserted in the left upper quadrant. Proper position was confirmed by aspiration and saline meniscus test, and then a 0-degree camera was used to insert a 5-mm optical port safely in the left upper quadrant.*

If optical trocar: *A skin incision in the left upper quadrant was made and the optical port was used to enter the abdomen safely under direct laparoscopic visualization using a 5-mm 0-degree camera.*

The patient's abdomen was insufflated to a pressure limit of ___ mmHg at a flow of ___ L/min of carbon dioxide. Once the abdomen was insufflated, the camera was used to confirm lack of iatrogenic injury from *Veress/optical trocar* insertion. The patient tolerated insufflation well. The 5-mm 0 degree camera was then switched to a 10-mm, 30-degree camera. The remaining ports were placed under direct vision and this included a 5-mm port in the left lateral position, a 12-mm port at the midline around 12–15 cm below the xiphoid process for the camera, a 15-mm port at the midclavicular line in the right side of the abdomen, and an additional 5-mm right lateral port.

The procedure was initiated by retracting the omentum cephalad over the transverse colon to identify the ligament of Treitz. The small bowel was then traced distally and it was divided at about 40 cm from the ligament of Treitz using endoscopic staplers ensuring that the distal small bowel could easily reach up to the level of the upper stomach. The mesentery at this point was also divided using *the endoscopic linear stapler/Ligasure vessel sealer/ultrasonic dissector*. In order to identify the Roux limb, a Penrose drain was sutured using a __-0 absorbable suture. The bowel was then traced 100 cm distally and was anastomosed in a side-to-side fashion to the end of the biliopancreatic limb creating the jejunojejunostomy.

[Choose One:]

If stapled anastomosis: Small enterotomies were made along the antimesenteric side of the proximal limb of the small bowel previously divided and the jejunum. A side-to-side stapled anastomosis was created using a 60-mm linear cutter endostapler (*purple/green/black* load). The edges of the enterotomy were transversely approximated and then closed with a firing of the endostapler.

If sutured anastomosis: Both limbs were fixed with interrupted seromuscular stitches, then small enterotomies were created and the posterior side of the anastomosis was sutured (single or two layers and in an interrupted or continuous fashion). Then the anterior side of the anastomosis was sutured in the same manner using a ___-0 absorbable suture.

The anastomosis was inspected for hemostasis and to ensure that it was patent. The mesenteric defect was then closed using a running nonabsorbable suture. Additionally, an antiobstruction stitch (Brolin stitch) was applied with a nonabsorbable suture to approximate the Roux limb to the biliopancreatic limb proximal to the anastomosis to avoid an obstruction from kinking of the bowel along the staple line.

Attention was then directed to the upper abdomen. The patient was positioned in a steep reverse Trendelenburg position and a liver retractor was inserted in the subxiphoid region through an additional 5-mm port site incision in order to retract the left lobe of the liver superiorly. The lesser omentum was opened and the lesser curvature of the stomach identified. The lesser omentum was divided with a firing of the linear endostapler (*white/blue/purple* load).

At this point, the distal part of the stomach was opened with an advanced bipolar device and the anvil of the *25/29*-mm EEA stapler was passed through the gastrotomy into the upper part of the stomach and brought out on the anterior surface of the upper gastric pouch remnant where we wished to perform the gastrojejunostomy. The stomach was then divided with the endostaplers along the anvil to create a small gastric pouch of approximately 30 ml. The enterotomy of the distal stomach was closed using the endostaplers. The staple lines were inspected to insure that the stomach was completely divided; the staple lines were hemostatic and intact.

Attention was directed back to the small bowel. The end of the Roux limb was identified with the Penrose drain. This was brought up to the level of the gastric remnant and the mesentery was inspected to ensure the limb was not twisted. The mesentery was further mobilized with the energy device and the end of the Roux limb was opened. The EEA stapler was passed through the RUQ port site and introduced into the open end of the small bowel. The spike was then brought out through the antimesenteric side of the Roux limb under direct vision and mated with the anvil. The anvil and stapler were brought together under direct vision ensuring there was no twisting, and no tissue was caught between the stapler and anvil. The EEA was fired and then removed and two complete donuts were identified. Using the endostapler (*blue/purple* load) the open end of the Roux limb was closed. *Absorbable suture was then placed at the gastrojejunostomy for reinforcement.*

At this point, the table was placed in neutral position and the gastrojejunostomy was submerged in warm sterile saline, a bowel clamp was placed on the Roux limb and an endoscope was inserted through the mouth into the esophagus, and the gastric pouch, gastrojejunostomy, and Roux limb were inspected. No leak was noted with insufflation. The EEA stapler line was noted to be intact and hemostatic. The endoscope was then removed. The 15- and 12-mm ports incisions were closed at the fascial level using a fascial suture device using 0-braided absorbable suture. All port sites were removed under direct vision. The liver retractor was also removed under direct vision. Pneumoperitoneum was released. The skin was closed using ___-0 braided absorbable suture. All incisions were locally anesthetized and sterile dressings were applied.

Upon completion of the procedure, a debriefing checklist was completed to share information critical to the postoperative care of the patient. The patient tolerated the procedure well, *was extubated in the operating room*, and was transported to the postanesthesia care unit in stable condition thereafter.

Jejunostomy Placement, Open and MIS Approaches

17

Frances C. Okolo, Paul K. Waltz, and Stefan Scholz

Indications and Benefits

- Inability to meet caloric needs via oral route/ oral aversion
- Failure to thrive
- Severe gastroesophageal reflux disease (GERD)
- Recurrent aspiration pneumonia
- Intolerance to gastric feeds
- Gastroparesis
- Need for durable postpyloric feeding access
- Inability to place gastrostomy tube/button
- No suitable stomach for gastric feeds (used for conduit)
- Benefits: Establish durable access for enteral feedings, avoid need for parenteral nutrition, and long-term vascular access

Risks and Alternatives

- Standard risks: Bleeding, infection, need for additional procedures, and risks of anesthesia
- Injury to small bowel, large bowel, stomach, or other organs
- Early tube/button dislodgement
- Postoperative bowel obstruction from tube, balloon, or adhesions
- Tube site leakage
- Anastomotic leak (in setting of Roux-en-Y jejunostomy)
- Intestinal volvulus around jejunostomy tube site
- Jejunal twisting around a narrow base insertion site
- Reflux into stomach if tube is placed too proximal with potential aspiration
- Malabsorption if tube is placed too distally
- Persisting enterocutaneous fistula after tube removal
- *Alternatives*: Nasoenteric tube placement, radiologic or endoscopic exchange of gastrostomy tube/button for gastrojejunostomy tube/ button that may obviate the need for separate surgically placed jejunostomy tube/button, parenteral nutrition

Essential Steps

Placement of Jejunostomy Tube (Adult Technique, Open or Laparoscopic)

1. Upper midline incision or laparoscopic umbilical port access.
2. Inspect for iatrogenic injuries and insert additional working ports.

F. C. Okolo · P. K. Waltz
University of Pittsburgh Medical Center, Department of General Surgery, Pittsburgh, PA, USA

S. Scholz (✉)
University of Pittsburgh School of Medicine, Children's Hospital of Pittsburgh, Department of Pediatric Surgery, Pittsburgh, PA, USA
e-mail: stefan.scholz@chp.edu

D. J. Papandria et al. (eds.), *Operative Dictations in Pediatric Surgery*,
https://doi.org/10.1007/978-3-030-24212-1_17

3. Perform abdominal exploration and lysis of adhesions (if present).
4. Place the patient in reverse Trendelenburg position.
5. Reflect the great omentum and transverse colon cranially and identify the ligament of Treitz.
6. Identify the jejunum approximately 10–20-cm distal to the ligament of Treitz that reaches the abdominal wall without tension.
7. Create a skin incision and fascial opening in the left upper quadrant and pass the jejunostomy tube through the abdominal wall.
8. Place a purse string suture on the antimesenteric border of the selected loop of jejunum.
9. Perform an enterotomy in the center of the purse string suture, insert the jejunostomy tube into the jejunum, and pass the tube toward the distal intestine.
10. Tie the purse string suture to secure the tube in place.
11. In older children, a serosal tunnel (Witzel) of approximately 4 cm may be created for the jejunostomy tube.
12. Secure the jejunum to the parietal peritoneum of the posterior abdominal wall at the site of tube insertion.
13. Pexy the jejunum to the posterior abdominal wall for several centimeters from the tube insertion site to create a broader base and prevent twisting at the site of tube insertion.
14. Flush the tube to ensure it is patent and functioning.
15. Remove ports, deflate the abdomen, and close the port sites or the fascia and the skin.
16. Suture a tube bolster to the skin exteriorly.

Laparoscopic Omega Loop Construction (Pediatric Technique for Jejunostomy Button) [1]

1. Follow steps 1 to 5 from above. Two right-sided working ports are typically used.
2. Identify the jejunum approximately 10–20 cm distal to the ligament of Treitz that reaches the abdominal wall without tension.
3. The selected loop of small intestine is exteriorized through the umbilical port site. A wound protector may be used in larger patients.
4. The loop is kinked over itself and approximated with a row of Lembert sutures in a side-to-side fashion.
5. An enterotomy is made at the apex of the loop in the antimesenteric aspect and a purse string suture placed around the enterotomy.
6. A 60-mm Endo GIA stapler is inserted through the enterotomy to create a jejunal pouch through a side-to-side anastomosis to accommodate the button balloon.
7. The location of the jejunostomy is marked on the abdominal wall in the left upper quadrant.
8. The bowel is reintroduced into the abdomen and pneumoperitoneum is reestablished.
9. The jejunal loop is secured to the abdominal wall below the marked jejunostomy site with transfascial sutures on either side of the purse string suture. Ensure there is no twisting of the jejunal loop.
10. Under direct vision, the gastrostomy dilator set is used percutaneously to introduce a needle and a wire into the created jejunal pouch through the center of the purse string suture.
11. This tract is then dilated up with consecutive dilators to 16 Fr and an appropriately sized button is placed into the jejunal pouch.
12. The purse string suture is then tied around the button before the balloon is completely inflated.
13. The balloon is then inflated with 5 ml of water.
14. Additional transfascial sutures should be placed to secure the jejunostomy site to the abdominal wall to create a broader base and prevent jejunal twisting at the site of tube insertion.
15. Close port sites and skin.

Laparoscopic Roux-en-Y Construction (Pediatric Technique for Jejunostomy Button) [2]

1. Follow steps 1 to 5 from above. Two right-sided working ports are typically used.
2. Identify a loop of jejunum 20 cm distal to the ligament of Treitz, make a window in the

mesentery, and divide the bowl with an Endo GIA stapler.
3. Further divide the mesentery proximally with cautery or energy device.
4. Exteriorize the bowel through the umbilical incision, extend the fascial incision as needed. A wound protector may be used.
5. Create a stapled side-to-side jejunojejunostomy of the proximal small intestine to the Roux limb (10–20 cm long).
6. Close the remaining enterotomy and the mesenteric defect.
7. Reintroduce the bowel into the abdomen, establish pneumoperitoneum, identify the stapled end of the Roux limb, and suture this to the marked site of the jejunostomy button in the left upper quadrant with transfascial sutures. Ensure the Roux limb is not twisted.
8. Place transabdominal sutures to secure the Roux limb to the posterior abdominal wall.
9. Under direct visualization utilize the percutaneous gastrostomy dilator set to introduce the button into the Roux limb and inflate the balloon.
10. Additional transfascial sutures should be placed to secure the jejunostomy site to the abdominal wall to create a broader base and prevent jejunal twisting at the site of tube insertion.
11. Close port sites and skin.

Note These Variations

- The 5-mm stapler may be utilized to create the jejunal pouch or the Roux limb in smaller patients.
- An intra-abdominal laparoscopic stapled jejunojejunostomy may be performed to create the Roux limb without exteriorization of the intestine.
- In larger patients, percutaneous T-fasteners may be used to suspend the jejunum to the abdominal wall.
- For laparoscopically assisted percutaneous placement of the jejunostomy tube or button, a peel-away sheath may be used for introduction into the bowel.
- The jejunum should be secured to the abdominal wall at some distance to prevent torsion of the jejunostomy tube site.
- A suture passer may be used in larger patients for fascia closure of the port sites or transfascial sutures.
- Ensure familiarity with all tubes, buttons, and percutaneous access kits before the procedure.
- A PEG tube may be used instead of a button.

Template Operative Dictation

Preoperative Diagnosis *Failure to thrive/malnutrition/intolerance to gastric feeds/aspiration pneumonia with need for durable enteral access*

Postoperative Diagnosis Same

Findings None

Procedure Performed *Laparoscopic/laparoscopically assisted/open* placement of jejunostomy *tube/button with Witzel tunnel/omega loop/Roux-en-Y limb construction/neither*

Anesthesia General anesthesia

Specimen None

Drains None

Implants *14 Fr jejunostomy tube/button/other*

Estimated Blood Loss Minimal

Indications This ___-*day/week/month/year*-old *male/female* with *malnutrition/failure to thrive/recurrent aspiration pneumonia/intolerance to gastric feeds/other* required durable access for enteral feeds. *Previous attempts at gastric feedings have failed. He/she* was deemed to be a suitable candidate for a feeding jejunostomy.

Procedure in Detail Following satisfactory induction of anesthesia, the patient was placed in supine position and appropriately padded. Time-outs were performed using both preinduction and preincision safety checklists with participation of all present in the operative suite. These confirmed the correct patient, procedure, operative site, instrumentation, and additional critical information prior to the start of the procedure. The abdomen was then prepped and draped in the usual sterile fashion and a broad-spectrum antibiotic was given intravenously.

Placement of Jejunostomy Tube (Adult Technique): A 5-cm vertical upper midline skin incision was performed. This was then carried down to the fascia using electrocautery. The peritoneum was identified and incised to enter the abdominal cavity. *A wound protector was placed and a wound retractor was applied for additional exposure.* Adhesions were lysed sharply under direct visualization with care to avoid injury to bowel or surrounding structures. The table was placed in reverse Trendelenburg position. The transverse mesocolon was then retracted superiorly to identify the ligament of Treitz at the base of the transverse mesocolon. A loop of jejunum about 20 cm distal to the ligament of Treitz was selected that reached the chosen jejunostomy site in the left upper quadrant abdominal wall without tension.

A 3-mm incision was made on the skin at this site and a Tonsil clamp was then passed from inside the abdomen through the fascia and the skin incision. The jejunostomy tube was grasped and passed into the abdomen using this clamp. Next, the chosen portion of jejunum was, again, verified to be about 20 cm distal to the ligament of Treitz and not twisted. A 3-0 *silk/Vicryl* purse string suture was placed at the antimesenteric border of the jejunum.

[Choose One:]

If laparoscopic: The percutaneous jejunostomy kit was used to gain transabdominal, intraluminal access with needle and guidewire through the site of the purse string. Intraluminal access was confirmed by air bolus injection. After sequential dilation and access with the tear-away sheath, the jejunostomy tube was introduced and passed distally.

If open: A small enterotomy was made in the center of the purse string using a needle for exposure and electrocautery. The jejunostomy tube was then passed through the enterotomy and directed about 5 cm into the distal jejunum. The purse string suture was tied down to secure the tube in place. (Optional: A 4-cm serosal Witzel tunnel was created with interrupted 3-0 silk/Vicryl sutures. Seromuscular bites of jejunum were taken in order to imbricate the jejunum over the feeding tube while always ensuring that the jejunal lumen was not narrowed.)

The jejunum was secured to the posterior abdominal wall at the tube insertion site with four 3-0 *silk/Vicryl* sutures oriented around the enterotomy. The jejunum was then confirmed to be without tension and the mesentery in correct orientation. Additional 3-0 *silk/Vicryl* sutures were placed distal to the tube insertion site to prevent jejunal torsion. Hemostasis was assured. The midline fascia was closed in a *running/interrupted* manner and the skin was closed with *staples/glue/subcuticular running stitch.* The tube site was appropriately dressed. The jejunal tube bolster was placed flush with the skin and sutured in place with 3-0 nylon sutures.

Upon completion of the procedure, a debriefing checklist was completed to share information critical to the postoperative care of the patient. The patient tolerated the procedure well, *was extubated in the operating room*, and transported to the postanesthesia care unit in stable condition.

Laparoscopic Omega Loop Construction (Pediatric Technique for Jejunostomy Button): A skin incision was made at the umbilicus and carried down to the fascia using electrocautery. The peritoneum was incised and entry into the peritoneal cavity was confirmed. Two stay sutures were placed through the fascia and a 12-mm trocar was inserted through the fascial opening into the peritoneal cavity. Carbon dioxide insufflation was performed with appropriate intra-abdominal pressure. A laparoscope was inserted and the peritoneal cavity was inspected for any injuries from abdominal access. Additional 5-mm working ports were placed in the abdomen and the patient placed in Trendelenburg position. Using atraumatic clamps, the omentum and transverse colon were retracted cranially to identify the ligament of Treitz at the base of the transverse mesocolon. A loop of jejunum about 20 cm distal to the ligament of Treitz was identified that reached the abdominal wall without tension. The loop of small intestine was extracted through the umbilical incision. The loop was folded on itself and a posterior row of 3-0 Lembert suture was placed to align the bowel. An enterotomy was made at the apex of the loop and a 60-mm Endo GIA stapler was introduced and fired to create a jejunal pouch. The enterotomy was then closed with a purse string suture. The bowel was reintroduced into the abdominal cavity and pneumoperitoneum reestablished. Correct orientation without twisting of the jejunal pouch at the jejunostomy site was assured. Two transabdominal traction sutures were placed around the apex and the purse string suture to secure the pouch to the jejunostomy site. The dilator set was then used to create and dilate a tract up to 16 Fr through the abdominal wall and the center of the purse string suture at the apex of the jejunal loop in a Seldinger technique. An appropriately sized button was then placed over the wire into the jejunal pouch and the balloon inflated. Correct intraluminal position was confirmed with insufflation. Additional transfascial stitches were placed to secure the jejunal loop to the abdominal wall to prevent jejunal torsion.

Upon completion of the procedure, a debriefing checklist was completed to share information critical to the postoperative care of the patient. The patient tolerated the procedure well, *was extubated in the operating room*, and was transported to the postanesthesia care unit in stable condition thereafter.

Laparoscopic Jejunostomy With Roux-en-Y Construction (Pediatric Technique for Jejunostomy Button): A skin incision was made at the umbilicus and carried down to the fascia using electrocautery. The peritoneum was incised and entry into the peritoneal cavity was confirmed. Two stay sutures were placed through the fascia and a 12-mm trocar was inserted through the fascial opening into the peritoneal cavity. Carbon dioxide insufflation was performed with appropriate intra-abdominal pressure. A laparoscope was inserted and the peritoneal cavity was inspected for any injuries from abdominal access. Additional 5-mm working ports were placed in the abdomen and the patient placed in Trendelenburg position. Using atraumatic clamps, the omentum and transverse colon were retracted cranially to identify the ligament of Treitz at the base of the transverse mesocolon. A loop of jejunum about 20 cm distal to the ligament of Treitz was identified that reached the abdominal wall without tension. The loop of small intestine was extracted through the umbilical incision.

A window was made in the mesentery and an Endo GIA stapler was introduced to divide the jejunum. The mesentery was divided proximally with the *hook cautery/energy device*. The staple lines were tagged with stitches and extracted through the umbilical port site. A side-to-side jejunojejunostomy was fashioned with the End GIA stapler. The mesenteric defect was closed with stitches. The bowel was reintroduced into the abdomen and pneumoperitoneum was reestablished. The stapled end of the Roux limb was identified and approximated to the abdominal wall at the site of the jejunostomy tube using two transabdominal sutures. Correct orientation was confirmed. A percutaneous dilator kit was utilized to gain access into the Roux limb. The button was then introduced into the Roux limb in a Seldinger technique and the balloon inflated. Correct intraluminal position was confirmed with insufflation. Additional transfascial stitches were placed to secure the jejunal loop to the abdominal wall to prevent jejunal torsion.

At the conclusion of the procedure, the jejunostomy *tube/button* was flushed and patency was confirmed. The peritoneal cavity was then inspected and hemostasis was confirmed. The mesentery was again confirmed to be in the appropriate configuration. The abdomen was then desufflated and all the ports were removed. All port sites and the umbilical incision were closed. The tube site was dressed and appropriately secured to the patient. A debriefing checklist was completed to share information critical to the postoperative care of the patient. The patient tolerated the procedure well, *was extubated in the operating room*, and was transported to the post-anesthesia care unit in stable condition.

References

1. Schalger A, Arps K, Siddharthan R, Rajdev P, Heiss K. The "omega" jejunostomy tube: a preferred alternative for postpyloric feeding access. J Pediatr Surg. 2016;51(2):260–3.
2. Neuman H, Phillips JD. Laparoscopic Roux-en-Y feeding jejunostomy: a new minimally invasive surgical procedure for permanent feeding access in children with gastric dysfunction. J Laparoendosc Adv Surg Tech. 2005;15(1):71–4.

18 Laparotomy for Midgut Volvulus

Lorraine I. Kelley-Quon

Indications and Benefits

- Bilious emesis in a child
- Benefits: salvage of midgut small bowel

Risks and Alternatives

- Standard risks: Bleeding, infection, need for additional procedures, and risks of anesthesia
- Injury to adjacent structures (liver)
- Need for bowel resection
- Need for second-look laparotomy
- *Alternatives*: None

Essential Steps

1. Counterclockwise derotation of the midgut
2. Assessment for bowel necrosis and bowel resection
3. Lysis of Ladd's bands of the duodenum and vascular pedicle
4. Appendectomy (optional)

L. I. Kelley-Quon (✉)
Children's Hospital Los Angeles, Division of Pediatric Surgery, Department of Surgery, Keck School of Medicine of University of Southern California, Los Angeles, CA, USA
e-mail: lkquon@chla.usc.edu

Template Operative Dictation (Open)

Preoperative Diagnosis Midgut volvulus

Postoperative Diagnosis Same as preoperative diagnosis

Findings Same as postoperative diagnosis

Procedure(s) Performed Laparotomy for midgut volvulus

Anesthesia General

Specimen *None/small bowel (__ cm)*

Drains None

Implants None

Estimated Blood Loss ___ mL

Indications This is a/an ___*-day/week/month/year*-old *male/female* with bilious emesis and an UGI consistent with midgut volvulus. He/she was deemed to be a suitable candidate for laparotomy for midgut volvulus.

Procedure in Detail Following satisfactory induction of anesthesia, the patient was placed supine and appropriately padded. Time-outs were

D. J. Papandria et al. (eds.), *Operative Dictations in Pediatric Surgery*,
https://doi.org/10.1007/978-3-030-24212-1_18

performed using both preinduction and preincision safety checklists with participation of all present in the operative suite. These confirmed the correct patient, procedure, operative site, and additional critical information prior to the start of the procedure. The abdomen was then prepped and draped in the usual sterile fashion.

A transverse laparotomy incision was made approximately 1 cm superior to the umbilicus. Electrocautery was used to dissect through the soft tissue and the abdomen was entered under direct vision. The falciform was identified, doubly ligated, and transected. Care was taken not to injure the liver, and the small bowel was inspected. The small bowel was noted to be dusky in appearance, was eviscerated in its entirety through the incision, and a midgut volvulus was confirmed. The bowel was then slowly derotated in a counterclockwise manner to improve perfusion. Of note, anesthesia was instructed to observe the EKG tracings during derotation to identify EKG changes consistent with hyperkalemia. After the volvulus was fully reduced, the bowel was inspected in its entirety from the duodenum to the ileum to identify any additional abnormalities or areas of frank necrosis.

If frank bowel necrosis is identified**:** *Surgical clips were placed/GIA staplers were fired proximal and distal to frankly necrotic bowel. The mesentery at the base of the necrotic bowel was taken using serial suture ligation/electrocautery/LigaSure vessel sealer. The bowel was passed off the field as specimen. In total, ____ cm of small bowel was resected leaving ___ remaining bowel from the duodenum to the terminal ileum. After lysis of Ladd's bands was completed, the bowel was left in discontinuity and the abdomen was left open with a temporary abdominal closure device for a planned second-look laparotomy.*

A warm, damp laparotomy pad was placed over the eviscerated bowel and attention was turned to the duodenum. Ladd's bands between the duodenum and cecum were lysed until the duodenum was able to lie free in a longitudinal fashion along the right abdominal wall. Ladd's bands along the pedicle of the small bowel were similarly lysed in order to open the vascular pedicle supplying the small bowel. Care was taken during dissection not to violate the mesentery of the small bowel.

The appendix was then identified and the mesoappendix was ligated. The base of the appendix was suture ligated, and the appendix transected with a 15 blade scalpel and passed off the field as specimen. The mucosal surface of the remaining appendiceal stump was cauterized.

The viscera were returned to the abdomen in the following order. The duodenum and jejunum were placed in the right upper and lower quadrants. The ileum was placed in the left lower quadrant followed by the cecum and remaining colon in the left upper quadrant. The fascial edges of the laparotomy incision were identified and reapproximated. Scarpa's fascia was similarly closed using interrupted sutures followed by skin closure in a running subcuticular fashion followed by a surgical dressing.

Upon completion of the procedure, a debriefing checklist was completed to share information critical to the postoperative care of the patient. The patient tolerated the procedure well, *was extubated in the operating room*, and was transported to the postanesthesia care unit in stable condition thereafter.

Ladd's Procedure

19

Courtney Pisano and Gail E. Besner

Indications and Benefits

- Midgut volvulus
- Intestinal malrotation
- Duodenal obstruction
- Incidental Ladd's bands found during another procedure

Risks and Alternatives

- Bleeding, infection, risks of anesthesia
- Postoperative intestinal obstruction
- *Conversion of laparoscopic to open procedure*

Essential Steps

Open Ladd's Procedure

1. A midline or transverse supraumbilical incision is made.
2. Deliver entire midgut onto the operative field.
3. Divide abnormal bands (Ladd's bands) which typically extend from a poorly fixated right colon to the right upper quadrant over the duodenum.
4. Mobilize and rotate the right colon.
5. Be vigilant not to divide the colonic mesentery during mobilization of the colon.
6. Place the entire right colon on the left side of the abdomen.
7. Mobilize and straighten the duodenum so that it is directed inferiorly.
8. Place small bowel on the right side of the abdomen.
9. Note that placing the colon on the left side of the abdomen and the small bowel in the right side of the abdomen will effectively broaden the base of the small bowel mesentery.
10. Divide any congenital bands along the superior mesenteric artery and vein, if present, to further broaden the base of the small bowel mesentery.
11. Perform appendectomy.
12. Irrigate abdomen.
13. Close abdomen.

Laparoscopic Ladd's Procedure

1. Induce pneumoperitoneum.
2. Inspect abdomen with laparoscope placed through umbilical port.
3. Place additional trocars under laparoscopic vision in the following sites: two in the right and one in left mid to low abdomen.

C. Pisano · G. E. Besner (✉)
Nationwide Children's Hospital, Department of Pediatric Surgery, Columbus, OH, USA
e-mail: gail.besner@nationwidechildrens.org

D. J. Papandria et al. (eds.), *Operative Dictations in Pediatric Surgery*,
https://doi.org/10.1007/978-3-030-24212-1_19

4. Divide abnormal bands (Ladd bands) which fix the bowel to the right upper quadrant retroperitoneal/intra-abdominal structures.
5. Mobilize the right colon fully.
6. Be vigilant not to divide the colonic mesentery during the colonic mobilization.
7. Place entire right colon on the left side of the abdomen.
8. Mobilize and straighten the duodenum so that it heads inferiorly.
9. Place small bowel on the right side of the abdomen.
10. Divide any congenital bands along the superior mesenteric artery and vein, if present, to further broaden the base of the small bowel mesentery.
11. Perform appendectomy.
12. Remove trocars under direct visualization.
13. Desufflate abdomen.
14. Close trocar sites.

Template Operative Dictation (Open)

Preoperative Diagnosis *Intestinal malrotation/ duodenal obstruction/other*

Postoperative Diagnosis *Malrotation without midgut volvulus*

Findings *Malrotation without midgut volvulus*

Procedure(s) Performed Ladd's procedure

Anesthesia General

Specimen None

Drains None

Implants None

Estimated Blood Loss ___ mL

Indications This is a/an ___-*day/week/month/ year*-old *male/female* presented with *abdominal pain/nausea/vomiting/fever/leukocytosis/other.* Diagnostic imaging and work up indicated *intestinal malrotation/other.* The patient was brought to the operating room for *Ladd's procedure/ exploratory laparotomy.*

Procedure in Detail The patient was brought to the operating room and placed on the operating table in the supine position. Following satisfactory induction of general endotracheal anesthesia, a time-out was completed verifying the patient by two identifiers, the procedure to be performed and the operative site. *A Foley catheter and a nasogastric tube were placed.* Appropriate perioperative antibiotics were administered and the abdomen was prepped and draped in the usual sterile fashion.

A *midline/transverse supraumbilical* incision was made and dissection was carried down through the subcutaneous tissue using electrocautery for hemostasis. The fascial and muscular layers were divided using electrocautery and the peritoneal cavity entered. The entire small bowel was delivered through the incision into the operative field to assess the rotation and fixation of the bowel. *Findings included intestinal malrotation/other with the presence of Ladd's bands fixing the bowel to the right upper quadrant retroperitoneal/intra-abdominal structures.* Ladd's bands draped over the duodenum were carefully divided. The right colon was mobilized taking care not to divide the colonic mesentery. The entire right colon was placed on the left side of the abdomen. The duodenum was mobilized and straightened so that it was directed inferiorly. The small bowel was placed on the right side of the abdomen. The base of the mesentery was further broadened using electrocautery and sharp dissection to divide congenital bands along the superior mesenteric artery and vein. Appendectomy was then performed using ligature/stapler to divide the mesoappendix and the appendix using ____ staple loads. Hemostasis was obtained using the electrocautery device. The abdomen was irrigated with normal saline. The *anterior rectus sheath/ posterior rectus sheath/midline fascia* was closed with *running/interrupted* __. The subcutaneous fat was approximated using *running/interrupted* __. The skin was closed using 5-0 vicryl in subcuticular fashion. The incision was dressed with *Steri-Strips/TegaDerm/topical skin adhesive.* All sponge, needle, and instrument counts were correct at the end of the procedure. Upon completion of the procedure, a debriefing checklist was completed to share information critical to the postoperative care of the patient. The patient tolerated the procedure well, *was extubated in the operating room*, and was transported to the postanesthesia care unit in stable condition thereafter.

Template Operative Dictation (Laparoscopic)

Preoperative Diagnosis *Intestinal malrotation/duodenal obstruction/internal hernia/other*

Postoperative Diagnosis *Malrotation without midgut volvulus*

Findings *Malrotation without midgut volvulus*

Procedure(s) Performed Laparoscopic Ladd's procedure

Anesthesia General

Specimen {Specimen}

Drains {Drains}

Implants {Implants}

Estimated Blood Loss ___

Indications This ___*-day/week/month/year* -old *male/female* presented with *abdominal pain/nausea/vomiting/fever/leukocytosis/other.* Diagnostic imaging and work up indicated *concern for intestinal malrotation/other.* The patient was brought to the operating room for *laparoscopic Ladd's procedure/exploratory laparoscopy.*

Procedure in Detail The patient was brought to the operating room and placed on the operating table in the supine position. Following satisfactory induction of general anesthesia, a time-out was completed verifying the patient by two identifiers, the procedure to be performed and the operative site. *A Foley catheter and a nasogastric tube were placed.* Appropriate perioperative antibiotics were administered and the abdomen was prepped and draped in the usual sterile fashion.

An *umbilical/infraumbilical* incision was made.

[Choose One:]

For Veress Needle: *The fascia was elevated and a Veress needle was inserted. Proper position of the needle was established using aspiration and the saline meniscus test.* Pneumoperitoneum was established using carbon dioxide to a pressure of *12–15 mmHg. A 5-/10-/12*-mm trocar was then inserted. A 5-mm laparoscope was introduced into the abdomen and the intraperitoneal contents were inspected. No traumatic sequelae of the initial trocar placement were noted.

For Hasson Cannula: *Using electrocautery, dissection was carried down to the level of the fascia. The fascia was divided with cautery and 2-0 vicryl traction sutures were placed on each side of the fascia. The Hasson 10–12-mm trocar was then advanced into the abdomen under direct supervision and secured to the fascia using the previously placed fascial sutures.* A 5-mm laparoscope was introduced into the abdomen and the intraperitoneal contents were inspected. No traumatic sequelae of the initial trocar placement were noted.

Local anesthetic infiltration was used and 5-mm incisions were made for additional trocar sites. Additional trocars were placed under laparoscopic visualization in the following sites: two in the right and one in left lower abdomen. Careful inspection of the abdomen was performed and the anatomy was delineated. Ladd's bands draped over the duodenum were carefully divided. Using atraumatic bowel graspers, the right colon was mobilized being vigilant not to open the colonic mesentery. The entire right colon was placed on the left side of abdomen. The duodenum was mobilized and straightened so that it was directed inferiorly. The small bowel was placed on the right side of the abdomen. The entire length of bowel was inspected for areas of ischemia. The base of the mesentery was broadened using hook electrocautery and sharp dissection to divide congenital bands along the superior mesenteric artery and vein. Appendectomy was performed using ligature/endostapler with _____ staple loads to divide the mesoappendix and the appendix. The appendix was placed in an EndoCatch bag and removed through the umbilical port. *The abdomen was irrigated with normal saline.* The 5-mm trocars were removed under direct laparoscopic vision and hemostasis confirmed at the trocar sites. Following desufflation of the abdomen, the umbilical trocar was removed and the site was closed at the fascial level with 2-0 vicryl figure-of-eight sutures. The fascia at the 5-mm port sites was closed with interrupted 2-0 vicryl sutures. The skin at all port sites was then closed with 5-0 vicryl in a subcuticular fashion. All sites were dressed with Steri-Strips/*TegaDerm*/*topic skin* adhesive/a folded 2 × 2 gauze placed at the umbilical incision. All sponge, needle, and instrument counts were correct at the end of the procedure. Upon completion of the procedure, a debriefing checklist was completed to share information critical to the postoperative care of the patient. The patient tolerated the procedure well, *was extubated in the operating room*, and was transported to the postanesthesia care unit in stable condition thereafter.

20 Repair of Duodenal Atresia (Open and MIS Approaches)

Afif Kulaylat and Karen A. Diefenbach

Indications and Benefits

- Duodenal atresia/stenosis/obstruction
- Benefits: Restoration of intestinal continuity

Risks and Alternatives

- Standard risks: Bleeding, infection, need for additional procedures, and risks of anesthesia
- Injury to adjacent structures (pancreas, bile duct/ampulla, stomach, liver, transverse colon, vena cava)
- Anastomotic stricture
- Anastomotic leak
- Persistent dysmotility
- *Alternatives*: Duodenojejunostomy

Essential Steps

Open and Laparoscopic Repair

1. Evaluate anatomy for malrotation, *rule out distal atresia.*
2. Kocherize duodenum.
3. Create transverse and longitudinal enterotomies on proximal and distal duodenum, respectively.
4. Rule out duodenal web.
5. Protect the ampulla.
6. Perform duodenoduodenostomy.

A. Kulaylat
Nationwide Children's Hospital, Department of Surgery, Columbus, OH, USA

K. A. Diefenbach (✉)
Nationwide Children's Hospital, Columbus, OH, USA
e-mail: Karen.Diefenbach@nationwidechildrens.org

Note These Variations

- Duodenoduodenostomy can be performed in Kimura/Diamond fashion, or side to side.
- Duodenojejunostomy can be performed in anatomy not amenable to duodenoduodenostomy.
- If laparoscopic approach is chosen and malrotation is identified, surgeon may consider advantages and disadvantages of conversion to complete both duodenoduodenostomy and Ladd's procedure laparoscopically.

Template Operative Dictation

Preoperative Diagnosis *Laparoscopic* repair duodenal atresia/duodenal obstruction/congenital duodenal stenosis

Postoperative Diagnosis *Same as preoperative diagnosis/annular pancreas/duodenal atresia/duodenal web*

Findings Same as postoperative diagnosis

D. J. Papandria et al. (eds.), *Operative Dictations in Pediatric Surgery*,
https://doi.org/10.1007/978-3-030-24212-1_20

Procedure(s) Performed *Laparoscopic* duodenoduodenostomy

Anesthesia General

Specimen None

Drains None

Implants None

Estimated Blood Loss ___ mL

Indications This is a/an ___-*day/week/month*-old *male/female* with findings consistent with a congenital duodenal obstruction. Based on preoperative assessment and imaging, *a complete/incomplete* duodenal obstruction is suspected. *He/she* was deemed to be a suitable candidate for *laparoscopic/open* repair of same.

Procedure in Detail Following satisfactory induction of anesthesia, the patient was placed in the supine position and appropriately padded. Time-outs were performed using both preinduction and preincision safety checklists with participation of all present in the operative suite. These confirmed the correct patient, procedure, operative site, and additional critical information prior to the start of the procedure. The abdomen was then prepped and draped in the usual sterile fashion.

[Choose One:]

If open approach: A/an ___-cm supraumbilical transverse incision was made from the midline across the right upper quadrant. This was extended through the fascia with electrocautery. The peritoneum was entered in a controlled fashion and opened the fill length of the incision. The umbilical vein was identified, ligated, and divided.

If laparoscopic approach: A/an ___-mm incision was made in an infraumbilical location and extended into the peritoneal cavity being careful to avoid injury to the umbilical vessels. A/an ___-mm port/Veress needle was passed through this incision. After intraperitoneal placement was confirmed, the abdomen was insufflated to a pressure of ___ mmHg. Two additional ports were placed lateral to the edge of the rectus muscle under direct vision, a/an ___-mm port in the right lower quadrant just below the level of the umbilicus and a/an ___-mm port in the left upper quadrant just above the level of the umbilicus. Liver retraction was achieved via a *transabdominal falciform stitch/a laparoscopic liver retractor placed through a lateral right upper quadrant incision.*

{Continue dictation}

The stomach, pylorus, and first portion of the duodenum were inspected. The first portion of the duodenum was bulbous consistent with duodenal obstruction. The position of the ligament of Treitz was evaluated to assess for the presence of malrotation. Normal rotation was noted with the ligament of Treitz in the left upper quadrant, normal fixation of the colon, and a wide-based mesentery. On further examination of the duodenum, the etiology of the duodenal obstruction was consistent with *duodenal atresia/annular pancreas/possible duodenal web.* The duodenum was mobilized and the distal, decompressed duodenum identified. This portion of the bowel was mobilized adequately to perform a tension-free anastomosis.

A transverse incision was made in the first portion of the duodenum. The distal duodenum was opened longitudinally. Care was taken to perform enterotomies of the same length.

If a web is suspected: A flexible catheter was inserted into the distal enterotomy and passed both proximally and distally to verify no web was present distal to this enterotomy.

{Continue dictation}

Of note, bile was encountered on opening the *proximal/distal/both* segment(s) of the duodenum. A/an ___-cm *side-to-side/diamond* duodenoduodenostomy was then completed with *interrupted/running* ___-0 *vicryl/PDS* sutures to close the posterior wall and then the anterior wall of the anastomosis.

[Choose One:]

For open approach: The abdomen was irrigated with saline. The fascia was closed with running/

interrupted ___-0 Vicryl/PDS sutures. The subcutaneous tissue was reapproximated with ___-0 Vicryl sutures. The skin was closed with a running 5-0 Vicryl/Monocryl suture in a subcuticular fashion. *Mastisol and Steri-Strips/Dermabond/a sterile dressing* was used over the incision.

For laparoscopic approach: The abdomen was deflated and all ports were removed. The fascia at the umbilical incision was closed using a ___-0 Vicryl suture. The fascia at the remaining port sites was closed using ___-0 Vicryl sutures. The skin at all incisions was closed using a subcuticular ___-0 *Vicryl/Monocryl* suture.

{Continue dictation}

All sponge and instruments counts were correct ×2. Upon completion of the procedure, a debriefing checklist was completed to share information critical to the postoperative care of the patient. The patient tolerated the procedure well, *was extubated in the operating room/remained intubated*, and was transported to the *postanesthesia care unit/neonatal intensive care unit* in *stable/guarded* condition thereafter.

21 Open Repair of Jejunoileal Atresia

Dominic J. Papandria and Karen A. Diefenbach

Indications and Benefits

- Jejunoileal atresia
- Benefits: restoration of intestinal continuity to permit enteral feeding

Risks and Alternatives

- Standard risks (bleeding, infection, need for additional procedures, risks of anesthesia)
- Injury to adjacent structures (stomach, small bowel, colon, associated nerves, arteries and veins)
- Stricture, stenosis, or leak at anastomosis
- Missed atresia necessitating reoperation
- Alternatives: Parenteral feeding

D. J. Papandria
Department of Surgery, Emory University,
Atlanta, GA, USA

K. A. Diefenbach (✉)
Nationwide Children's Hospital,
Columbus, OH, USA
e-mail: Karen.Diefenbach@nationwidechildrens.org

Essential Steps

Resection

1. Exploratory laparotomy
2. Inspection of the large and small bowel, with careful attention directed by preoperative radiographs and contrast studies
3. Resection of atretic segment(s)

Reconstruction

1. Anastomosis
2. Placement of diverting enterostomy (if needed)

Note These Variations

- Hand-sewn anastomosis may be required in cases of diminutive defunctionalized postatretic bowel segment, but stapled anastomosis is acceptable, if the device can be accommodated.
- Bowel tapering and end-to-side anastomoses may be employed to address discordant bowel caliber between the proximal and distal segments.
- Extensive or multiple atretic segments may predispose to short gut syndrome and dependence on TPN; in such cases, preservation of bowel length is crucial to future efforts at intestinal rehabilitation.

D. J. Papandria et al. (eds.), *Operative Dictations in Pediatric Surgery*,
https://doi.org/10.1007/978-3-030-24212-1_21

Template Operative Dictation (Open)

Preoperative Diagnosis Small bowel atresia

Postoperative Diagnosis *Jejunal/Ileal/Multiple sites of small bowel* atresia

Findings Same as postoperative diagnosis, with residual ___ cm of small bowel

Procedure(s) Performed Repair of jejunoileal atresia

Anesthesia General

Specimen Small bowel to pathology

Drains None

Implants None

Estimated Blood Loss *minimal/___ mL*

Indications This is a/an ___*-day/week/month-*old *male/female* with small bowel atresia identified on preoperative contrast studies. *He/she* was deemed to be a suitable candidate for open repair of jejunoileal atresia.

Procedure in Detail Following satisfactory induction of anesthesia, the patient was placed in supine position and appropriately padded. Timeouts were performed using both preinduction and preincision safety checklists with participation of all present in the operative suite. These confirmed the correct patient, procedure, operative site, and additional critical information prior to the start of the procedure. The abdomen was then prepped and draped in the usual sterile fashion.

A/an __-cm transverse epigastric incision was placed and carried down through the skin and subcutaneous tissues using monopolar electrocautery. The anterior fascia and abdominal musculature likewise divided, and the peritoneum was secured between DeBakey forceps and sharply divided with a Metzenbaum scissor. The peritoneal defect was then extended for the length of the incision and the small bowel delivered into the operative field. A cursory inspection of the intraperitoneal structures demonstrated no evidence of traumatic sequelae of abdominal access. The bowel was then run and closely examined in its entirety, with particular attention paid to the discontinuity noted on preoperative imaging at the *proximal/middle/distal* portion of the *jejunum/ileum.*

[Choose One:]
If single atresia: The atretic segment was clearly identified at ___ cm from the ligament of Treitz and the remainder of the exam and small bowel was found to be competent. The defunctionalized distal small bowel was carefully inspected and palpated to confirm this.

If multiple atresias: Multiple atretic segments were identified at ___, ___, … and ___ cm from the ligament of Treitz, and the remainder of the small bowel was found to be unaffected.

The colon was similarly assessed, and no areas of narrowing were noted.

The small bowel was then divided proximal to the aforementioned area of atresia using *a 2-0 silk ligature, followed by monopolar cautery/a linear stapler cutter.* This was repeated distally, and the resected specimen passed off the field for delivery to pathology.

If proximal tapering required: The discordant caliber of the proximal jejunum/ileum as compared with the defunctionalized distal bowel necessitated small bowel tapering. This was performed using *a linear stapler cutter/monopolar cautery and interrupted 3-0/4-0 Vicryl sutures* to longitudinally resect the redundant antimesenteric small bowel prior to anastomosis. The resulting taper reduced the small bowel diameter from approximately ___ cm to ___ cm over a length of ___ cm. Upon completion of this, reinspection of the bowel demonstrated no ischemia or overt narrowing of the lumen concerning for potential stricture.

[Choose One:]

If sutured anastomosis: Primary anastomosis was then performed using sutured technique. And *end-to-end/end-to-side*, *single/double-layer* hand-sewn anastomosis was performed using interrupted *3-0/4-0* Vicryl sutures. *The narrowed distal small bowel was opened along its antimesenteric aspect to "spatulate" the end-to-side anastomosis to ensure a broadly patent lumen.*

If stapled anastomosis: Primary anastomosis was then performed using stapled technique. The jaws of the *5/3*-mm endoscopic stapler were introduced into each lumen, with the anvil inserted into the distal segment and the cartridge into the proximal. The stapler was then closed, and correct alignment of the antimesenteric aspect of each segment within the jaws of the device was confirmed prior to firing. Upon firing, a broadly patent side-to-side, functional end-to-end anastomosis was created, and this was noted to be hemostatic. The residual common channel was then closed with *an additional staple firing/ with a single/double layer of interrupted 3-0/4-0 Vicryl sutures. Additional reinforcement sutures were placed at the crossing of the two staple lines and at the anastomotic crotch at the apex of the initial staple fire.*

If multiple atresias: The remaining atretic segments were resected with primary anastomosis performed in fashion identical to that described above.

Upon completion of anastomosis, the small bowel was inspected and palpated to assess for any focal ischemia or narrowing. *Meconium/ Succus entericus* and gas were gently milked across *the/each* anastomosis to ensure that it was sufficiently patent. No leaks were observed during these tests, and the bowel appeared healthy and well-perfused. No significant additional morphologic abnormalities involving the bowel were noted. Small bowel in continuity was measured as noted in findings above.

If enterostomy placed: To affected decompression of the distal bowel and protect the anastomoses, it was decided to divert the small bowel proximally. A/an ___-mm incision was placed sharply anterior to the rectus on the *right/left* side and then carried down through the skin and subcutaneous taste issues with monopolar cautery. The anterior fascia was opened with cautery, and the muscle of the rectus was split bluntly and the peritoneum entered with a hemostat. The jejunum/ileum was then brought out per this incision, maintaining its anatomic orientation to prevent torsion. At its terminus, this proximal segment measured ___ cm from the ligament of Treitz. *The bowel was then and tacked to the posterior fascia with interrupted 3-0 Vicryl sutures.*

If mucus fistula placed: The proximal limb of the defunctionalized bowel was then brought out as a mucous fistula at ___ cm from the ileocecal valve. It was directed into the *right/left* lateral corner of the laparotomy incision *and tacked to the fascia with interrupted 3-0 Vicryl sutures.*

Following completion of resection and anastomosis, the residual contiguous small bowel was measured and found to total ___ cm from the ligament of Treitz to the ileocecal valve. The abdomen was then irrigated with sterile saline until aspirates were clear. Turning attention to abdominal closure, the fascia was closed using *interrupted/running* 2-0 *Vicryl/PDS* sutures, followed by running subcuticular closure of the skin with 5-0 *Vicryl/Monocryl*. The incision was then dressed with *Steri-Strips, 2 × 2 gauze, and Medipore tape.*

If enterostomy placed: The *ileostomy/jejunostomy* was then opened with monopolar cautery and *left to mature spontaneously/matured with interrupted 4-0 Vicryl to fashion a Brooke ileostomy*. Upon completion of this, *the/each* ostomy was healthy in appearance and well-perfused. The *site was/sites were* dressed with *Xeroform* and covered with *2 × 2 gauze and Medipore tape.*

Upon completion of the procedure, a debriefing checklist was completed to share information critical to the postoperative care of the patient. The patient tolerated the procedure well, *was extubated in the operating room,* and was transported to the post-anesthesia care unit in stable condition thereafter.

22 Resection of Meckel's Diverticulum

Courtney Pisano and Gail E. Besner

Indications and Benefits

- Bleeding
- Volvulus
- Intussusception
- Littre's hernia
- Incidental finding during laparotomy

Risks and Alternatives

- Bleeding, infection, and risks of anesthesia
- Anastomotic leak
- Enterocutaneous fistula
- Small-bowel obstruction
- Abscess
- *Conversion of laparoscopic to open procedure*

Essential Steps

Open Meckel's Resection

1. Lower midline/transverse infraumbilical incision.
2. Mobilize the Meckel's diverticulum and adjacent ileum.
3. Inspect the diverticulum for the presence of ectopic mucosa.
4. Clamp, transect, and ligate the mesentery of the Meckel's diverticulum near the ileal mesentery.
5. *Apply stapler obliquely to the base of the Meckel's diverticulum and transect it. If sutured instead of stapled, close enterotomy in two layers with running __sutures and interrupted 3-0 silk Lembert sutures.*
6. If the base of the diverticulum is very wide, and simple transection would narrow the adjacent ileum, an ileal sleeve resection may be required.
7. Check *staple/suture* line for integrity and inspect the terminal ileum for adequate lumen.
8. Check hemostasis.
9. Irrigate abdomen.
10. Close abdomen.

Laparoscopic Meckel's Resection

1. Induce pneumoperitoneum.
2. Inspect abdomen with laparoscope placed through an umbilical port.
3. Place additional trocars under laparoscopic vision in following sites: one in the left lower abdomen and one in the right lower abdomen.
4. Mobilize the Meckel's diverticulum and ileum using blunt graspers.

C. Pisano · G. E. Besner (✉)
Nationwide Children's Hospital, Department of Pediatric Surgery, Columbus, OH, USA
e-mail: gail.besner@nationwidechildrens.org

D. J. Papandria et al. (eds.), *Operative Dictations in Pediatric Surgery*,
https://doi.org/10.1007/978-3-030-24212-1_22

5. Apply an endostapler obliquely to the base of the Meckel's diverticulum; transect the diverticulum.
6. If the base of the diverticulum is very wide, and simple transection would narrow the adjacent ileum, an ileal sleeve resection may be required.
7. Check for hemostasis at staple line.
8. Examine patency of the ileum lumen.
9. Remove Meckel's diverticulum.
10. Remove trocars under direct visualization.
11. Desufflate abdomen.
12. Close trocar sites.

Note These Variations

If discovered incidentally during an unrelated procedure, the decision to resect should be based on the appearance of the diverticulum as well as the condition of the patient and nature of the primary procedure.

Template Operative Dictation (Open)

Preoperative Diagnosis *Meckel's diverticulum/Bleeding/peritonitis/small-bowel obstruction/conversion from laparoscopic procedure/other*

Postoperative Diagnosis Same as preoperative diagnosis

Findings *Meckel's diverticulum with/without ectopic mucosa*

Procedure(s) Performed Resection of Meckel's diverticulum

Anesthesia *General/Regional/Procedural Sedation*

Specimen *Meckel's diverticulum/small-bowel segment with Meckel's diverticulum*

Drains None

Implants None

Estimated Blood Loss ___

Indications This is a/an ___*-day/week/month/year*-old *male/female* presented with *abdominal pain/bleeding/nausea/vomiting/fever/leukocytosis/other.* Diagnostic imaging and workup indicated *concern for Meckel's diverticulum with small-bowel obstruction/peritonitis/other.* The patient was brought to the operating room for exploratory laparotomy.

Procedure in Detail The patient was brought to the operating room and placed on the operating table in the supine position. Following satisfactory induction of general anesthesia, a time out was completed verifying the patient by two identifiers, the procedure to be performed and the operative site. *A Foley catheter and nasogastric tube were placed.* Appropriate perioperative antibiotics were administered, and the abdomen was prepped and draped in the usual sterile fashion.

A *vertical lower midline/transverse infraumbilical* abdominal incision was made. Dissection was carried down through subcutaneous tissue using electrocautery for adequate hemostasis. The *linea alba/muscular layers* were identified and divided, and the peritoneal cavity entered. The abdomen was explored and findings included ___, including a Meckel's diverticulum, approximately __ cm from the ileocecal valve.

The Meckel's diverticulum and ileum were mobilized. The blood supply to the diverticulum was identified, ligated, and divided. A stapler was then applied obliquely to the base of the diverticulum and the diverticulum was transected.

[Choose One:]

If stapler not used: The enterotomy was closed in two layers, an inner layer of running __ sutures and an outer layer of interrupted 3-0 *silk* Lembert sutures.

If stapler used to excise diverticulum: A linear stapler cutter (*blue/purple*) load was then used to transect the diverticulum at its base, which did not result in any significant narrowing of the ileal lumen.

For a wide-mouthed diverticulum: The base of the diverticulum was sufficiently broad that transection would lead to stenosis of the ileal lumen, and a segmental resection was, therefore, performed. Linear stapler cutter (*blue/purple*) loads were used to divide the bowel ___ cm proximal and __ cm distal to the border of the diverticulum, and the mesentery was *taken with a vessel sealing device/clamped and ligated in stepwise fashion using 2-0/3-0 silk ties.*

The integrity of the *staple/suture line* was examined and the patency of the lumen of the ileum confirmed. Hemostasis was confirmed *and the abdomen was irrigated with normal saline.* The peritoneum and the *fascial/muscular layers* were approximated using *running/interrupted* __. The subcutaneous fat was approximated using *running/interrupted* __. The skin was closed using 5-0 Vicryl in a subcuticular fashion. The incision was dressed with *Steri-strips/TegaDerm/topical skin adhesive.* All sponge, needle, and instrument counts were correct at the end of the procedure. Upon completion of the procedure, a debriefing checklist was completed to share information critical to the postoperative care of the patient. The patient tolerated the procedure well, *was extubated in the operating room*, and was transported to the post-anesthesia care unit in stable condition thereafter.

Template Operative Dictation (Laparoscopic)

Preoperative Diagnosis *Meckel's diverticulum/Bleeding/small-bowel obstruction/other*

Postoperative Diagnosis Same as preoperative diagnosis

Findings *Meckel's diverticulum with/without ectopic mucosa*

Procedures Performed Laparoscopic Resection of Meckel's diverticulum

Anesthesia General

Specimen None

Drains None

Implants None

Estimated Blood Loss ___ mL

Indications This is a/an ___-*day/week/month/year*-old *male/female* presented with *abdominal pain/bleeding/nausea/vomiting/other.* Diagnostic imaging and workup indicated *concern for Meckel's diverticulum with small-bowel obstruction/volvulus/other.* The patient was brought to the operating room for exploratory laparoscopy.

Procedure in Detail The patient was brought to the operating room and placed on the operating table in the supine position. Following satisfactory induction of general anesthesia, a time out was completed verifying the patient by two identifiers, the procedure to be performed and the operative site. *A Foley catheter and nasogastric tube were placed.* Appropriate perioperative antibiotics were administered, and the abdomen was prepped and draped in the usual sterile fashion.

An infraumbilical incision was made.

[Choose One:]

For Veress needle: *The fascia was elevated and the Veress needle was inserted. Proper position of the needle was established using aspiration and the saline meniscus test.* Pneumoperitoneum was established using carbon dioxide to a pressure of *12–15 mmHg.* ***A*** 5-mm/*10/12*-mm trocar was then inserted. A 5-mm laparoscope was introduced into the abdomen, and the intraperitoneal contents were inspected. No traumatic sequelae of the initial trocar placement were noted.

For Hasson cannula: *Using electrocautery, dissection was carried down to the level of the fas-*

cia. The fascia was divided with cautery, and 2-0 Vicryl traction sutures were placed on each side of the fascia. The Hasson 10- to 12-mm trocar was then advanced into the abdomen under direct supervision and secured using the previously placed fascial sutures. A 5-mm laparoscope was introduced into the abdomen, and the intraperitoneal contents were inspected. No traumatic sequelae of the initial trocar placement were noted.

Local anesthetic infiltration was used, and 5-mm incisions were made for additional trocar sites. Two additional trocars were placed, one in the left lower abdomen and one in the right lower abdomen under direct visualization. Careful inspection of the abdomen was performed, and *Meckel's diverticulum/small-bowel obstruction/ volvulus/other findings were noted.* Using blunt laparoscopic graspers, the Meckel's diverticulum was mobilized along with the ileum. The Meckel's diverticulum was located approximately __ cm from the ileocecal valve.

[Choose One:]

If stapler used to excise diverticulum: The blood supply to the diverticulum was identified. An endostapler was introduced through the *10/12-mm* trocar, and a (*white/gray*) load was used to ligate the blood supply to the diverticulum. A (*blue/purple*) load was then used to transect the diverticulum at its base, which did not result in any significant narrowing of the ileal lumen.

For a wide-mouthed diverticulum: The base of the diverticulum was sufficiently broad that transection would lead to stenosis of the ileal lumen, and a segmental resection was, therefore, performed. An endostapler was introduced through the *10/12-mm* trocar and (*blue/purple*) loads were used to divide the bowel ___ cm proximal and __ cm distal to the border of the diverticulum, and the mesentery was *taken with a vessel sealing device.*

The staple line was checked for hemostasis, and the patency of the ileal lumen was confirmed. The specimen was placed in an EndoCatch bag and removed through the umbilical port. The 5-mm trocars were removed under direct laparoscopic vision, and hemostasis confirmed at the trocar sites. Following desufflation of the abdomen, the umbilical trocar was removed and the site was closed at the fascial level with 2-0 Vicryl figure-of-eight sutures. The fascia at the 5-mm port sites was closed with interrupted 2-0 Vicryl sutures. The skin at all port sites was then closed with 5-0 Vicryl in a subcuticular fashion. All sites were dressed with Steri-*strips/ TegaDerm/topic skin adhesive/a folded 2 × 2 gauze placed at the umbilical incision.*

All sponge, needle, and instrument counts were correct at the end of the procedure. Upon completion of the procedure, a debriefing checklist was completed to share information critical to the postoperative care of the patient. The patient tolerated the procedure well, *was extubated in the operating room,* and was transported to the post-anesthesia care unit in stable condition thereafter.

Resection of Omphalomesenteric Duct Remnant

23

Lorraine I. Kelley-Quon

Indications and Benefits

- Persistent omphalomesenteric duct
- Benefits: Removal of duct

Risks and Alternatives

- Standard risks (bleeding, infection, need for additional procedures, risks of anesthesia)
- Injury to adjacent structures ({small bowel})
- Alternatives: None

Essential Steps

1. Cannulate duct (if possible)
2. Curvilinear incision circumscribing the edges of duct
3. Carry dissection along duct edges
4. Free duct from fascia
5. Eviscerate base attached to small bowel
6. Excise omphalomesenteric duct
7. Close fascia
8. Umbilicoplasty

L. I. Kelley-Quon (✉)
Children's Hospital Los Angeles, Division of Pediatric Surgery, Department of Surgery, Keck School of Medicine of University of Southern California, Los Angeles, CA, USA
e-mail: lkquon@chla.usc.edu

Template Operative Dictation (Open)

Preoperative Diagnosis Omphalomesenteric duct remnant

Postoperative Diagnosis Same as preoperative diagnosis

Findings Same as postoperative diagnosis

Procedure(s) Performed Resection of omphalomesenteric duct remnant

Anesthesia General

Specimen {Omphalomesenteric duct}

Drains {None}

Implants {None}

Estimated Blood Loss ___

Indications This is a/an ___-*day/week/month/year*-old *male/female* with an omphalomesenteric duct remnant. He/she was deemed to be a suitable candidate for resection of omphalomesenteric duct remnant.

Procedure in Detail Following satisfactory induction of anesthesia, the patient was placed

D. J. Papandria et al. (eds.), *Operative Dictations in Pediatric Surgery*,
https://doi.org/10.1007/978-3-030-24212-1_23

in the supine position and appropriately padded. Timeouts were performed using both pre-induction and pre-incision safety checklists with participation of all present in the operative suite. These confirmed the correct patient, procedure, operative site, and additional critical information prior to the start of the procedure. The abdomen was then prepped and draped in the usual sterile fashion.

The umbilicus was inspected and a small probe was placed in the orifice of the patent duct. A curvilinear circumferential incision was made lateral to the edges of the duct. Dissection was carried down through the subcutaneous tissue along the edge of the duct to the level of the fascia. A right angle was placed on the right edge of the fascia–duct interface, and the fascia was opened under direct vision. The same maneuver was performed on the left side of the duct. This allowed the intestinal base of the duct to be eviscerated and inspected. The base of the duct was transected longitudinally with an EndoGIA stapler, and the bowel was returned to the intra-abdominal cavity. The duct was passed off the field as specimen. The fascia was then closed in an interrupted fashion using PDS. The edges of the umbilical incision were reapproximated using Vicryl in an inverted dermal fashion to complete the umbilicoplasty. A sterile pressure dressing was placed on the umbilicus.

Upon completion of the procedure, a debriefing checklist was completed to share information critical to the postoperative care of the patient. The patient tolerated the procedure well, *was extubated in the operating room*, and was transported to the post-anesthesia care unit in stable condition thereafter.

Reduction of Intussusception

24

Courtney Pisano and Gail E. Besner

Indications and Benefits

- Ileocolic intussusception
- Failed enema reduction
- *Conversion of laparoscopic to open procedure*

Risks and Alternatives

- Bleeding, infection, risks of anesthesia
- Recurrent intussusception

Essential Steps

Open Reduction of Ileocolic Intussusception

1. Infraumbilical transverse right-sided incision.
2. Deliver intussusception through incision.
3. Use gentle continuous pressure at the site of intussusception to reduce it.
4. Check bowel for serosal tears.
5. Examine bowel for signs of ischemia or perforation.
6. *Remove ischemic segments/ileocecectomy/ right hemicolectomy.*
7. Examine for an obvious pathologic lead point.
8. Note that there will be thickening and edema at the site of reduction. This should not be mistaken for a pathologic lead point.
9. *Remove pathologic lead point.*
10. *Perform appendectomy.*
11. Examine for adequate hemostasis.
12. Irrigate abdomen.
13. Close abdomen.

Laparoscopic Reduction of Ileocolic Intussusception

1. Induce pneumoperitoneum.
2. Inspect abdomen with laparoscope placed through umbilical port.
3. Place additional trocars under laparoscopic vision in locations based on location of intussusception.
4. With atraumatic graspers, use gentle squeezing pressure distally and gentle traction proximally to reduce the intussusception.
5. Check bowel for serosal tears.
6. Examine bowel for signs of ischemia or perforation.
7. *Remove pathologic lead point.*
8. *Perform appendectomy.*

C. Pisano · G. E. Besner (✉)
Nationwide Children's Hospital, Department of Pediatric Surgery, Columbus, OH, USA
e-mail: gail.besner@nationwidechildrens.org

D. J. Papandria et al. (eds.), *Operative Dictations in Pediatric Surgery*,
https://doi.org/10.1007/978-3-030-24212-1_24

9. Examine for adequate hemostasis.
10. Remove trocars under direct visualization.
11. Desufflate abdomen.
12. Close trocar sites.

Template Operative Dictation (Open)

Preoperative Diagnosis Ileocolic intussusception

Postoperative Diagnosis Same as preoperative diagnosis

Findings *Intussusception with/without lead point*

Procedure(s) Performed Reduction of intussusception

Anesthesia *General/regional/procedural sedation*

Specimen None

Drains None

Implants None

Estimated Blood Loss ___

Indications This is a/an___-*day/week/month/year*-old *male/female* presented with *abdominal pain/nausea/vomiting/fever/bloody stools/other.* Diagnostic imaging and workup indicated *ileocolic intussusception/other. Enema reduction was unsuccessful.* The patient was brought to the operating room for *open reduction of ileocolic intussusception/exploratory laparotomy.*

Procedure in Detail The patient was brought to the operating room and placed on the operating table in the supine position. Following satisfactory induction of general anesthesia, a time out was completed verifying the patient by two identifiers, the procedure to be performed and the operative site. *A Foley catheter and nasogastric tube were placed.* Appropriate perioperative antibiotics were administered, and the abdomen was prepped and draped in the usual sterile fashion.

An infraumbilical transverse right-sided incision was made. Dissection was carried down through the subcutaneous tissue using electrocautery for adequate hemostasis. The fascia, muscular layers, and peritoneum were divided and the peritoneal cavity entered. Upon entering the peritoneal cavity, the intussusception was delivered through the incision. *The right colon was mobilized.* Starting at the most distal end, gentle squeezing of the intussusceptum from within the intussuscipiens was performed. After several minutes of continuous pressure, the intussusception was reduced. The bowel was examined for serosal tears *which were present/were not present. If transmural tears are present, the intussusception is not reducible, and ileocecectomy/right hemicolectomy may be performed. Describe procedure here.* The bowel was examined for ischemic areas and none were found. Further inspection showed *no pathologic lead point/lead point caused by Meckel's diverticulum/polyp/other was found. If pathological lead point found, dictate removal here. If appendectomy is performed for concern it may act as a lead point, dictate procedure here.* The abdomen was irrigated with normal saline. The peritoneum and the posterior rectus sheath were approximated using *running/interrupted* __. The anterior rectus sheath was approximated using *running/interrupted* __. The subcutaneous fat was closed with _____. The skin was closed using a 5-0 Vicryl subcuticular closure. The incision was dressed with *Steri-strips/topical skin adhesive.* All sponge, needle, and instrument counts were correct at the end of the procedure. Upon completion of the procedure, a debriefing checklist was completed to share information critical to the postoperative care of the patient. The patient tolerated the procedure well, *was extubated in the operating room*, and was transported to the post-anesthesia care unit in stable condition thereafter.

Template Operative Dictation (Laparoscopic)

Preoperative Diagnosis Ileocolic intussusception

Postoperative Diagnosis Same as preoperative diagnosis

Findings *Intussusception with/without lead point*

Procedure(s) Performed Laparoscopic Reduction of intussusception

Anesthesia General

Specimen None

Drains None

Implants None

Estimated Blood Loss ___

Indications This is a/an ___*-day/week/month/ year*-old *male/female* presented with *abdominal pain/nausea/vomiting/fever/bloody stools/other.* Diagnostic imaging and workup indicated *ileocolic intussusception/other. Enema reduction was unsuccessful.* The patient was brought to the operating room for laparoscopic reduction of ileocolic intussusception/*exploratory laparoscopy.*

Procedure in Detail The patient was brought to the operating room and placed on the operating table in the supine position. Following satisfactory induction of general anesthesia, a time out was completed verifying the patient by two identifiers, the procedure to be performed and the operative site. *A Foley catheter and nasogastric tube were placed.* Appropriate perioperative antibiotics were administered, and the abdomen was prepped and draped in the usual sterile fashion.

A 5-mm infraumbilical incision was made.

[Choose One:]

For Veress needle: *The fascia was elevated and the Veress needle was inserted. Proper position of the needle was established using aspiration and the saline meniscus test.* Pneumoperitoneum was established using carbon dioxide to a pressure of *12–15 mmHg. A 5-mm/10/12*-mm trocar was then inserted. A 5-mm laparoscope was introduced into the abdomen, and the intraperitoneal contents were inspected. No traumatic sequelae of the initial trocar placement were noted.

For Hasson cannula: *Using electrocautery, dissection was carried down to the level of the fascia. The fascia was divided with cautery, and 2-0 Vicryl traction sutures were placed on each side of the fascia. A Hasson 10-mm trocar was then advanced into the abdomen under direct vision and secured using the previously placed fascial sutures.* A 5-mm laparoscope was introduced into the abdomen, and the intraperitoneal contents were inspected. No traumatic sequelae of the initial trocar placement were noted.

Local anesthetic infiltration was used, and incisions were then created for additional trocar sites *Placement of trocar sites depends on location of the intussusception.* Upon further inspection of the abdomen, an ileocolic intussusception was identified. Using atraumatic graspers, the bowel was carefully handled with continue gentle traction applied just proximal to the intussusception and constant gentle pressure applied just distal to the intussusception. Once the intussusception was reduced, the bowel was examined for any serosal tears or signs of ischemia or perforation. *No signs of ischemia were seen/no serosal tears/other specific findings. If appendectomy is performed for concern, it may act as a lead point, dictate procedure here. The abdomen was irrigated with normal saline.* The 5-mm trocars were removed under direct laparoscopic vision and hemostasis confirmed at the trocar sites. Following desufflation of the abdomen, the umbilical trocar was removed and site was closed at the fascial level with 2-0 Vicryl figure-of-eight sutures. The fascia at the 5-mm port sites was closed with 2-0 Vicryl sutures. The skin at all port sites was closed with 5-0 Vicryl subcuticular closures. All sites were dressed with *Steri-strips/TegaDerm/topic skin adhesive/a folded 2 × 2 gauze placed at the umbilical incision.*

All sponge, needle, and instrument counts were correct at the end of the procedure. Upon completion of the procedure, a debriefing checklist was completed to share information critical to the postoperative care of the patient. The patient tolerated the procedure well, *was extubated in the operating room*, and was transported to the post-anesthesia care unit in stable condition thereafter.

25 Resection of Enteric Duplication or Mesenteric Cyst

Mitchell R. Ladd and Daniel Rhee

Indications and Benefits

- Presence of enteric or mesenteric cyst.
- Symptomatic enteric or mesenteric cyst (e.g., pain, distention, small-bowel obstruction, volvulus).
- Benefits: Reduce the risk of infection, bleeding, small-bowel obstruction, intestinal volvulus, or development of malignancy.

Risks and Alternatives

- Standard risks (bleeding, infection, need for additional procedures, risks of anesthesia)
- Injury to adjacent structures (liver, gallbladder, spleen, stomach, small and large intestine)
- Injury to uninvolved mesentery resulting in bowel ischemia/necrosis
- Alternatives: Sclerotherapy, image-guided cyst aspiration, observation

M. R. Ladd
Johns Hopkins Hospital, Department of General Surgery, Baltimore, MD, USA

D. Rhee (✉)
Johns Hopkins School of Medicine, Department of Surgery, Baltimore, MD, USA
e-mail: drhee1@jhmi.edu

Essential Steps

1. Abdominal exploration (via open or laparoscopic technique)
2. Evaluate the entire small bowel with its mesentery from ligament of Treitz to the terminal ileum and the colon with its mesentery
3. Identification of the cyst(s)
4. Decompress the cyst if needed with needle aspiration or partial opening
5. Resect the cyst (or enucleation/marsupialize depending on the situation) with bowel resection if needed
6. If bowel was resected, perform primary anastomosis; if marsupialized or partially resected, sclerose the remaining cyst lining
7. Abdominal closure

Note These Variations

- Laparoscopic access can be obtained with Veress or Hasson technique.
- Trocar sizes used will depend on the age of the child.
- Trocar number will depend on the complexity of cyst resection.
- The cyst will either be resected alone, included with a bowel resection, enucleated, or if not able to safely resect will be partially resected and marsupialized followed by sclerosing the cyst lining depending on the scenario.

D. J. Papandria et al. (eds.), *Operative Dictations in Pediatric Surgery*,
https://doi.org/10.1007/978-3-030-24212-1_25

Template Operative Dictation (Open)

Preoperative Diagnosis *Presence of enteric/mesenteric cyst/symptomatic enteric/mesenteric cyst*

Postoperative Diagnosis Same as preoperative diagnosis

Findings *Enteric/mesenteric* cyst

Procedure(s) Performed Resection of enteric duplication or mesenteric cyst

Anesthesia General

Specimen *Enteric/mesenteric cyst*

Estimated Blood Loss ___

Indications This is a/an ___*-day/week/month/year*-old *male/female* with an *enteric/mesenteric* cyst. *He/she* was deemed to be a suitable candidate for resection of enteric duplication or mesenteric cyst.

Procedure in Detail Following satisfactory induction of anesthesia, the patient was placed in the supine position and appropriately padded. Timeouts were performed using both pre-induction and pre-incision safety checklists with participation of all present in the operative suite. These confirmed the correct patient, procedure, operative site, and additional critical information prior to the start of the procedure. The abdomen was then prepped and draped in the usual sterile fashion.

A *midline/transverse* laparotomy was performed to enter the abdomen. All four quadrants of the abdomen were explored to identify the cyst. The small bowel and its mesentery were examined from the ligament of Treitz to the terminal ileum, and the colon and its mesentery were inspected to rule out the presence of other cysts or pathology.

[Choose One:]

If enteric duplication cyst or mesenteric cyst requiring bowel resection: The identified cyst was brought into the operative field. *The cyst fluid was then aspirated to better define the anatomy.* The amount of *overlying/connected* bowel to be resected was determined. At the proximal aspect of the bowel, a mesenteric defect was created and the intestine divided with *electrocautery/a gastrointestinal stapler*. At the distal aspect of the bowel, a mesenteric defect was created and the bowel divided. The mesentery of the bowel to be resected, which included the cyst, was then carefully divided with *electrocautery/vessel sealing device/clamps and suture ligation*. The specimen was then removed. Next, the two ends of the bowel were anastomosed in an *end-to-end/side-to-side hand-sewn/stapled fashion*.

If mesenteric cyst not requiring bowel resection: The identified cyst was brought into the operative field. The cyst was then carefully dissected from the mesentery using electrocautery being careful to avoid injury to the nearby mesenteric vessels. The specimen was then removed.

If mesenteric cyst requiring marsupialization: The identified cyst was brought into the operative field and was deemed *too large/too close to critical structures* to safely resect. Thus, the decision was made to do a partial resection with marsupialization. The boundaries of the cyst were identified to the extent possible, and the maximum amount of cyst that could be safely resected was removed using electrocautery being careful to avoid nearby mesenteric vessels. The remaining cyst was opened as much as possible so that it could adequately drain. Next, the lining of the cyst was sclerosed with *10% glucose solution/electrocautery/tincture of iodine* to prevent recurrence.

If enteric duplication cyst with long common wall: The identified duplication cyst was brought into the field and deemed to involve too long of an intestinal segment for resection.

[Choose One:]

If proximal communication exists: A communication was seen at the entrance of the proximal end of the duplication cyst. The decision was made to fenestrate the common wall on the distal end. At the distal end of the cyst, the *duplication cyst/intestine* was opened and the common wall was opened using *electrocautery/a gastrointestinal stapler.* The common channel was hemostatic, and the *duplication cyst/intestine* was closed using sized ___-0 absorbable suture in a *continuous/interrupted* fashion.

If no proximal communication exists: A longitudinal seromuscular incision was made over the duplication, taking care to avoid the mesenteric vessels, and the submucosal lining was stripped from the duplication cyst. This was repeated along the length of the cyst until the submucosa was removed.

The abdomen was irrigated with warm saline. Then, the abdominal fascia was closed with sized ___ *absorbable suture in a/an continuous/interrupted* fashion. The skin was then closed with ___-0 *absorbable sutures using a subcuticular stitch and skin glue was applied.* All needle and sponge counts were verified and correct.

Upon completion of the procedure, a debriefing checklist was completed to share information critical to the postoperative care of the patient. The patient tolerated the procedure well, *was extubated in the operating room,* and was transported to the post-anesthesia care unit in stable condition thereafter.

Template Operative Dictation (Laparoscopic)

Preoperative Diagnosis *Presence of enteric/mesenteric cyst/symptomatic enteric/mesenteric cyst*

Postoperative Diagnosis Same as preoperative diagnosis

Findings *Enteric/mesenteric* cyst

Procedure(s) Performed Laparoscopic resection of enteric duplication or mesenteric cyst

Anesthesia General

Specimen *Enteric/mesenteric* cyst

Estimated Blood Loss ___

Indications This is a/an ___*-day/week/month/year*-old *male/female* with an *enteric/mesenteric* cyst. *He/she* was deemed to be a suitable candidate for laparoscopic resection of enteric duplication or mesenteric cyst.

Procedure in Detail Following satisfactory induction of anesthesia, the patient was placed in the supine position and appropriately padded. Timeouts were performed using both pre-induction and pre-incision safety checklists with participation of all present in the operative suite. These confirmed the correct patient, procedure, operative site, and additional critical information prior to the start of the procedure. The abdomen was then prepped and draped in the usual sterile fashion.

The abdomen is entered near the umbilicus using the *Hasson/Veress* technique and placement of size ___ trocar. The abdomen was then insufflated with carbon dioxide to ___ mm Hg. Safe entry into the abdomen was confirmed with visual inspection. The abdomen was then inspected in all four quadrants looking for the cyst and for sites of safe placement of additional trocars. An additional *2–3 trocars* were placed under direct visualization in order to triangulate the cyst and allow for full evaluation of the bowel. After trocar placement, atraumatic graspers were used to evaluate the bowel and its mesentery by running the small bowel from the ligament of Treitz to the terminal ileum and inspection of the entire colon to rule out the presence of additional cysts or pathology. *Due to the size of the cyst, adequate visualization was not initially obtained and the cyst was laparoscopically aspirated to allow for better inspection of the abdomen and subsequent dissection.*

[Choose One:]

If enteric duplication cyst or mesenteric cyst requiring bowel resection: After fully defining the extent of the cyst, the amount of *overlying/*

connected bowel to be resected was determined. At the proximal aspect of the bowel, a mesenteric defect was created using a *Maryland dissector* and the intestine divided with scissors/*electrocautery/a gastrointestinal stapler*. At the distal aspect of the bowel, a mesenteric defect was created in a similar fashion and the bowel divided. Then, the mesentery of the bowel to be resected, which included the cyst, was carefully divided with *hook electrocautery/vessel sealing device/clamps and suture ligation*. The specimen was then placed in a laparoscopic specimen bag and removed from the umbilical port. Next, the two ends of the bowel were anastomosed in an *end-to-end/side-to-side intra-corporeally sewn/stapled fashion*.

If mesenteric cyst not requiring bowel resection: After fully defining the extent of the cyst, it was carefully dissected from the mesentery using hook electrocautery being careful to avoid injury to the nearby mesenteric vessels. The specimen was then placed in a laparoscopic specimen bag and removed from the umbilical port.

If mesenteric cyst requiring marsupialization: After evaluating the cyst, it was deemed *too large/too close to critical structures* to safely resect. Thus, the decision was made to do a partial resection with marsupialization. The boundaries of the cyst were identified to the extent possible, and the maximum amount of cyst that could be safely resected was removed using hook electrocautery being careful to avoid nearby mesenteric vessels. The specimen was then placed in a laparoscopic specimen bag and removed from the umbilical port. The remaining cyst was opened as much as possible using *hook electrocautery/laparoscopic scissors* so that it could adequately drain. Next, the lining of the cyst was sclerosed with *10% glucose solution/hook electrocautery/tincture of iodine* to prevent recurrence.

The abdomen was irrigated with warm saline. The trocars were removed under direct visualization. The laparoscope was removed and the abdomen desufflated. The periumbilical fascia was then closed using sized ___ absorbable suture in an *interrupted/figure-of-eight fashion*. The skin at each port site was then closed with ___ *absorbable sutures using a subcuticular stitch, and skin glue was applied*. All needle and sponge counts were verified and correct.

Upon completion of the procedure, a debriefing checklist was completed to share information critical to the postoperative care of the patient. The patient tolerated the procedure well, *was extubated in the operating room*, and was transported to the post-anesthesia care unit in stable condition thereafter.

26 Serial Transverse Enteroplasty (STEP)

Afif Kulaylat and Karen A. Diefenbach

Indications and Benefits

- Short-bowel syndrome
- Failure to thrive
- Poor weight gain
- Inability to advance enteral feeds
- Large segment dilation with dysmotility
- Small intestinal bacterial overgrowth (SIBO)
- Benefits: Improved mucosal absorptive surface area, facilitates enteral autonomy, addresses areas of stasis associated with SIBO

Risks and Alternatives

- Standard risks (bleeding, infection, need for additional procedures, risks of anesthesia)
- Anastomotic/staple line leak
- Anastomotic/segmental stricture
- Alternatives: Bianchi procedure or alternative bowel lengthening techniques

A. Kulaylat
Nationwide Children's Hospital, Department of Surgery, Columbus, OH, USA

K. A. Diefenbach (✉)
Nationwide Children's Hospital, Columbus, OH, USA
e-mail: Karen.Diefenbach@nationwidechildrens.org

Essential Steps

Preoperative Assessment

1. Upper GI with small bowel follow through to assess bowel dilation (generally >6 cm) and general estimate of length

Operative

2. Complete lysis of adhesion such that no kinks present in bowel or mesentery
3. Creation of serial transverse enteroplasties at 2-cm intervals from alternating sides of the bowel

Template Operative Dictation (Open)

Preoperative Diagnosis *Short-bowel syndrome*

Postoperative Diagnosis Same as preoperative diagnosis

Findings Same as postoperative diagnosis

Procedure(s) Performed
1. Exploratory laparotomy
2. Extensive lysis of adhesions (___ hours)

D. J. Papandria et al. (eds.), *Operative Dictations in Pediatric Surgery*,
https://doi.org/10.1007/978-3-030-24212-1_26

3. Serial transverse enteroplasty x ___ enteroplasties performed
4. *Tru-Cut Liver Biopsy*

Anesthesia General

Specimen *Liver biopsy*

Drains None

Implants None

Estimated Blood Loss ___ mL

Indications This is a/an ___*-month/year-*old *male/female* with short-bowel syndrome associated with *failure to thrive/poor weight gain/inability to advance enteral feeds/repeated bouts of bacterial overgrowth. He/she* was assessed with upper GI with small bowel follow through, and dilated segments of small bowel exceeding ____ cm for a length of _____ cm were noted. *He/she* was found to be a suitable candidate for exploration and serial transverse enteroplasty.

Procedure in Detail Following satisfactory induction of anesthesia, the patient was placed in the supine position and appropriately padded and secured. Timeouts were performed using both pre-induction and pre-incision safety checklists with participation of all present in the operative suite. These confirmed the correct patient, procedure, operative site, and additional critical information prior to the start of the procedure. The abdomen was then prepped and draped in the usual sterile fashion.

An incision was made along the previous *transverse/midline* incision. The incision was extended through the fascia down the peritoneum using electrocautery for hemostasis. The peritoneum was entered and opened the full length of the incision being careful to avoid injury to the underlying bowel. An *extensive* lysis of adhesions was performed which took approximately ____ hours to free the entirety of the small bowel. Once completed, the bowel could be completely straightened and there with no kinks present along the length of the small bowel or its mesentery. The length of the small bowel was measured at ___ cm. The liver was then examined; it appeared grossly *normal/abnormal. A Tru-Cut liver biopsy was performed and hemostasis achieved using electrocautery. The specimen was sent to pathology.*

Further inspection of the small bowel identified approximately _____ cm that was dilated to a diameter of at least ___ cm. There *was no* evidence of stricture distal to this dilated bowel. Attention was then turned to performing serial transverse enteroplasties. The midline of the antimesenteric border was marked along the length of the dilated segment(s) of small bowel. In 2-cm intervals, alternating perpendicular or transverse marks were made from the edge of the bowel to map out the intended enteroplasties. Serial transverse enteroplasties were then performed in an alternating fashion at the previously marked 2-cm intervals by creating defects in the mesentery and then using a *GIA/EndoGIA* ______ staple load at a 90-degree angle to the mesentery and reinforcing them with 3-0 *Vicryl/PDS interrupted/Figure-of-8* suture at the crotch of the staple line. This process was repeated until the intestine was less than 4 cm in diameter. In total, _____ serial transverse enteroplasties were created. The luminal small intestine was then remeasured at _____ cm. The bowel was carefully returned to the abdomen, ensuring that there were no twists and that the hemostasis was achieved.

The abdomen was irrigated with saline. The fascia was closed with *running/interrupted* ____-0 *Vicryl/PDS* suture. The subcutaneous tissue was irrigated. The subcutaneous tissue/scar was reapproximated with ___-0 Vicryl sutures. A ___-0 *Vicryl/Monocryl* suture was then used to close the skin. *Mastisol and Steri-Strips/Dermabond/A sterile dressing* was used over the incision.

All sponges and instruments counts were correct ×2. Upon completion of the procedure, a debriefing checklist was completed to share information critical to the postoperative care of the patient. The patient tolerated the procedure well, *was extubated in the operating room/remained intubated,* and was transported to the *post-anesthesia care unit/intensive care unit* in *stable/guarded* condition thereafter.

27 Stricturoplasty and Small-Bowel Stricture Bypass (Open and MIS Approaches)

Lea Wehrli and Stefan Scholz

Indications

- Symptomatic partial small-bowel obstruction due to stricture as diagnosed by small-bowel contrast study, CT, or MRI enterography
- Weight loss, intolerance of feeds, abdominal cramping, most commonly patients with known inflammatory bowel disease such as Crohn's disease

Benefits

- Correction of obstruction
- Preservation of bowel length and absorptive surface

Risks and Alternatives

- Standard risks (bleeding, infection, need for additional procedures, risks of anesthesia).
- Injury to major vessels, stomach, small or large bowel, injury to bladder, liver or spleen or other organs.
- Post-operative bowel obstruction from adhesions or inflammation.
- Anastomotic leak of side-to-side bypass or from stricturoplasty site.
- Bacterial overgrowth in cases with side-to-side antiperistaltic bypass (Finney stricturoplasty).
- Alternatives: Small-bowel resection in case of a long-segment stricture. If multiple resections are performed, the patient may be at risk for short-bowel syndrome.
- If the stricture is located too close to the ileocecal valve, an ileocecectomy may be safer due to increased risk of postoperative leakage.

Essential Steps

1. Place a 12-mm umbilical port and induce pneumoperitoneum.
2. Perform standard general inspection of the abdomen.
3. Depending on the location of the expected stricture site, place two additional 5-mm working ports.

L. Wehrli
Children's Hospital of Pittsburgh of UPMC, Department of Pediatric Surgery, Pittsburgh, PA, USA

S. Scholz (✉)
University of Pittsburgh School of Medicine, Children's Hospital of Pittsburgh, Department of Pediatric Surgery, Pittsburgh, PA, USA
e-mail: stefan.scholz@chp.edu

D. J. Papandria et al. (eds.), *Operative Dictations in Pediatric Surgery*,
https://doi.org/10.1007/978-3-030-24212-1_27

4. Run the small bowel with two bowel graspers from the ileocecal valve to the ligament of Treitz.
5. Identify the site with strictures and stenosis.
6. Perform stricturoplasty, either with a laparoscopic intra-abdominal technique or open extra-abdominal by extending the small umbilical incision. Then, place a wound retractor and eviscerate the small bowel for an outside stricturoplasty.
    1. A *Heineke–Mikulicz* stricturoplasty is usually performed if a short stricture is found. Two stay sutures (e.g., silk 4-0) are placed in the center of the incision in the area of the stricture; these are going to be the most lateral sutures of the stricturoplasty. A longitudinal enterotomy is then made along the antimesenteric border across the stricture using electrocautery or scissors. The incision should extend at least 1–2 cm proximal and distal beyond the stricture. The enterotomy is then closed in a transverse fashion with interrupted vicryl or silk sutures. Additional interrupted seromuscular sutures (Lembert sutures) as a second row are optional.
    2. In case of medium length strictures (up to 20 cm), a *Finney* stricturoplasty is a better option. The bowel is brought into a U-shaped fashion, and a total of three stay sutures are placed at the base and the end of the U. Two enterotomies at the base of the U are used to perform a side-to-side stapled anastomosis along the length of the bowel. Alternatively, a longitudinal antimesenteric incision is made extending 1–2 cm beyond the stricture. A side-to-side anastomosis is then fashioned with either interrupted or running Vicryl sutures along the backwall. Additionally, interrupted seromuscular sutures (Lembert suture) are placed with Vicryl 4-0.
    3. A *side-to-side isoperistaltic stricturoplasty* is performed for long-segment strictures or in case of multiple strictures in close proximity. The bowel and its mesentery are divided in the middle of the segment with the stricture. The proximal bowel is positioned to overlay the distal bowel loop in a side-to-side fashion. Multiple interrupted seromuscular nonabsorbable sutures that approximate the two bowel loops are placed. The bowel loops are opened longitudinally with cautery on its antimesenteric border. Both ends are spatulated and anastomosed in a tapered fashion. Alternatively, a stapled anastomosis can be performed.
7. Check the intestinal closure or anastomosis for adequate patency and leak.
8. If extra-abdominal, reposition the small bowel into the abdominal cavity.
9. Assure hemostasis.
10. Irrigate abdominal cavity and suction all fluid.
11. Remove all ports under vision and deflate abdomen.
12. Close port sites.

Note These Variations:

- Stricturoplasty can either be accomplished by intra-abdominal suturing or stapling or through an extended umbilical incision with a wound retractor (minilaparotomy) and evisceration of the small bowel for extra-abdominal stricturoplasty.
- The three different techniques (Heineke–Mikulicz or Finney stricturoplasties as well as isoperistaltic side-to-side small-bowel bypass) can either be performed open, completely laparoscopic, or laparoscopically assisted with an extra-abdominal anastomosis. The anastomosis can either be performed with a hand-sewn or stapled technique. A number of mostly retrospective studies that reported on surgical recurrences showed recurrent stricture to occur less likely with a stapled anastomosis in comparison to a hand-sewn technique.

Template Operative Dictation

Preoperative Diagnosis Small-bowel obstruction due to stricture

Postoperative Diagnosis Same

Findings Small (or large)-bowel obstruction due to short- or long-segment stricture

Procedure Performed Exploratory laparotomy and stricturoplasty of small (or large) bowel

Anesthesia General

Specimen None

Drains None

Implants None

Estimated Blood Loss Minimal

Indications Partial obstructive symptoms due to small (or large)-bowel stricture with weight loss and intolerance of oral feeds

Procedure in Detail Following induction of general anesthesia, the patient was placed in supine position. All exposed bony sites have been padded appropriately. Timeouts were performed using both pre-induction and pre-incision safety checklists with participation of all present in the operative suite. These confirmed the correct patient, procedure, operative site, instrumentation, and additional critical information prior to the start of the procedure. The abdomen was prepped and draped in the usual sterile fashion. A single shot antibiotic (coverage for aerobic and anaerobic bacteria) was given intravenously 30 min prior to the incision.

Diagnostic laparoscopy (with conversion to minilaparotomy) and laparoscopic Heineke–Mikulicz stricturoplasty: A 12-mm trocar was placed through an umbilical midline incision into the abdominal cavity and pneumoperitoneum established. A laparoscope was inserted, and a screening diagnostic laparoscopy performed. We then placed two additional 5-mm trocars under direct vision in the left (*right*) abdomen. The small bowel was then run from the ileocecal valve to the ligament of Treitz using two atraumatic bowel graspers. The location of the stricture was identified, and additional strictures of the intestine excluded.

(a) *The umbilical incision was then extended, and a wound retractor placed into the minilaparotomy. The small bowel with the strictured segment was then eviscerated in front of the abdominal wall. Two antimesenteric 4-0 silk stay sutures were placed well proximal and distal to the stricture. A longitudinal enterotomy was made extending 2 cm beyond the strictured segment. The enterotomy was then closed in a transverse fashion using interrupted* (running) *Vicryl 4-0 sutures. Additional interrupted seromuscular Lembert sutures were placed with Vicryl 4-0.*
(b) *Laparoscopically, the longitudinal enterotomy was extended beyond the intestinal stricture. We then closed the enterotomy in a transverse fashion using interrupted sutures starting with the most distant corner stitch.*

We then checked the stricturoplasty for patency and leak and assured hemostasis. *The bowel was then returned to the abdominal cavity.* We then irrigated the abdominal cavity with warm saline and removed all laparoscopic ports under direct vision. The fascia at the umbilicus was closed with Vicryl 0 sutures. The skin was re-approximated with Vicryl Rapide 5-0. Steri-strips were applied to the wound site as well as a strike dressing.

Diagnostic laparoscopy (with conversion to minilaparotomy) and laparoscopic Finney stricturoplasty: A 12-mm trocar was placed through an umbilical midline incision into the abdominal cavity and pneumoperitoneum established.

A laparoscope was inserted, and a screening diagnostic laparoscopy performed. We then placed two additional 5-mm trocars under direct vision in the left (right) abdomen. The small bowel was then run from the ileocecal valve to the ligament of Treitz using two atraumatic bowel graspers. The location of the stricture was identified, and additional strictures of the intestine excluded.

(a) *The umbilical incision was then extended and a wound retractor placed into the minilaparotomy. The small bowel with the strictured segment was then eviscerated in front of the abdominal wall. The small bowel with the stricture was brought together in a U-shaped fashion, and a total of three stay sutures were placed at the base and the end of the U. A longitudinal enterotomy was made extending 2 cm beyond the strictured intestinal segment. A hand-sewn, side-to-side anastomosis was made starting initially at the back wall with interrupted* (running) *4-0 vicryl sutures before completing the front wall. Additional interrupted seromuscular Lembert sutures were placed using 4-0 Vicryl.*
(b) *A laparoscopic enterotomy was opened at the base of the U, and a 60-mm intestinal endostapler was fired along both limbs of the U across the strictured small bowel. The enterotomy was then closed with a second load of the endostapler.*

We then checked the anastomosis for patency and leak and assured hemostasis. *The bowel was then returned to the abdominal cavity.* We then irrigated the abdominal cavity with warm saline and removed all laparoscopic ports under direct vision. The fascia at the umbilicus was closed with Vicryl 0 sutures. The skin was reapproximated with Vicryl Rapide 5-0. Steri-strips were applied to the wound site as well as a strike dressing.

Diagnostic laparoscopy (with conversion to minilaparotomy) and performing an isoperistaltic side-to-side small-bowel bypass: A 12-mm trocar was placed through an umbilical midline incision into the abdominal cavity and pneumoperitoneum established. A laparoscope was inserted, and a screening diagnostic laparoscopy performed. We then placed two additional 5-mm trocars under direct vision in the left (right) abdomen. The small bowel was then run from the ileocecal valve to the ligament of Treitz using two atraumatic bowel graspers. The location of the stricture was identified, and additional strictures of the intestine excluded. The umbilical incision was then extended and a wound retractor placed into the minilaparotomy. The small bowel with the strictured segment was then eviscerated in front of the abdominal wall.

(a) *The umbilical incision was then extended and a wound retractor placed into the minilaparotomy. The small bowel with the strictured segment was then eviscerated in front of the abdominal wall. The bowel and its mesentery were then divided in the center of the strictured segment. The proximal 50% of the affected bowel was then positioned to overlay the distal 50% in an isoperistaltic side-to-side fashion. Multiple interrupted seromuscular nonabsorbable sutures were placed. A longitudinal, antimesenteric enterotomy was opened with cautery 2 cm beyond the strictured intestinal segment. Both ends were spatulated.*
(b) *The strictured bowel was aligned in an isoperistaltic fashion and a proximal stay suture was placed. A laparoscopic enterotomy was opened at the proximal end of the aligned bowel, and a 60-mm intestinal endostapler was fired along both limbs of the strictured small bowel. The enterotomy was then closed with a second load of the endostapler* (closed with interrupted sutures).

We then checked the anastomosis for patency and leak and assured hemostasis. *The bowel was then returned to the abdominal cavity.* We then irrigated the abdominal cavity with warm saline and removed all laparoscopic ports under direct vision. The fascia at the umbilicus was closed with Vicryl 0 sutures. The skin was re-approximated with Vicryl Rapide 50. Steri-strips were applied to the wound site as well as a strike dressing.

Upon completion of the procedure, a debriefing checklist was completed to share information critical to the postoperative care of the patient. The patient tolerated the procedure well, was extubated in the operating room, and was transported to the post-anesthesia care unit in a stable condition [1–4].

References

1. Spitz L, Coran AG, Teitelbaum DH, Tan HL, Pierro A. Operative pediatric surgery: CRC press, Taylor & Francis Group, Boka Ratan, London, New York; 2013. p. 583.
2. Potter DD, Moir CR. Chapter 49: Inflammatory bowel disease. In: Ziegler MM, Azizkhan RG, von Allmen D, Weber TR, editors. Operative pediatric surgery. 2nd ed. New York: McGraw-Hill Education/Medical; 2014.
3. Lee EC, Papaioannou N. Minimal surgery for chronic obstruction in patients with extensive or universal Crohn's disease. Ann R Coll Surg Engl. 1982;64(4):229–33.
4. Michelassi F, Hurst RD, Melis M, Rubin M, Cohen R, Gasparitis A, Hanauer SB, Hart J. Side-to-side isoperistaltic strictureplasty in extensive Crohn's disease. A prospective longitudinal study. Ann Surg. 2000;232(3):401–8.

28 Ileostomy Creation (Open and MIS Approaches)

Justin T. Huntington and Karen A. Diefenbach

Indications and Benefits

- Fecal diversion for high-risk anastomoses/leak
- Hirschsprung's disease in small neonates or high transition zone
- Inflammatory bowel disease
- Necrotizing enterocolitis
- Provides a fecal conduit for diversion or treatment of many disease processes and is typically reversible (depending on underlying disorder)

Risks and Alternatives

- Standard risks (bleeding, infection, need for additional procedures, risks of sedation/anesthesia)
- Injury to adjacent structures (small bowel, intra-abdominal contents)
- Procedure specific risks: parastomal hernia, small-bowel ischemia, prolapse, wound issues, pouching issues, dehydration, electrolyte derangements
- Alternatives: anastomosis without ileostomy

Essential Steps

1. Ensuring a good position on the abdominal wall for pouching issues. Ideally, the patient will be marked for potential stoma locations in the preoperative area by an experienced enterostomal nurse.
2. Proper orientation and maturation of proximal (afferent) limb in loop ileostomy (not maturing the incorrect side of the bowel).
3. Using a Brooke technique for formation of a spout type ileostomy to help with skin protection.
4. Proper alignment of stoma without mesenteric twisting.
5. Ensuring good anatomy for future ileostomy takedown in terms of bowel length, blood supply, and accessibility of mucous fistula.
6. Closing the port sites or laparotomy and keeping these areas sterile prior to and during stoma creation to reduce incidence of surgical site infections.

Note These Variations

- Loop versus end ileostomy variations

J. T. Huntington
Nationwide Children's Hospital, Department of Pediatric Surgery, Columbus, OH, USA

K. A. Diefenbach (✉)
Nationwide Children's Hospital, Columbus, OH, USA
e-mail: Karen.Diefenbach@nationwidechildrens.org

D. J. Papandria et al. (eds.), *Operative Dictations in Pediatric Surgery*,
https://doi.org/10.1007/978-3-030-24212-1_28

Operative Dictation (Open)

Preoperative Diagnosis *Inflammatory bowel disease/colitis/Hirschsprung's disease/anastomotic leak/necrotizing enterocolitis*

Postoperative Diagnosis *Same as preoperative diagnosis*

Findings *Same as postoperative diagnosis*

Procedure Performed Placement of *loop/end* ileostomy

Anesthesia General anesthesia

Specimen None/small bowel/colon

Drains *None*

Implants None

Estimated Blood Loss None or minimal

Indication This is a/an __-*day/week/month/year*-old *male/female* who presents to the operative suite for __ due to concern for *colitis/Hirschsprung's disease/need for fecal diversion/necrotizing enterocolitis*. Informed consent was obtained from the *patient/caregiver* after all risks, benefits, and alternatives were discussed.

Procedure in Detail Following satisfactory induction of anesthesia/sedation, the patient was placed in a supine position and padded appropriately. A timeout was performed using both pre-induction and pre-incision safety checklists with participation of all present in the operative/endoscopy suite. These confirmed the correct patient, procedure, operative site, and additional critical information prior to the start of the procedure. Preoperative antibiotics were required and administered prior to and within 1 hour of incision.

[Choose One:]

If neonatal patient: A transverse laparotomy was carried out, and the abdomen was safely entered. The diseased small bowel was identified. A small-bowel resection was performed by ligating the healthy extents of the small bowel with 3-0 Vicryl and then using cautery to transect the small-bowel mesentery close to the small bowel. This was passed off for permanent pathology. The length of small bowel from ligament of Treitz to the proximal transection was measured and recorded. Similarly, the distance from the distal transection to the ileocecal valve was measured and recorded. The abdomen was irrigated with warm saline and then the proximal stoma was secured to the fascia with 3-0 Vicryl in four locations at the left most portion of the transverse incision. Inspection confirmed adequate distal bowel above the level of the skin to allow for future pouching. The mucous fistula was then matured at the corner of the right aspect of the incision in a similar manner. Fascia was then closed with interrupted 3-0 Vicryl, and then, skin was loosely approximated with deep dermal 5-0 Vicryl sutures. A sterile dressing was applied to the incision, and nonadherent dressings were applied to the stomas.

If older patient: A laparotomy was carried out, and the small bowel was run to identify the proper orientation of the small intestine and the abdomen surveyed to identify all intra-abdominal processes. The location of the ileostomy was identified by ensuring that it was proximal to the pathologic process and at least 10 cm proximal to the ileocecal valve to ensure easier future takedown. One of the preoperatively marked areas for stoma creation was selected (typically in the right abdomen just below the level of the umbilicus). A circular incision was carried out above the rectus sheath, and the subcutaneous tissue below this was cored out down to the level of the fascia. A cruciate incision was carried out on the fascia and to just above the rectus muscles which were then bluntly split and the posterior sheath identified. The intra-abdominal contents were protected with a malleable retractor covered with a lap pad, and a cruciate incision was carried out through the posterior rectus sheath and the peritoneum. Once this full-thickness tract was created, it was dilated to approximately two fingerbreadths (depending on patient size and surgeon finger size in relation to the small bowel). The small bowel at the area of the stoma to be created was then grasped with a Babcock and externalized. It was ensured to not have significant tension, and the underlying mesentery was ensured to have proper orientation without any twisting. The small bowel was then secured to the fascia with four quadrant 3-0 Vicryl sutures using seromuscular bites. Attention was then turned to closing the laparotomy with interrupted 2-0 Vicryl sutures, and then, skin was closed with 5-0 Vicryl in a running subcuticular manner. A sterile dressing was placed on top of this, and then attention was turned to maturing the ileostomy.

[Choose One:]
If loop ileostomy: Care was taken to ensure that the proximal small bowel was matured as an ileostomy, and the distal end was brought out beside this as a mucous fistula. The bowel was divided using cautery along the antimesenteric portion to divide approximately 50% circumference. The proximal small bowel was matured in a Brooke manner by using 3-0 Vicryl in the superior and lateral aspects of the bowel with full-thickness bites of the divided bowel, seromuscular bites of proximal small bowel, and then deep dermal bites. These were tied, and then interrupted full-thickness bowel bites to the corresponding deep dermis were performed with 3-0 Vicryl until there were no significant gaps. The mucous fistula was then matured flush to the skin inferior to the ileostomy by taking full-thickness bowel bites to the corresponding deep dermis with 3-0 Vicryl until there were no significant gaps. *A 3-0 chromic/PDS purse-string suture was used to close the mucous fistula to prevent spillage of stool into the distal bowel.*

If end ileostomy: The end of the ileum was opened by removing the entire staple line and then matured in a Brooke manner by using 3-0 Vicryl in four quadrants of the bowel with full-thickness bites of the end of the bowel, seromuscular bites of proximal small bowel, and then deep dermal bites. These were tied, and then, interrupted full-thickness bowel bites to the corresponding deep dermis were performed with 3-0 Vicryl until there were no significant gaps.

A stoma appliance was then cut to size and placed over the completed ileostomy.

Upon completion of the procedure, a debriefing checklist was completed to share information critical to the postoperative care of the patient. The patient tolerated the procedure well, was extubated in the operating room, and was transported to the post-anesthesia care unit in stable condition thereafter.

Operative Dictation (Laparoscopic)

Preoperative Diagnosis *Inflammatory bowel disease/colitis/Hirschsprung's disease/anastomotic leak/necrotizing enterocolitis*

Postoperative Diagnosis *Same as preoperative diagnosis*

Findings *Same as postoperative diagnosis*

Procedure Performed Laparoscopic placement of *loop/end* ileostomy

Anesthesia General anesthesia

Specimen None/small bowel/colon

Drains *None*

Implants None

Estimated Blood Loss None or minimal

Indication This is a/an __*-day/week/month/year*-old *male/female* who presents to the operative suite for __ due to concern for *colitis/Hirschsprung's disease/need for fecal diversion/necrotizing enterocolitis*. Informed consent was obtained from the *patient/caregiver* after all risks, benefits, and alternatives were discussed.

Procedure in Detail Following satisfactory induction of anesthesia/sedation, the patient was placed in a supine position and padded appropriately. A timeout was performed using both pre-induction and pre-incision safety checklists with participation of all present in the operative/endoscopy suite. These confirmed the correct patient, procedure, operative site, and additional critical information prior to the start of the procedure. Preoperative antibiotics were required and administered prior to and within 1 hour of incision.

A curvilinear incision was carried out at the inferior aspect of the umbilicus, and dissection was carried down to the base of the umbilicus to the level of the fascia. The fascia was grasped, and a Veress needle inserted. A saline drop test was reassuring, and the abdomen was insufflated. The abdomen was surveyed and an iatrogenic injury from initial trocar placement was not discovered. An additional 5-mm port was placed under direct visualization in the right lower quadrant at the location marked for a stoma. An additional 5-mm port was placed in the left lower quadrant (as necessary) to help with running the small bowel. The location of the ileostomy was identified by ensuring that it was proximal to the pathologic process and at least 10 cm proximal to the ileocecal valve to ensure easier future takedown. The small bowel was grasped at this site with an atraumatic laparoscopic grasper in the right lower quadrant and this was locked. A circular incision was created at the site of the right lower quadrant trocar of adequate size to mature a stoma. The subcutaneous tissue was cored out down to the level of the fascia. A cruciate incision was carried out on the fascia and to just above the rectus muscles which were then bluntly split and the posterior sheath identified. It was incised in a cruciate manner while watching laparoscopically to ensure no intra-abdominal thermal injury was created. Two small hernia retractors were then used to spread the fascial incision to an adequate size to mature the stoma without creating tension on the small bowel. The trocar and grasper were backed out until the small bowel was externalized and not under undue tension. The correct orientation was ensured laparoscopically. Four quadrant fascial sutures were placed using seromuscular bites with 3-0 Vicryl. The previously placed trocars were removed. Fascia at the trocar sites were closed with 3-0 Vicryl, and then skin was closed with 5-0 Vicryl in a deep dermal buried manner. Sterile dressings were applied, and then attention was turned to maturing the ileostomy.

[Choose One:]

If loop ileostomy: Care was taken to ensure that the proximal small bowel was matured as an ileostomy, and the distal end was brought out beside this as a mucous fistula. The bowel was divided using cautery along the antimesenteric portion to divide approximately 50% circumference. The proximal small bowel was matured in a Brooke manner by using 3-0 Vicryl in the superior and lateral aspects of the bowel with full-thickness bites of the divided bowel, seromuscular bites of proximal small bowel, and then deep dermal bites. These were tied and then interrupted; full-thickness bowel bites to the corresponding deep dermis were performed with 3-0 Vicryl until there were no significant gaps. The mucous fistula was then matured flush to the skin inferior to the ileostomy by taking full-thickness bowel bites to the corresponding deep dermis with 3-0 Vicryl until there were no significant gaps. *A 3-0 chromic/PDS purse-string suture was used to close the mucous fistula to prevent spillage of stool into the distal bowel.*

If end ileostomy: The end of the ileum was opened by removing the entire staple line and then matured in a Brooke manner by using 3-0 Vicryl in four quadrants of the bowel with full-thickness bites of the end of the bowel, seromuscular bites of proximal small bowel, and then deep dermal bites. These were tied and then interrupted; full-thickness bowel bites to the corresponding deep dermis were performed with 3-0 Vicryl until there were no significant gaps.

A stoma appliance was then cut to size and placed over the completed ileostomy.

Upon completion of the procedure, a debriefing checklist was completed to share information critical to the postoperative care of the patient. The patient tolerated the procedure well, was extubated in the operating room, and was transported to the post-anesthesia care unit in stable condition thereafter.

Appendectomy

29

Melissa Vanover and Payam Saadai

Indications and Benefits

- Acute appendicitis
- Interval appendectomy
- Benign tumor of the appendix
- Benefits: Control of infection, removal of tumor

Risks and Alternatives

- Standard risks (bleeding, infection, need for additional procedures, risks of anesthesia)
- Injury to adjacent structures (colon, small bowel, bladder, vascular)
- Abscess
- Stump leak
- Small-bowel obstruction
- Alternatives: Antibiotics alone for simple appendicitis

Essential Steps

Open Appendectomy

1. Right lower quadrant *transverse/oblique* incision over McBurney's point or the point of maximal tenderness that was marked prior to anesthesia. *Rarely, the incision is made in the lower midline or right paramedian aspect.*
2. Divide parallel to fibers of each muscular and aponeurotic layer to achieve a muscle splitting incision.
3. Enter the peritoneum, noting any malodorous or discolored peritoneal fluid. Send peritoneal fluid for gram stain and culture.
4. Expose the cecum, elevating it into the wound with a moist pad.
5. *Divide the lateral peritoneal attachments of the cecum (if required to improve exposure).*
6. Deliver the appendix into the wound. *If having difficulty locating appendix, track tenia along the cecum to the base of the appendix.*
7. *If the appendix appears normal, examine the terminal ileum and pelvis. Check for fluid in the right paracolic gutter, which may arise from other intra-abdominal pathology (convert to laparotomy, if necessary).*
8. Divide and ligate the appendiceal mesentery.
9. Crush the base of the appendix just distal to the cecum with a clamp; then move the clamp 1 cm distally.

M. Vanover
University of California, Davis, Department of Pediatric General, Thoracic and Fetal Surgery, Sacramento, CA, USA

P. Saadai (✉)
UC Davis Medical Center/Shriners Hospital for Children, Division of Pediatric Surgery, Sacramento, CA, USA
e-mail: psaadai@ucdavis.edu

D. J. Papandria et al. (eds.), *Operative Dictations in Pediatric Surgery*,
https://doi.org/10.1007/978-3-030-24212-1_29

10. Ligate the proximal edge of the crushed appendix.
11. *Take a purse-string suture/z-stitch in the wall of the cecum at the base of the appendix if planning to invert the appendiceal stump.*
12. Transect the appendix distal to the ligature and remove it from the operative field.
13. *Invaginate the appendiceal stump and tie the purse-string suture/z-stitch.*
14. Aspirate any purulent material. Cautiously irrigate and gently suction to minimize bleeding.
15. *If a well-formed abscess cavity is encountered, place a closed-suction drain. Remove all fibrinous material lining the abscess cavity and send for culture.*
16. Check for hemostasis.
17. Close the incision in three layers: peritoneum, external oblique, and Scarpa's fascia.
18. *Close the subcutaneous tissue and skin/pack the wound open.*

Laparoscopic Appendectomy

1. Tuck the left arm.
2. Monitor at the patient's *right side/foot.*
3. *Foley catheter to decompress the bladder.*
4. Induce pneumoperitoneum using a *Veress needle/Hassan cannula superior to/inferior to/through the base of the* umbilicus.
5. *If Veress needle used: Insert the initial 5/12-mm cannula.*
6. Introduce the laparoscope and inspect the abdomen for pathology or injury.
7. Place a 5-mm cannula above the symphysis pubis, taking care to avoid the bladder.
8. Place a second 5-mm cannula in the left lower quadrant lateral to the rectus muscle and between the umbilicus and the left anterior superior iliac spine.
9. Trendelenburg position with table rotated right side up.
10. Gently grasp the appendix with an atraumatic grasper and retract anteriorly.
11. *If the appendix is not readily identified, trace the tenia of the cecum to the base of the appendix. Carefully dissect away omentum as necessary.*
12. *If the appendix is retrocecal, the lateral peritoneal attachments can be incised to mobilize the cecum and improve exposure.*
13. Develop a window in the appendiceal mesentery at the base of the appendix.
14. ***If stapled***: *Endoscopic linear cutting stapler across the base of the appendix, then across the mesoappendix, using two separate cartridges.*
15. ***If pretied ligature***: *Serially divide the mesentery with clips/electrocautery/ultrasonic shears. Doubly ligate the base of the appendix with pretied ligatures, then transect distally with endoscopic shears.*
16. *Place the appendix into an endoscopic retrieval pouch.*
17. Remove the *appendix/endoscopic retrieval pouch* through the *10/12*-mm port.
18. *Short bursts of electrocautery may be used on the appendiceal stump, if needed.*
19. *Aspirate any purulent material and send for culture. Cautiously irrigate and gently suction to minimize bleeding. Place a closed suction drain if a well-formed abscess cavity is encountered.*
20. Check for hemostasis.
21. Desufflate the abdomen and close the *10/12*-mm port site fascia.
22. Close the skin.

Note These Variations

- Incision
- Mobilization of the cecum
- Location of the appendix (retrocecal)
- Stump inversion
- Veress needle or Hassan cannula
- Stapler or pretied ligature
- Endoscopic retrieval pouch
- Drain placement
- Skin closure

Template Operative Dictation (Open)

Preoperative Diagnosis Acute appendicitis

Postoperative Diagnosis *Same as preoperative diagnosis/mesenteric adenitis/Crohn's disease/ Meckel's diverticulitis/pelvic inflammatory disease/other*

Findings Same as postoperative diagnosis

Procedure(s) Performed Appendectomy

Anesthesia *General/regional/procedural sedation*

Specimen Appendix, to pathology*; abscess fluid to microbiology*

Drains *None/closed suction drain*

Implants None

Estimated Blood Loss ___mL

Indications: [Choose one:]
If acute appendicitis: This is a/an ___-year-old *male/female* presented with right lower quadrant pain of ___ duration. *Physical exam/ultrasound/ computed tomography scan* was consistent with acute appendicitis.

If interval appendectomy: This is a/an ___-year-old *male/female* had perforated appendicitis treated with percutaneous drainage and antibiotics ___ weeks ago and now presents for interval appendectomy.

Procedure in detail Following satisfactory induction of anesthesia, the patient was placed in supine position and appropriately padded. Timeouts were performed using both pre-induction and pre-incision safety checklists with participation of all present in the operative suite. These confirmed the correct patient, procedure, operative site, and additional critical information prior to the start of the procedure. *A nasogastric tube/Foley catheter was/were placed.* The abdomen was then prepped and draped in the usual sterile fashion. Perioperative antibiotics were *administered/confirmed.*

A(n) *oblique/transverse* skin incision was made in *the right lower quadrant over McBurney's point/the point of maximal tenderness.* Subcutaneous tissues were divided until the aponeurosis of the external oblique was encountered. This was incised in a direction parallel to its fibers, extended medially toward the rectus sheath and laterally toward the iliac crest. The internal oblique and transversus abdominis muscles were bluntly split to expose the peritoneum. The peritoneum was lifted and entered, taking care not to injure the bowel below. *Turbid fluid was encountered and cultured.* The cecum was identified and gently pulled into the wound with a moist pad. *The appendix came readily into view/It was necessary to incise the lateral peritoneal attachments to mobilize the cecum and expose the appendix.* The appendix was noted to be *free/retrocecal* and *inflamed/suppurative/gangrenous/perforated/ normal.* [*If normal:* The terminal ileum was run for ___ ft and found to be *normal/inflamed.* Pelvic viscera were inspected and found to be *unremarkable/___.* A presumptive diagnosis of *acute appendicitis/mesenteric adenitis/Crohn's disease/ Meckel's diverticulitis/pelvic inflammatory disease/___* was made. The decision was made to proceed with appendectomy].

[Choose One:]
Sharp transection of the appendix with purse-string: The mesentery of the appendix was divided between clamps and ligated with *3-0 silk.* The base of the appendix was crushed in a clamp and the clamp then advanced 1 cm distally. The appendix was then ligated at the proximal edge of the crushed portion with a 0 Vicryl suture. *A purse-string suture/z-stitch was taken in the wall of the cecum.* The appendix was held upward, cut distal to the ligature, and removed. *The stump was (cauterized and) then invaginated into the cecum using forceps. The purse-string suture/z-stitch was tied to completely invert and cover the appendiceal stump.* Hemostasis was confirmed.

Sharp transection of the appendix with Endoloop: *All purulent material was aspirated, and the field gently irrigated with antibiotic infused/normal saline.* The incision was closed in layers with absorbable sutures. A *dry gauze* dressing was applied.

Upon completion of the procedure, a debriefing checklist was completed to share information critical to the postoperative care of the patient. The patient tolerated the procedure well, *was extubated in the operating room,* and was transported to the post-anesthesia care unit in stable condition thereafter.

Template Operative Dictation (Laparoscopic)

Preoperative Diagnosis Acute appendicitis

Postoperative Diagnosis *Same as preoperative diagnosis/mesenteric adenitis/Crohn's disease/ Meckel's diverticulitis/pelvic inflammatory disease/other*

Findings Same as postoperative diagnosis

Procedure(s) Performed Laparoscopic appendectomy

Anesthesia General

Specimen Appendix

Drains *None/closed suction drain*

Implants None

Estimated Blood Loss ___ mL

Indications: [Choose One:]
If acute appendicitis: This is a/an ___-year-old *male/female* presented with right lower quadrant pain of ___ duration. *Physical exam/ultrasound/ computed tomography scan* was consistent with acute appendicitis.

If interval appendectomy: This is a/an ___-year-old *male/female* had perforated appendicitis treated with percutaneous drainage and antibiotics ___ weeks ago and now presents for interval appendectomy.

Procedure in detail Following satisfactory induction of anesthesia, the patient was placed in supine position and appropriately padded. Timeouts were performed using both pre-induction and pre-incision safety checklists with participation of all present in the operative suite. These confirmed the correct patient, procedure, operative site, and additional critical information prior to the start of the procedure. A Foley catheter *and nasogastric/orogastric tube was/were* placed. The abdomen was then prepped and draped in the usual sterile fashion. Perioperative antibiotics were *administered/confirmed.*

An incision was made *supraumbilical/infra-umbilical/through the base of the umbilicus.*

[Choose One:]
If Veress needle: The fascia was elevated and the Veress needle inserted. Proper position was confirmed by aspiration and saline drop test. The abdomen was insufflated to and a *5/12*-mm port was inserted.

If Hasson cannula: The fascia was elevated and incised. Entry into the peritoneum was confirmed visually and noted to be clear of any bowel loops. Two figure-of-eight sutures were placed, and the Hassan cannula inserted under direct vision. The sutures were then anchored around the cannula and the abdomen was insufflated.

The laparoscope was introduced, and the peritoneal cavity inspected. There *was/was no* evidence of injury from initial port placement. Two 5-mm ports were placed under direct vision in the suprapubic region and left lower quadrant.

The appendix *was/was not readily* identified. *The lateral peritoneal attachments were incised to mobilize the cecum and expose the appendix.* The appendix was noted to be *free/retrocecal* and *inflamed/suppurative/gangrenous/perforated/normal.* [*If normal*: The terminal ileum was run for ___ ft and found to be *normal/ inflamed.* Pelvic viscera were inspected and found to be ___. A presumptive diagnosis of *mesenteric adenitis/Crohn's disease/Meckel's diverticulitis/pelvic inflammatory disease/___* was made. The decision was made to proceed with appendectomy. (Detail any other procedures performed.)]

The appendix was carefully grasped and retracted anteriorly. Dissection was carried out using a combination of blunt technique and electrocautery, identifying the mesoappendix and appendiceal base, as well as the ileocecal valve. A defect was developed bluntly between the appendix and mesoappendix at the base.

[Choose One:]

Division with endostapler: The base of the appendix was divided using an endoscopic linear cutting stapler with a *blue/purple* cartridge. The appendiceal mesentery was then divided with a *white/gray* cartridge.

Division with pretied ligature: The mesentery was serially divided with *clips/electrocautery/ultrasonic shears/a vessel sealer.* The base of the appendix was then doubly ligated with pretied endoscopic ligatures and transected distally.

The appendix *was placed in an endoscopic retrieval pouch and* withdrawn through the umbilical port site. The *appendiceal stump/staple line* was inspected and hemostasis was confirmed.

If an abscess was encountered: A contained purulent fluid collection was entered and drained in the course of the procedure. *Swab/fluid* was sent for gram stain and culture. *The abscess was well formed; its entire lining of fibrinous material was removed and sent for culture.* A closed suction drain was placed in the abscess cavity and brought out through the left lower quadrant port site/a separate stab incision, and secured with a *3-0 Nylon* suture.

The secondary trocars were removed under direct vision. *No bleeding was noted/trocar site bleeding was controlled with electrocautery/suture placement.* The laparoscope was removed and the abdomen desufflated. The *5/12*-mm port site fascia was closed with interrupted absorbable suture. The skin of each port site was closed with subcuticular sutures. Dry, sterile dressings were applied.

Upon completion of the procedure, a debriefing checklist was completed to share information critical to the postoperative care of the patient. The patient tolerated the procedure well, *was extubated in the operating room*, and was transported to the post-anesthesia care unit in stable condition thereafter.

30 Cecal Volvulus

Andrew Yeh and Stefan Scholz

Indications

- Cecal volvulus
- Distal bowel obstruction with characteristic radiographic findings

Risks

- Standard risks (bleeding, infection, need for additional procedures, risks of anesthesia)
- Injury to adjacent structures (small bowel, ureter, colon)
- Anastomotic leak
- Recurrence of cecal volvulus

Alternatives

- Instead of resection, cecostomy tube placement is an alternative for unstable or frail patients that do not have bowel ischemia. The tube provides a fixation point for the colon and for decompression. This procedure carries a relatively higher risk of recurrence than a right hemicolectomy. Wound infections are more common and a larger chronic colocutaneous fistula could develop.
- Cecopexy is a second alternative to right hemicolectomy when the bowel is viable. In patients that are unstable and may not tolerate a bowel resection and anastomosis, a cecopexy is a potential option. However, recurrence rates are high. Extensive fixation of the colon may reduce the recurrence risk but also prolongs operative time. For these reasons, cecopexy is generally not recommended.

Essential Steps

1. Place patient in the supine position.
2. Make a low midline abdominal incision.
3. Explore the abdomen. The cecum will likely be very distended and be encountered early.
4. Exteriorize cecum and terminal ileum if possible without detorsion.
5. Evaluate for bowel compromise and direction of torsion before deciding on detorsion.
6. If the bowel appears viable, detorse the volvulus in a counter-clockwise fashion (most often). If the bowel appears necrotic, do not detorse the bowel to prevent reperfusion injury and release of inflammatory mediators.

A. Yeh
University of Pittsburgh, Department of Surgery, Pittsburgh, PA, USA

S. Scholz (✉)
University of Pittsburgh School of Medicine, Children's Hospital of Pittsburgh, Department of Pediatric Surgery, Pittsburgh, PA, USA
e-mail: stefan.scholz@chp.edu

D. J. Papandria et al. (eds.), *Operative Dictations in Pediatric Surgery*,
https://doi.org/10.1007/978-3-030-24212-1_30

Right Hemicolectomy

1. Mobilize the right colon and terminal ileum sufficiently to allow for division of the terminal ileum and the transverse colon immediately proximal to the middle colic artery. Incise the lateral peritoneal attachments by rotating the cecum anteriorly and medially and divide the hepatic flexure. Incise the medial and inferior attachments of the cecum and terminal ileum toward the duodenum.
2. Clamp the terminal ileum distally and proximally to the transection point.
3. Transect the terminal ileum using staplers.
4. Clamp the transverse colon distally and proximally to the desired transection point. The colon should be transected proximal to the middle colic artery.
5. Transect the transverse colon with staplers.
6. Divide the colon mesentery between clamps, with energy device or staplers, the ligament attachments (gastrocolic ligament), and the peritoneal attachments of the right colon to deliver the specimen.
7. Perform a tension-free anastomosis of the ileum to the colon using hand-sewn or stapled techniques.
8. Close the mesenteric defect.
9. Close the abdominal incision in the standard fashion.

Cecostomy Tube Placement

1. Cecostomy is a fast alternative to a right hemicolectomy in the unstable or frail patient with viable bowel.
2. Evaluate the viability of the bowel. If viable, detorse the volvulus in a counter-clockwise fashion. If the bowel is not viable, cecostomy tube placement is not appropriate and a right hemicolectomy should be performed.
3. Evaluate the viability of the bowel after detorsion. Bowel should be viable to proceed with a cecostomy tube.
4. Make a small incision in the skin to the right of the midline incision for where the cecostomy tube will exit using electrocautery.
5. Tunnel the tube or button through the incision using a long clamp.
6. Using 2-0 silk or Vicryl suture, make a purse-string stitch in the cecum surrounding the location of the future cecostomy tube.
7. Make a small colotomy at the site of the future cecostomy tube to accommodate the tube in the center of your purse-string stitch.
8. Use the colotomy to decompress the very distended bowel with pool suction.
9. Insert the tube or button into the colotomy.
10. Tie down purse-string stitch to secure the tube in the cecum being careful not to occlude the tube.
11. Suture the seromuscular layer of the cecum surrounding the tube to the parietal peritoneum surrounding the abdominal wall exit site of the tube.
12. Close the abdominal incision in your preferred standard fashion.

Note These Variations

- The cecostomy tube placement can be done percutaneously.
- A button may be used primarily instead of a cecostomy tube.
- A cecostomy tube can be useful for colonic decompression or integrate enemas in cases of reduced colonic motility.
- Cecal bascule can lead to intermittent large bowel obstruction through flooding of the cecum anteriorly over the ascending colon or distal closed loop obstruction between the ascending colon and the ileocecal valve.
- There are two types of cecal volvulus depending on the mechanism and direction of rotation: cecal bascule and axial ileocolic.

Template Operative Dictation

Preoperative Diagnosis Cecal volvulus

Postoperative Diagnosis Same as preoperative diagnosis

Findings Cecal volvulus, bowel *viable/ischemic*

Procedure(s) Performed Exploratory laparotomy with detorsion of cecal volvulus and right hemicolectomy

Anesthesia General

Specimen {Specimen}

Drains {Drains}

Implants {Implants}

Estimated Blood Loss ___mL

Indications This is a/an ___-day/week/month/year-old male/female with a cecal volvulus. He/she was deemed to be a suitable candidate for an exploratory laparotomy with possible right hemicolectomy.

Procedure in Detail Following satisfactory induction of anesthesia, the patient was placed in the supine position. Timeouts were performed using both pre-induction and pre-incision safety checklists with participation of all present in the operative suite. These confirmed the correct patient, procedure, operative site, and additional critical information prior to the start of the procedure. The abdomen was then prepped and draped in the usual sterile fashion. A low midline abdominal incision was made. The incision was carried down through the subcutaneous tissue where the linea alba was identified and incised. Care was taken to establish hemostasis using electrocautery.

The abdomen was entered carefully and explored. A cecal volvulus was apparent on examination. The bowel appeared to be massively dilated.

[Choose One:]
If the cecum is necrotic: The cecum was noted to be necrotic. Detorsion was avoided to prevent reperfusion injury and release of inflammatory mediators.

If the cecum is potentially viable: The cecum appeared viable with no obvious evidence of frank necrosis. The cecum was then detorsed in a *clockwise/counter-clockwise fashion*. The bowel was then again evaluated for viability.

[Choose One:]
If performing a right hemicolectomy: Attention was then turned to mobilizing the terminal ileum and right colon sufficiently to perform a right hemicolectomy. The lateral, medial, and inferior peritoneal attachments of the right colon were incised taking care to not injure the ureter and duodenum. Once the mobilization was adequate, the terminal ileum was *divided with a stapler/doubly clamped and incised*. The transverse colon was also *divided with a stapler/doubly clamped and incised*. Care was taken to ensure the middle colic artery was distal to the transection point and not included in the future specimen. The bowel mesentery of the specimen was divided using *a vessel sealant device/vascular staplers*. Attention was then turned to fashioning the ileocolic anastomosis using a stapler technique. The antimesenteric corner of the staple line of the ileum and colon were removed using electrocautery. A stapler was then introduced and stapled on the antimesenteric border. The enterotomy was then appropriately aligned with Allis clamps and closed with a TA stapler. An anti-obstruction stitch was placed proximal to the anastomosis. The mesenteric defect was then closed with absorbable sutures.

If performing a cecostomy tube placement (bowel should be viable): Due to the patient's instability and concern that the patient may not tolerate a bowel resection, the decision was made to place a cecostomy tube. A small incision was made in the skin in the right lower quadrant for the cecostomy tube. The incision was carried down through the abdominal wall using electrocautery. A ballooned *catheter//button* was tunneled through this incision using a long clamp. A purse-string stitch was placed on the cecum surrounding the future site of the cecostomy tube. The colotomy was then made using electrocautery. The suction device with a pool tip was used for decompression of the massively dilated bowel. The tip of the catheter was then introduced into the cecum, and the purse-string stitch was tied being careful to secure the tube without occluding it. The seromuscular layer of the cecum was then sutured to the abdominal wall at the exit site of the cecostomy *tube/button*. The bowel was again inspected and appeared viable.

The abdomen was irrigated with warmed saline. The midline fascia was closed with a running suture. The skin was closed with running fine absorbable sutures, and a sterile dressing was placed. Upon completion of the procedure, a debriefing checklist was completed to share information critical to the postoperative care of the patient. The patient tolerated the procedure well, *was extubated in the operating room,* and was transported to the post-anesthesia care unit in stable condition thereafter.

31 Percutaneous Peritoneal Drain Placement for Necrotizing Enterocolitis

William B. Rothstein and Laura A. Boomer

Indications and Benefits

- Pneumoperitoneum
- Necrotizing enterocolitis with suspected perforation
- Hemodynamically unstable or VLBW infants
- Benefits: Preserves intestinal length, can be placed at bedside, may be used as a temporizing procedure to allow for resuscitation and stabilization before laparotomy, and can be successful as a primary procedure alone

Risks and Alternatives

- Standard risks (bleeding, infection, need for additional procedures, risks of anesthesia)
- Injury to adjacent structures (abdominal viscera)
- Failure of improvement with drain alone
- Alternatives: Laparotomy with or without bowel resection

W. B. Rothstein
Virginia Commonwealth University Health System, Department of Surgery, Richmond, VA, USA

L. A. Boomer (✉)
Children's Hospital of Richmond, Virginia Commonwealth University, Department of Pediatric Surgery, Richmond, VA, USA
e-mail: Laura.boomer@vcuhealth.org

Essential Steps

1. Place the patient supine. The procedure is most often performed in the NICU.
2. Infiltrate local anesthetic and make a small left lower quadrant incision in the skin.
3. Carefully open the fascia and peritoneum. This may be done sharply with scissors or bluntly with hemostats, taking caution to enter in a controlled manner.
4. Using hemostats, carefully advance a penrose drain along the anterior abdominal wall.
5. Take extra caution to avoid inadvertent liver injury.
6. Suture the penrose drain in place to the skin to facilitate drainage and eventual fistula formation.

Note These Variations

- Holes may be placed in the penrose drain to facilitate drainage, although there is a risk of bowel becoming trapped in these holes.
- A counter-incision may be made and the drain advanced out of the abdomen opposite to its entry point.
- The abdomen may be irrigated prior to placement of the drain.
- If there is no improvement (ongoing acidosis, ongoing drainage, hemodynamic instability),

D. J. Papandria et al. (eds.), *Operative Dictations in Pediatric Surgery*,
https://doi.org/10.1007/978-3-030-24212-1_31

laparotomy may need to be performed in 24–72 hours.
- If the patient improves with drain placement, and primary drain therapy is desired, the drain can be slowly pulled back each day either after a prescribed number of days or after there is no longer meconium draining from the incision.

Template Operative Dictation

Preoperative Diagnosis Pneumoperitoneum, suspected perforated viscus, and necrotizing enterocolitis

Postoperative Diagnosis Pneumoperitoneum, suspected perforated viscus, and necrotizing enterocolitis

Findings
1. Air *was/was not* expressed from the abdomen after entry into the peritoneal cavity.
2. A *small/large* amount of *meconium/clear fluid/blood* drained.

Procedure(s) Performed Peritoneal drain placement

Anesthesia *Local anesthesia/Procedural sedation*

Specimen *None*

Estimated Blood Loss None

Indications This is a/an ___*-day/week/month/year*-old *male/female* with a/an ___*-day/hour/week* history of abdominal distension after initiation of enteric feeds, with worsening organ dysfunction requiring resuscitation and hemodynamic support. A diagnosis of suspected perforated viscus and necrotizing enterocolitis with intraperitoneal air was confirmed radiographically. *He/she* was deemed too unstable for transport and unlikely to tolerate laparotomy, and thus a good candidate for peritoneal drainage.

Procedure in Detail The patient was placed in supine position in their NICU incubator. Their abdomen was prepped and draped in the usual sterile fashion. A timeout was performed using a pre-incision safety checklist with participation of all present. These confirmed the correct patient, procedure, operative site, and additional critical information prior to the start of the procedure. The liver was palpated prior to incision. ___ mL of local anesthetic was infiltrated in the lower right quadrant. A small incision was made in the skin layer with a scalpel. The peritoneum was lifted and incised sharply under direct visualization with *scissors/a knife*. A Penrose drain was grasped in hemostats and gently introduced into the peritoneal cavity. The drain and hemostats were advanced against the anterior abdominal wall, with special care to avoid contacting the liver. Once the drain was advanced, the hemostats were withdrawn, and the drain was sutured to the skin edge with ___ suture. A small gauze dressing was placed over the end of the drain.

Upon completion of the procedure, a debriefing checklist was completed to share information critical to the postoperative care of the patient. The patient tolerated the procedure well and remains in the NICU under close observation.

32 Laparotomy for Necrotizing Enterocolitis

William B. Rothstein and Laura A. Boomer

Indications and Benefits

- Necrotizing enterocolitis with suspected gangrenous bowel or intraperitoneal air
- Relative indications for surgery include ongoing organ failure, persistent acidosis despite maximum resuscitation, persistent hemodynamic instability, abdominal wall erythema, palpable mass, portal venous gas, thrombocytopenia, fixed loop, or failure of clinical status to improve after a period of treatment with a peritoneal drain
- Benefits: removes gangrenous tissue and provides source control for sepsis

Risks and Alternatives

- Standard risks (bleeding, infection, need for additional procedures, risks of anesthesia)
- Liver capsular hemorrhage
- Short bowel syndrome from excessive resection
- Alternatives: Peritoneal drain placement

W. B. Rothstein
Virginia Commonwealth University Health System, Department of Surgery, Richmond, VA, USA

L. A. Boomer (✉)
Children's Hospital of Richmond, Virginia Commonwealth University, Department of Pediatric Surgery, Richmond, VA, USA
e-mail: Laura.boomer@vcuhealth.org

Essential Steps

1. Place the patient supine and prep and drape the abdomen.
2. Make a transverse laparotomy.
3. Eviscerate the entire length of bowel and gently examine from stomach to rectum.
4. Evaluate intestine for viability. Disease is considered focal, multifocal (>50% viable), or panintestinal (<25% viable). The decision to resect bowel must be made in consideration of the length of remaining bowel.
5. Focal disease can be treated with a limited resection. Ligate the mesenteric vessels and divide proximal and distal bowel. Exteriorize the proximal and distal intestine through the lateral aspect of the incision to create a proximal enterostomy and mucus fistula, taking seromuscular bites of intestine to the abdominal fascia.
6. Primary reanastamosis after focal resection may be appropriate in well-selected patients; well resuscitated, without progression of sepsis, with bowel that appears viable and well perfused.
7. Multifocal disease must be resected for source control while preserving intestinal length. Exteriorize proximal intestine as above for a proximal enterostomy.
8. Multiple diseased segments may be resected and primarily reanastamosed. Alternatively, multiple stomas may be created.

D. J. Papandria et al. (eds.), *Operative Dictations in Pediatric Surgery*,
https://doi.org/10.1007/978-3-030-24212-1_32

9. Panintestinal involvement presents few viable surgical options. You may elect to proximally divert and drain the peritoneal cavity. Alternatively, a silo may be used for ongoing assessment of intestinal viability during continued resuscitation.
10. Close the abdominal incision in layers.

Note These Variations

- The patch technique is an alternative technique for multifocal disease when intestinal length is a concern. Bowel perforations are closed with single-layer suture closures. Gangrenous bowel is not resected. A gastrostomy tube is placed for gastric decompression. Penrose drains are left in the abdomen and TPN is initiated.
- The clip and drop technique is another alternative for multifocal disease. Gangrenous bowel is resected, and the lumens of remaining segments are closed with clips, staples, or ties and left in discontinuity. The patient then returns to the operating room after 48–72 hours of resuscitation, and the remaining segments are primarily reanastamosed or proximal ostomies created.
- An additional option is to resect frankly necrotic bowel, and leave the intestine in discontinuity and the bowel placed in a silo. The portions of bowel with questionable viability can then directly visualized, rather than resected. Additional resection can be performed at repeat laparotomy in the event that the disease progresses.

Template Operative Dictation

Preoperative Diagnosis Necrotizing enterocolitis

Postoperative Diagnosis Necrotizing enterocolitis

Findings
1. ___ frank perforation was identified.
2. ___ cm of small bowel is remaining proximal to the enterostomy, and ____ cm of small bowel is remaining from mucus fistula to ileocecal valve.

Procedure(s) Performed Laparotomy, bowel resection, proximal enterostomy, and mucus fistula creation

Anesthesia *General anesthesia/sedation as provided by the NICU*

Specimen *Small bowel/none*

Estimated Blood Loss ___ mL

Indications This is a/an ___*-day/week/month/year*-old *male/female* with a/an ___*-day/hour/week* history of abdominal distension after initiation of enteric feeds, with worsening organ dysfunction requiring resuscitation and hemodynamic support. A diagnosis of necrotizing enterocolitis with intraperitoneal air was confirmed radiographically. *He/she* was stable for transport and able to tolerate laparotomy, and thus was taken to the operating room for surgical treatment.

Procedure in Detail The patient was placed in supine position. Their abdomen was prepped and draped in the usual sterile fashion. A timeout was performed using a pre-incision safety checklist with participation of all present. These confirmed the correct patient, procedure, operative site, and additional critical information prior to the start of the procedure. The liver was palpated prior to incision. A transverse supraumbilical incision was made, and the fascia and peritoneum were opened *sharply/with electrocautery*. The abdominal cavity was inspected, with no iatrogenic bowel injury detected. The intestines were eviscerated and gently explored manually, with care taken to avoid direct contact with the liver. An approximately ___-cm segment of gangrenous ___ was encountered with a perforation of the antimesenteric wall. There *was/was not* frank perforation. {There was significant contamination of the peritoneal cavity.} The remaining intestine was viable.

The mesenteric vessels entering the diseased segment of intestine were *suture ligated sequentially/divided with electrocautery*. The proximal and distal portions of diseased intestine were transected and the specimen sent to pathology. At this point, the proximal segment was brought up through the right lateral aspect of the abdominal incision. A stoma was created using four quadrant seromuscular intestinal stitches to the abdominal fascia. The distal intestine was brought through the left end of the incision, and a mucus fistula stoma was created using a similar technique. After irrigating the abdominal cavity, the abdominal wall was closed in layers.

Upon completion of the procedure, a debriefing checklist was completed to share information critical to the postoperative care of the patient. The patient tolerated the procedure well, was extubated in the operating room, and was transported to the post-anesthesia care unit in stable condition.

Malone Continent Appendicostomy

33

Devin R. Halleran, Richard J. Wood, and Marc A. Levitt

Indications and Benefits

- Intractable constipation or fecal incontinence despite maximal medical therapy
- Inability to tolerate rectal enemas
- Benefits: Antegrade enema access that allows flushes to be performed by the patient, and thereby renders them socially continent

Risks and Alternatives

- Standard risks (bleeding, infection, need for additional procedures, risks of anesthesia)
- Injury to adjacent structures (cecum)
- Stenosis
- Prolapse
- Leakage
- Alternatives: Cecostomy, retrograde enemas

Essential Steps

In situ Appendicostomy

1. Mobilize the cecum and right colon from their retroperitoneal attachments.
2. Vertically incise the infraumbilical fascia approximately 4 cm.
3. Bring the cecum and appendix through the umbilical incision.
4. Plicate the cecum around the appendix using nonabsorbable suture to create a valve mechanism.
5. Transect the distal appendix.
6. Close the fascia with long-term absorbable suture.
7. Perform anastomosis of the appendix to the umbilical skin.

Neoappendicostomy

1. Mobilize the right colon and cecum from their retroperitoneal attachments.
2. Vertically incise the infraumbilical fascia approximately 2 cm.
3. Bring the cecum through the umbilical incision.
4. Incise a U-shaped flap of cecum over a single vessel.
5. Tubularize the flap over a feeding tube.
6. Close the cecal defect in two layers.
7. Plicate the cecum around the neoappendix using nonabsorbable sutures to create a valve mechanism.
8. Close the fascia with long-term absorbable suture.
9. Perform anastomosis of the appendix to the umbilical skin.

D. R. Halleran · R. J. Wood · M. A. Levitt (✉)
Nationwide Children's Hospital, Center for Colorectal and Pelvic Reconstruction, Columbus, OH, USA
e-mail: marc.levitt@nationwidechildrens.org

D. J. Papandria et al. (eds.), *Operative Dictations in Pediatric Surgery*,
https://doi.org/10.1007/978-3-030-24212-1_33

Note These Variations

- This procedure may be performed at the time of colonic resection in children with intractable functional constipation or severe colonic dysmotility.
- This procedure may be performed at the time of an appendicovesicostomy (Mitrofanoff) in patients with coinciding urologic dysfunction, and the need for simultaneous urologic reconstruction should be considered prior to appendicostomy as the appendix may be utilized in both procedures.
- Note that a split-appendix technique may be used in patients with concomitant urologic dysfunction.
- Note that the appendicostomy can be anastomosed to the skin in the umbilicus or the right lower quadrant as dictated by the patient's anatomy and need for urologic reconstruction.
- Note that a neoappendicostomy may be created in patients with prior appendectomy or in cases where the appendix is needed for appendicovesicostomy.
- Note that if an abdominal incision is desired, a prior scan (such as an old colectomy site) can be used.

Template Operative Dictation (Open)

Preoperative Diagnosis *Constipation/fecal incontinence*

Postoperative Diagnosis Same as preoperative diagnosis

Findings Same as postoperative diagnosis

Procedure(s) Performed Malone continent appendicostomy

Anesthesia *General*

Specimen *Appendix/none*

Estimated Blood Loss ___

Indications This is a/an ___-year-old *male/female* with *constipation/fecal incontinence*. He/she was deemed to be a suitable candidate for Malone continent appendicostomy.

Procedure in Detail Following satisfactory induction of anesthesia, the patient was placed in the supine position and appropriately padded. Timeouts were performed using both pre-induction and pre-incision safety checklists with participation of all present in the operative suite. These confirmed the correct patient, procedure, operative site, and additional critical information prior to the start of the procedure. The abdomen was then prepped and draped in the usual sterile fashion.

An __ incision was made in the abdomen and carried down to the underlying fascia, which was incised, exposing the peritoneum. The peritoneum was then incised with care to not injure the underlying abdominal contents. After inspection of the abdominal cavity and confirmation that the viscera was uninjured, we turned our attention to the right colon. We then mobilized the right colon and cecum, taking down their retroperitoneal attachments so that the cecum was freely mobile. We then plicated the cecum around the appendix *with an 8 Fr. catheter in the lumen* without interfering with the appendiceal blood supply in four positions with nonabsorbable suture, creating a valve-like mechanism for the base of the appendix. The distal portion of the appendix was transected. We brought the tip of the appendix to the prepared umbilical skin. We then closed the fascia inferior to the umbilicus with *interrupted* long-term absorbable suture. We then performed a Y to V anastomosis from the appendix to the umbilical skin and then closed the umbilical dermis to itself, making the appendiceal mucosa hidden. This recreated the umbilical ring, and the orifice was hidden nicely within it. A __ French tube was placed through the appendix. It passed easily and was sutured in place. A sterile dressing was applied. The patient tolerated the procedure without complications.

Upon completion of the procedure, a debriefing checklist was completed to share information critical to the postoperative care of the patient. The patient tolerated the procedure well, *was extubated in the operating room*, and was transported to the post-anesthesia care unit in stable condition thereafter.

Template Operative Dictation (Laparoscopic)

Preoperative Diagnosis *Constipation/fecal incontinence*

Postoperative Diagnosis Same as preoperative diagnosis

Findings Same as postoperative diagnosis

Procedure(s) Performed Laparoscopic Malone continent appendicostomy

Anesthesia General

Specimen *Appendix/none*

Estimated Blood Loss ___

Indications This is a/an ___-*year*-old *male/female* with *constipation/fecal incontinence*. He/she was deemed to be a suitable candidate for laparoscopic Malone continent appendicostomy.

Procedure in Detail Following satisfactory induction of anesthesia, the patient was placed in supine position and appropriately padded. Timeouts were performed using both pre-induction and pre-incision safety checklists with participation of all present in the operative suite. These confirmed the correct patient, procedure, operative site, and additional critical information prior to the start of the procedure. The abdomen was then prepped and draped in the usual sterile fashion.

For Veress technique A small V skin incision was made at the umbilicus and the Veress needle inserted. Appropriate position within the abdominal cavity by aspiration and saline meniscus test.

For Hasson technique An infraumbilical skin incision was made and carried down to the fascia which was elevated and incised. A V incision was made at the umbilicus for the later Y to V appendix to skin anastomosis. The peritoneum was identified and incised with care not to injure the underlying abdominal contents. Two anchoring sutures were placed laterally through the fascia. The Hasson cannula was then inserted under direct visualization and secured with stay sutures.

The abdomen was then insufflated with CO_2 through a/an __-mm trocar. A __ camera was placed into the abdominal cavity and the contents inspected, verifying no injury to the abdominal viscera upon entry. Two additional __-mm trocars were then placed in the __ and __. We then mobilized the right colon and cecum taking down its retroperitoneal attachments so that the cecum was freely mobile. The infraumbilical fascia was incised for 2 cm, and the cecum was brought through the incision. We then plicated the cecum around the appendix without interfering with the appendiceal blood supply *with an 8 Fr. catheter in the lumen* in four positions using permanent suture, creating a valve-like mechanism for the base of the appendix. The distal portion of the appendix was transected. We then closed the fascia with interrupted long-term absorbable suture. The tip of the appendix lay just at the prepared umbilical skin. We then performed a Y to V anastomosis from the appendix to the umbilical skin and then closed the umbilical dermis to itself, making the appendiceal mucosa hidden. This recreated the umbilical ring, and the orifice was hidden nicely within it. A __ French tube was placed through the appendix. It passed easily and was sutured in place. A sterile dressing was applied. The patient tolerated the procedure without complications.

Upon completion of the procedure, a debriefing checklist was completed to share information critical to the postoperative care of the patient. The patient tolerated the procedure well, *was extubated in the operating room*, and was transported to the post-anesthesia care unit in stable condition thereafter.

Total Abdominal Colectomy with End-Ileostomy

34

Benedict C. Nwomeh, Jeremy G. Fisher, and Jason Zakko

Indications and Benefits

- Indications:
  - Inflammatory bowel disease
  - Trauma
  - Familial adenomatous polyposis (when combined with proctectomy +/− reconstruction)
- Benefits:
  - Resolution of disease

Risks and Alternatives

- Standard risks (bleeding, infection, need for additional procedures, risks of anesthesia)
- Injury to adjacent structures: Rectal stump leak, ureteral transection/injury, splenic capsule tear, injury to duodenum during mobilization of right colon and hepatic flexure, stoma complications
- Alternatives: Combined proctocolectomy

B. C. Nwomeh (✉) · J. G. Fisher
Nationwide Children's Hospital, Department of Pediatric Surgery, Columbus, OH, USA
e-mail: Benedict.Nwomeh@nationwidechildrens.org

J. Zakko
Ohio State University Medical Center/Nationwide Children's Hospital, Department of Pediatric Surgery, Columbus, OH, USA

Essential Steps

1. *Place patient in supine position.*
2. *Establish exposure (Vertical midline incision vs port placement).*
3. *Explore all quadrants of the abdomen.*
4. ***Mobilize the splenic flexure and left colon:***
   (a) *Incise White Line of Toldt from sigmoid colon to splenic flexure.*
   (b) *Reflect the colon medially while identifying and protecting the left ureter.*
5. Divide greater omentum to mobilize transverse colon.
6. ***Mobilize the right colon:***
   (a) *Incise White Line of Toldt from the cecum to the hepatic flexure.*
   (b) *Divide retroperitoneal adhesions to the colon.*
   (c) *Identify and protect right ureter and second portion of the duodenum.*
7. Divide the sigmoid colon with a linear cutting stapler (*Note: may be performed earlier in sequence*).
8. Divide the terminal ileum with a linear cutting stapler (*Note: may be performed earlier in sequence*).
9. Divide the mesentery (suture ligation or sealing device).
10. Create an end-ileostomy.
11. Close the abdomen.
12. Mature the stoma.

D. J. Papandria et al. (eds.), *Operative Dictations in Pediatric Surgery*,
https://doi.org/10.1007/978-3-030-24212-1_34

Template Operative Dictation (Open)

Preoperative Diagnosis *Ulcerative colitis/ Crohn's colitis* refractory to medical management

Postoperative Diagnosis Same as preoperative diagnosis

Findings Same as postoperative diagnosis

Procedure(s) Performed Total abdominal colectomy with end-ileostomy

Anesthesia *General*

Specimen ___ colon, to Pathology

Drains None

Implants {None}

Estimated Blood Loss ___

Indications This is a/an ___-year-old *male/ female* with inflammatory bowel disease refractory to medical management. *He/she* was deemed to be a suitable candidate for total abdominal colectomy with end-ileostomy with end-ileostomy.

Procedure in Detail Following satisfactory induction of anesthesia, the patient was placed in supine position and appropriately padded. Timeouts were performed using both preinduction and pre-incision safety checklists with participation of all present in the operative suite. These confirmed the correct patient, procedure, operative site, and additional critical information prior to the start of the procedure. The abdomen and perineum was then prepped and draped in the usual sterile fashion. The patient was seen preoperatively by an enterostomal care nurse and the planned ileostomy site was marked.

We began by making a vertical midline incision, followed by dissection to the fascia using electrocautery. The linea alba was identified, incised, and the peritoneal cavity was entered. The abdomen was explored for gross abnormalities and iatrogenic injuries.

Mobilization of the left colon began by using blunt dissection and the LigaSure electrocautery device to incise the white line of Toldt up to the level of the splenic flexure, followed by division of the associated mesentery using the LigaSure. The ascending colon was then mobilized in a similar fashion, taking care to preserve the ileocolic artery. The transverse colon was then freed from its cephalad attachments, with care taken to avoid injuring the duodenum. The greater omentum was *mobilized off the transverse colon/divided and taken en bloc with the specimen.* The right colic, branches of the middle colic, and left colic arteries were each identified and taken with the LigaSure at the level of the bowel wall. Our attention then turned to the sigmoid colon, where we identified the convergence of taenia coli and divided the distal aspect of the sigmoid colon using a GIA stapler (*blue load*). After inspecting the distal staple line looking for hemostasis and an adequate staple bite, a *Prolene* suture was placed through the staple line and left long to identify the rectal stump for possible future procedures.

We then turned our attention to the proximal resection site. A window was developed using blunt dissection in the mesentery adjacent to the terminal ileum at the level of the ileocecal valve and a GIA stapler was used to divide the bowel, followed by division of the remaining mesocolon using the LigaSure device. The specimen was then passed off for pathology. Final examination of the abdomen revealed a hemostatic field and expected orientation of the bowel.

We then began with creating our ileostomy. At the previously marked stoma site, a disk of skin was excised and the incision was deepened through subcutaneous tissue using electrocautery. Using blunt dissection to spread the rectus musculature, the anterior and posterior fascia was incised *in cruciate fashion*, and an opening in the abdominal wall was created to pass two fingers. The ileum was passed through this opening, ensuring that it was not strangulated or under significant tension.

At this point, we turned our attention to closing our midline laparotomy. The fascia was closed with a running *0 PDS* suture, followed by running a *3–0 Vicryl* deep dermal stitch, and finally closing skin (*staples/subcuticular sutures*). A sterile dressing was placed over this incision. We then matured our ileostomy with multiple circumferential 3–0 Vicryl interrupted sutures to fashion a typical Brooke ileostomy. A stoma appliance was placed.

Upon completion of the procedure, a debriefing checklist was completed to share information critical to the postoperative care of the patient. The patient tolerated the procedure well, *was extubated in the operating room* and was transported to the postanesthesia care unit in stable condition.

Template Operative Dictation (Laparoscopic)

Preoperative Diagnosis *Ulcerative colitis/ Crohn's colitis* refractory to medical management

Postoperative Diagnosis Same as preoperative diagnosis

Findings Same as postoperative diagnosis

Procedure(s) Performed Laparoscopic total abdominal colectomy with end-ileostomy

Anesthesia General

Specimen Colon

Drains None

Implants None

Estimated Blood Loss ___

Indications This is a/an ___-*month/year*-old *male/female* with inflammatory bowel disease. He/she was deemed to be a suitable candidate for three-stage laparoscopic colectomy with ileostomy, with future plans for completion of proctectomy with ileal pouch-anal anastomosis.

Procedure in Detail Following satisfactory induction of anesthesia, the patient was placed in supine position and appropriately padded. Timeouts were performed using both preinduction and pre-incision safety checklists with participation of all present in the operative suite. These confirmed the correct patient, procedure, operative site, and additional critical information prior to the start of the procedure. The patient was seen preoperatively by an enterostomal care nurse and the planned ileostomy site was marked. The abdomen was then prepped and draped in the usual sterile fashion.

A 4-cm transverse incision was placed at the planned ileostomy site and carried down to the level of the fascia using electrocautery. The fascia and rectus abdominis were divided and a small Alexis wound protector was then placed in the incision and fitted with a port cap, through which a 12 mm trocar was introduced into the abdomen. The abdomen was then insufflated to a pressure of 15 mm Hg, which was well tolerated. A cursory survey of the abdominal contents revealed no traumatic sequelae of abdominal access. Local anesthetic infiltration and stab incisions were then placed at *2/3/4* additional trocar sites. 5-mm ports were placed in the right upper quadrant, left lower quadrant, and left upper quadrant. Trocars were introduced under direct laparoscopic vision.

A window was created in the sigmoid mesocolon using the LigaSure. The sigmoid colon was then divided over the iliac vessels with the EndoGIA stapler with a *purple* load. Mobilization of the left colon was initiated using a combination of blunt technique and electrocautery using the LigaSure. This mobilized the descending colon along the white line of Toldt to the level of the splenic flexure. We then divided the associated mesentery. The splenic flexure peritoneal attachments were isolated and divided taking care not to place excess tension on the spleen. The transverse colon was then mobilized: the omentum was *mobilized off the transverse colon/ divided and taken en bloc with the specimen* and the transverse mesocolon was divided along the bowel wall with the LigaSure. The hepatic flexure was similarly mobilized, taking care to avoid injuring the duodenum. This left only the right colon in situ.

The Alexis cap was then removed. The appendix was identified and used to pull the cecum into the wound. A window was made in the mesentery of the ileum at the ileocecal valve and an EndoGIA *purple* load stapler was used to divide the ileum. The cecum was then mobilized from lateral attachments and mesocolon using the LigaSure. The remaining right colon was similarly mobilized. Once complete, the entire specimen was then delivered through the wound and passed off for pathology.

The fascia at the incision was partially closed with interrupted *0 Vicryl* suture. The terminal ileum was then affixed to the fascia using 3–0 Vicryl in an interrupted fashion.

Final laparoscopic examination of the abdomen revealed a hemostatic field and expected orientation of the ileostomy. All trocars were then removed and sites were likewise noted to be hemostatic. The fascia was closed where visible with *3–0 Vicryl* sutures and the skin at all port sites was then closed with *5–0 Vicryl* subcuticular stitches. All sites were dressed with *Dermabond*. The extracorporeal bowel was then matured in standard fashion with interrupted *3–0 Vicryl* to create a Brooke ileostomy. A stoma appliance was then placed.

Upon completion of the procedure, a debriefing checklist was completed to share information critical to the postoperative care of the patient. The patient tolerated the procedure well, *was extubated in the operating room*, and was transported to the post anesthesia care unit in stable condition.

35 Completion Proctectomy and Ileal Pouch-Anal Anastomosis, Diverting Loop Ileostomy

Benedict C. Nwomeh, Jeremy G. Fisher,
and Jason Zakko

Indications and Benefits

- Indication: Ulcerative colitis (usually with complication or refractory to medical management), classic second of three stages for proctocolectomy and reconstruction
- Benefits: Removal of UC-containing rectum and restoration of anal stooling after total colectomy with end ileostomy

Risks and Alternatives

- Standard risks (bleeding, infection, need for additional procedures, risks of anesthesia).
- Injury to adjacent structures: Injury to the urethra (male), hemorrhage from the presacral venous plexus, sexual dysfunction (pelvic autonomic nerves), infertility (female), urinary retention
- Alternatives: Proctectomy with end ileostomy

B. C. Nwomeh (✉) · J. G. Fisher
Nationwide Children's Hospital, Department of Pediatric Surgery, Columbus, OH, USA
e-mail: Benedict.Nwomeh@nationwidechildrens.org

J. Zakko
Ohio State University Medical Center/Nationwide Children's Hospital, Department of Pediatric Surgery, Columbus, OH, USA

Essential Steps

1. Combined lithotomy-supine position.
2. Takedown end ileostomy (dissect free from abdominal wall).
3. Construct J-pouch ileal reservoir (may be done after laparotomy incision if open).
4. Gain exposure (low vertical midline incision or place laparoscopic ports).
5. Incise pelvic peritoneum and dissect along rectal wall.
6. Carefully dissect circumferentially to levators.
7. Divide rectum.
8. Perform stapled/sutured anastomosis from below.
9. Temporary diverting loop ileostomy.
10. Close abdomen/ports.

Note These Variations

- Combined colectomy and proctocolectomy followed by staged ileal pouch-anal anastomosis (classic 2-stage).
- Proctectomy with ileal pouch-anal anastomosis without diverting loop ileostomy (alternative 2-stage).

D. J. Papandria et al. (eds.), *Operative Dictations in Pediatric Surgery*,
https://doi.org/10.1007/978-3-030-24212-1_35

Template Operative Dictation (Open)

Preoperative Diagnosis Ulcerative colitis

Postoperative Diagnosis Same as preoperative diagnosis

Findings Same as postoperative diagnosis

Procedure(s) Performed Completion proctectomy, ileal pouch-anal anastomosis, diverting loop ileostomy

Anesthesia *General*

Specimen Rectum

Drains *None / __ Fr Blake / Jackson-Pratt*

Implants None

Estimated Blood Loss ___

Indications This is a/an ___-year-old *male/female* with history of ulcerative colitis refractory to medical management. He/she has previously undergone a total colectomy with end ileostomy and now presents for *his/her* second (of three) stages: completion proctectomy, ileal pouch-anal anastomosis, diverting loop ileostomy.

Procedure in Detail Following satisfactory induction of anesthesia, the patient was placed in *lithotomy* position and appropriately padded. Timeouts were performed using both pre-induction and pre-incision safety checklists with participation of all present in the operative suite. These confirmed the correct patient, procedure, operative site, and additional critical information prior to the start of the procedure. Perioperative antibiotics were administered and the ileostomy was closed with 3–0 silk sutures. The abdomen was then prepped and draped in the usual sterile fashion. A Foley catheter was placed under sterile conditions and the urimeter passed off the field.

We began by making an incision circumferentially around the ileostomy, and using electrocautery, carried this incision down into the subcutaneous space adjacent to the bowel. We continued this dissection down to the fascia, and then entered the peritoneal space. The bowel was completely mobilized from the abdominal wall and was then allowed to drop into the abdomen.

A vertical midline incision was made sharply. Using Bovie electrocautery, this incision was deepened through the subcutaneous tissues through the linea alba, and the peritoneal cavity was entered. Adhesions were lysed sharply under direct vision. The abdominal cavity was inspected for gross abnormalities, and the rectal stump from the previous procedure was identified. The inferior mesenteric artery and superior rectal artery were then identified and divided near the root. Dissection then followed on both sides of the rectosigmoid to the cul-de-sac, taking great care to stay close to the rectum to avoid injuring the pelvic neurovasculature, ureters, and gonadal vessels. The rectum was mobilized along the rectal wall by using a combination of blunt and electrocautery dissection. The rectum was carefully elevated until the endopelvic fascia and the levator sling was identified. The anterior dissection proceeded after positively identifying all pelvic structures anterior to the rectum (including the bladder, *prostate/vagina, uterus*) and preserving them. Following complete circumferential exposure of the levators, a sponge forceps was introduced per rectum and used to secure the proximal aspect of the rectum, which was then everted. Inspection of the anus and perineum revealed satisfactory dissection and full exposure of the rectum to the anal verge. Two *3–0 Prolene* stay sutures were placed at the lateral edges *1* cm above the dentate line, and just proximal to this a TA stapler *blue load* was affixed and fired across the bowel. The rectal specimen was then excised sharply and passed off the field. *(Note: Rectum may be stapled intra-corporeally instead of the described eversion technique.)*

The terminal ileum (ileostomy) was then identified and the peritoneum overlying its mesentery was divided back to the first major vascular pedicle (*and fenestrated*) to gain additional length. Adhesion to the ileum was lysed and the peritoneum at the base of the small bowel mesentery was incised to fully mobilize the ileum.

We then again turned our attention to creating the pouch. The midpoint of the planned J-pouch reached the pubis without tension on the mesentery and a *3–0 Vicryl* stay suture was placed at the proximal boundary of the ileal pouch. A longitudinal enterotomy was then made at the distal border of the pouch, into which a GIA stapler *blue load* was inserted, with the anvil and cartridge directed up each lumen. The stapler was fired along the antimesenteric aspect of the bowel, which resulted in a generous pouch lumen.

Using *3–0 Prolene,* a purse-string suture was then placed around the enterotomy and the anvil for a *19/21/25/27/29* mm EA stapler was placed within the pouch. The purse string was tied, allowing only the anvil post through the opening. Orienting stay sutures were placed on the lateral and anterior aspect of the pouch using *3–0 silk* sutures. The GIA stapler *blue load* was then used to resect the distal ileum (previous ileostomy site) flush with the border of the pouch to minimize the blind tip length. The specimen was then passed off to pathology. The visible staple line was then imbricated with *3–0 Vicryl* suture in running fashion.

Next, the proper orientation of the terminal ileum and pouch were re-confirmed. The anvil post was grasped, being careful to maintain the proper alignment of the bowel to avoid twisting the mesentery. The EA stapler was then used to restore the rectal stump to its anatomic position. The stapler trocar deployed until the orange marker was clearly visible and the anvil post was then anchored securely onto the stapler, which was then fired without difficulty. Two complete anastomotic rings of tissue were recovered following removal and disassembly of the stapler. The anastomosis and pouch staple lines were airtight on submersion/insufflation testing *with a colonoscope in the rectum.* Rectal stay sutures were removed.

A loop of ileum was identified approximately *20* cm proximal to the pouch that easily reached the ileostomy incision. This was delivered into the incision and marked with stay sutures at its proximal and distal extent. Proper position and orientation were confirmed, and the bowel wall was then affixed to the fascia using *3–0 Vicryl* suture in interrupted fashion. At this point, we closed our vertical midline incision. Using a *looped 0 PDS*, the fascia was closed in standard running fashion. We then placed a wet to dry dressing and covered the incision with sterile towels prior to turning our attention to maturing the ileostomy.

The extracorporeal bowel was opened along its inferior border using electrocautery and a *3–0 PDS* purse-string suture was placed to exclude the distal segment, which was then affixed to the skin along its inferior border using interrupted *3–0 Vicryl.* The proximal lumen was then matured in a standard fashion with interrupted *3–0 Vicryl* to create a Brooke ileostomy. A stoma appliance was then placed.

Upon completion of the procedure, a debriefing checklist was completed to share information critical to the postoperative care of the patient. The patient tolerated the procedure well, *was extubated in the operating room*, and was transported to the postanesthesia care unit in stable condition.

Template Operative Dictation (Laparoscopic)

Preoperative Diagnosis Ulcerative colitis

Postoperative Diagnosis Same as preoperative diagnosis

Findings Same as postoperative diagnosis

Procedure(s) Performed Laparoscopic-assisted completion proctectomy, ileal pouch-anal anastomosis, diverting loop ileostomy

Anesthesia General

Specimen Rectum

Drains *None / __ Fr Blake / Jackson-Pratt*

Implants None

Estimated Blood Loss ___

Indications This is a/an ___ -*year*-old *male/female* with ulcerative colitis refractory to medical management. He/she was deemed to be a suitable candidate for laparoscopic-assisted completion proctectomy, ileal pouch-anal anastomosis, diverting loop ileostomy.

Procedure in Detail Following satisfactory induction of anesthesia, the patient was placed in *lithotomy* position and appropriately padded. Timeouts were performed using both pre-induction and pre-incision safety checklists with the participation of all present in the operative suite. These confirmed the correct patient, procedure, operative site, and additional critical information prior to the start of the procedure. Perioperative antibiotics were administered and the ileostomy was closed with 3–0 silk sutures. The abdomen was then prepped and draped in the usual sterile fashion. A Foley catheter was placed under sterile conditions and the urimeter passed off the field.

We began by making an incision circumferentially around the ileostomy, and using electrocautery, carried this incision down into the subcutaneous space adjacent to the bowel. We continued this dissection down to the fascia, and then entered the peritoneal space. The bowel was completely mobilized at the incision and the peritoneum overlying its mesentery was divided back to the first major vascular pedicle (*and fenestrated*) to gain additional length. Adhesions to the ileum were lysed and the peritoneum at the base of the small bowel mesentery was incised to fully mobilize the ileum.

We then again turned our attention to creating the pouch. The midpoint of the planned J-pouch reached the pubis without tension on the mesentery and a *3–0 Vicryl* stay suture was placed at the proximal boundary of the ileal pouch. A longitudinal enterotomy was then made at the distal border of the pouch, into which a GIA stapler *blue load* was inserted, with the anvil and cartridge directed up each lumen. The stapler was fired along the antimesenteric aspect of the bowel, which resulted in a generous pouch lumen.

Using *3–0 Prolene,* a purse-string suture was then placed around the enterotomy and the anvil for a *19/21/25/27/29*-mm EA stapler was placed within the pouch. The purse string was tied, allowing only the anvil post through the opening. Orienting stay sutures were placed on the lateral and anterior aspect of the pouch using *3–0 silk* sutures. The GIA stapler *blue load* was then used to resect the distal ileum (previous ileostomy site) flush with the border of the pouch to minimize the blind tip length. The specimen was then passed off to pathology. The visible staple line was then imbricated with *3–0 Vicryl* suture in running fashion.

A small Alexis wound protector was then placed in the ileostomy incision and fitted with a port cap, through which a 10–12-mm trocar was introduced into the abdomen. The abdomen was then insufflated to a pressure of *15* mmHg, which was well tolerated. A cursory survey of the abdominal contents revealed no traumatic sequelae of abdominal access. Local anesthetic infiltration and stab incisions were then placed at three additional trocar sites, reusing old incisions where possible. 5-mm ports were placed in the right lower quadrant, left lower quadrant, and left upper quadrant, each under direct laparoscopic vision. The ileum and pouch were examined and additional mobilization was accomplished using a combination of blunt technique and electrocautery using the LigaSure device to ensure adequate mobility into the pelvis.

Dissection of the rectum was initiated in similar fashion in the plane immediately adjacent to the bowel, dividing the posterior attachments until the levators were encountered. Careful division of the lateral attachments was used to ensure hemostasis and to maintain a safe distance from the bilateral ureters. The anterior dissection proceeded after positively identifying all pelvic structures anterior to the rectum (including the bladder, *prostate/vagina, and uterus*) and preserving them. Following complete circumferential exposure of the levators, a sponge forcep was introduced per rectum and used to secure the proximal aspect of the rectum, which was then everted. Inspection of the anus and perineum revealed satisfactory dissection and full exposure of the rectum to the anal verge. Two *3–0 Prolene* stay sutures were placed at the lateral edges *1* cm above the dentate line and just proximal to this, a TA stapler *blue load* was affixed and fired across the bowel. The rectal specimen was then excised sharply and passed off the field. *(Note: Rectum may be stapled intra-corporeally instead of the described eversion technique.)*

Attention was then turned back to the abdomen and proper orientation of the terminal ileum and pouch were re-confirmed. The anvil post was grasped using the anvil grasper, being careful to maintain the proper alignment of the bowel to avoid twisting the mesentery. The EA stapler was then used to restore the rectal stump to anatomic position under laparoscopic visualization. The stapler trocar deployed until the orange marker was clearly visible and the anvil post was then anchored securely onto the stapler, which was then fired without difficulty. Two complete anastomotic rings of tissue were recovered following removal and disassembly of the stapler. The anastomosis and pouch staple lines were air-tight on submersion/insufflation testing *with a colonoscope in the rectum*. Rectal stay sutures were removed.

A loop of ileum was identified approximately *20* cm proximal to the pouch that easily reached the ileostomy incision. This was delivered into the incision and marked with stay sutures at its proximal and distal extent. Proper position and orientation was confirmed laparoscopically and the bowel wall was then affixed to the fascia using *3–0 Vicryl* suture in interrupted fashion.

After aspirating all irrigation fluid and inspecting the abdomen, trocars were removed under direct laparoscopic vision and the laparoscope was removed. The skin at all port sites was closed with *5–0 Vicryl* in subcuticular fashion. All sites were then dressed with DermaBond.

The extracorporeal bowel was then opened along its inferior border using electrocautery and a *3–0 PDS* purse-string suture was placed to exclude the distal segment, which was then affixed to the skin along its inferior border using interrupted *3–0 Vicryl*. The proximal lumen was then matured in a standard fashion with interrupted *3–0 Vicryl* to create a Brooke ileostomy. A stoma appliance was then placed.

Upon completion of the procedure, a debriefing checklist was completed to share information critical to the postoperative care of the patient. The patient tolerated the procedure well, *was extubated in the operating room*, and was transported to the postanesthesia care unit in stable condition.

Swenson-Like Transanal Pull-Through

36

Devin R. Halleran, Richard J. Wood, and Marc A. Levitt

Indications and Benefits

- Hirschsprung disease
- Benefits: Removal of aganglionic bowel

Risks and Alternatives

- Standard risks (bleeding, infection, need for additional procedures, risks of anesthesia)
- Injury to adjacent structures (anal sphincter, dentate line, posterior urethra, posterior vagina, nervi erigentes)
- Fecal, urinary, and sexual dysfunction
- Transition zone pull-through
- Anastomotic stricture
- Anastomotic twist
- Alternatives: Soave, Duhamel

D. R. Halleran · R. J. Wood · M. A. Levitt (✉)
Nationwide Children's Hospital, Center for Colorectal and Pelvic Reconstruction, Columbus, OH, USA
e-mail: marc.levitt@nationwidechildrens.org

Essential Steps

Combined Abdominal and Transanal Approach

1. Gain laparoscopic or open access to the abdominal cavity
2. Perform full-thickness biopsy to determine the level of the normal ganglionic bowel.
3. Mobilize the descending and sigmoid colon from its peritoneal attachments.
4. Begin circumferential dissection down into the pelvis right at the bowel wall in a Swenson fashion.
5. Ligate the inferior mesenteric artery while preserving the sigmoid arcade.
6. When intraabdominal dissection is complete, place the patient in a legs up position.
7. Place Lone Star pins to hide dentate line.
8. Place circumferential interrupted silk sutures 1.0 cm proximal to dentate line.
9. Using electrocautery, perform full-thickness rectal dissection until reaching the previous dissection from the level of the peritoneum.
10. Pull through the rectum and sigmoid colon at least 5 cm proximal to the biopsy demonstrating normal ganglion cells.
11. Place deep layer of sutures circumferentially at the resection margin from muscle to colonic serosa, 1 cm proximal to dentate line.

D. J. Papandria et al. (eds.), *Operative Dictations in Pediatric Surgery*,
https://doi.org/10.1007/978-3-030-24212-1_36

12. Resect aganglionic segment of rectum and colon.
13. Perform second layer of anastomosis from mucosa to mucosa.

Transanal Approach Only

1. Place Lone Star pins to hide the dentate line.
2. Place circumferential interrupted silk sutures 1.0 cm proximal to dentate line.
3. Using electrocautery, perform full-thickness rectal dissection along retraction line to the level of the peritoneum.
4. Extract sigmoid once anterior plane breaks through the peritoneal reflection.
5. Perform full-thickness biopsy to verify the level of normal ganglionic bowel.
6. Push sigmoid back into the pelvis.
7. Continue posterior rectal dissection.
8. Pull out rectum and sigmoid and ligate branches of the sigmoid mesentery transanally.
9. Pull through the rectum and sigmoid colon at least 5 cm proximal to the biopsy demonstrating normal ganglion cells and nerves that are less than 40 microns.
10. Place deep layer of sutures circumferentially at the resection margin from muscle to colonic serosa, 1 cm proximal to dentate line.
11. Resect aganglionic segment of rectum and colon.
12. Perform second layer of anastomosis from mucosa to mucosa.

Note These Variations

- Note that depending on the prior surgical procedures performed and the length of segment of aganglionic bowel, an abdominal portion may be needed in addition to the transanal approach.

Template Operative Dictation

Preoperative Diagnosis Hirschsprung disease

Postoperative Diagnosis Same as preoperative diagnosis

Findings Same as postoperative diagnosis

Procedure(s) Performed Swenson-like transanal pull-through

Anesthesia *General*

Specimen Rectal biopsy x __, *sigmoid colon*, and rectum

Estimated Blood Loss ___

Indications This is a/an ___-*day/week/month/year*-old *male/female* with Hirschsprung disease. *The child underwent previous suction/full-thickness rectal biopsy which showed absence of ganglion cells and hypertrophic nerve cells. The child to this point has been managed with rectal irrigations. The prior contrast enema is compatible with a transition zone at the level of the rectosigmoid.* He/she was deemed to be a suitable candidate for Swenson-like transanal pull-through *with laparoscopic assistance.*

Procedure in Detail Following satisfactory induction of anesthesia, the patient was placed in the *supine/prone* position and appropriately padded. Timeouts were performed using both preinduction and pre-incision safety checklists with participation of all present in the operative suite. These confirmed the correct patient, procedure, operative site, and additional critical information prior to the start of the procedure. The child underwent a total body preparation and was then draped in the usual sterile fashion.

[Choose One]
If Abdominal dissection required: The patient was placed in the supine position. An incision was made through the umbilicus and carried down to the umbilical stalk where the fascia was incised, revealing the peritoneum, which was carefully opened so as to avoid causing injury to the underlying abdominal viscera. A *4-mm* port was placed and secured with a *3–0 silk* suture.

The abdomen was then insufflated using CO_2. Additional *3-mm* incisions were then made through the *right upper quadrant*, *right lower quadrant*, and *left upper quadrant* through which we placed our additional ports under direct visualization.

We inspected the abdominal cavity, which revealed no evidence of traumatic injury. We focused our attention on the colon, where we noted a dilated segment of *sigmoid colon which tapered to a smaller diameter as it reached the pelvis, suggesting that this was the transition zone*. A full-thickness biopsy was taken at the level of bowel in the sigmoid colon proximal to the abrupt change in caliber and sent to pathology for frozen section. We began to mobilize the splenic flexure using *hook cautery/energy device which we continued down the white line of Toldt*. Once the colon was mobilized, the left side of the gastrocolic ligament was divided to allow adequate length to reach the pelvis. At this point, we were informed that our biopsy demonstrated normal ganglion cells with no evidence of hypertrophic nerves. *The sigmoid and distal descending colon was then separated from the left retroperitoneal attachments up to just distal to the splenic flexure. The sigmoid mesenteric arcade was preserved proximally to the level of the mid-descending colon, including the marginal branch that parallels the sigmoid colon.* This level of bowel reached the peritoneal reflection easily. The peritoneal reflection was then opened circumferentially and dissection along the bowel wall carried out to *approximately 2 cm* below the reflection. We then focused our attention to the transanal portion of the procedure.

With the patient still in the supine position, the legs were placed up and secured to either screen, and a bump was placed under the buttocks. We examined the anus, which was noted to be in the correct anatomical position. The Lone Star retractor was then brought into the field and initially placed at the level of the mucocutaneous junction. Once this was accomplished, we then further retracted at the level of the dentate line circumferentially, so that the dentate line was no longer visible and therefore could not be damaged during the dissection. We then placed circumferential interrupted silk sutures, approximately 1.0 cm proximal to the dentate line, to provide uniform circumferential tension. We then used electrocautery to perform a Swenson-type full-thickness dissection along our retraction line of silk sutures. This was continued circumferentially all the way through down to the level of the peritoneum with care to remain intimately close to the rectum to avoid any adjacent structures. We continued the dissection of the rectum up until we reached the distal most point of our previous abdominal dissection.

At this point, we pulled the *sigmoid colon forth and we ligated any remaining branches of the sigmoid mesentery transanally and we were able to pull through the rectum and sigmoid colon to 5 cm above the biopsy site*. At this level, we placed a deep layer of sutures circumferentially at the level of the resection margin, from muscle to colonic serosa, which was once again 1.0 cm proximal to the dentate line. Once this was accomplished, the distal pulled through bowel was resected utilizing electrocautery and passed off the table as specimen. We then completed our second layer of the anastomosis at the level of the previous resection using interrupted absorbable sutures, from mucosa to mucosa. Finally, we closed our trocar sites, using interrupted absorbable sutures to close the umbilical fascial defect, and absorbable subcuticular sutures to close our skin incisions.

If transanal only: The patient was placed in the *prone* position. The anus was examined and noted to be in the correct anatomical position. The Lone Star retractor was then brought into the field and initially placed at the level of the mucocutaneous junction. Once this was accomplished, we then further retracted at the level of the dentate line circumferentially, so that the dentate line was no longer visible and therefore could not be damaged during the dissection. We then placed circumferential interrupted silk sutures, approximately 1.0 cm proximal to the dentate line, to provide uniform circumferential tension. We then utilized electrocautery to perform a Swenson-type full-thickness dissection along our retraction line of silk sutures. This was continued circumferentially all the way through down to the level of the peritoneum with care to avoid any adjacent structures. We continued the dissection of the rectum up until we reached the peritoneal reflection. At this point, we pulled the sigmoid colon forth and took a full-thickness biopsy which we sent to pathology for frozen section. Dissection then continued proximally. We ligated the *distal branches of the sigmoid mesentery transanally and we were able to pull through the rectum and sigmoid colon*. We were then informed that our prior biopsy contained normal ganglion cells without hypertrophic nerves. At 5 cm above this level, we placed a deep layer of sutures circumferentially at the level of the resection margin, from muscle to colonic serosa, which was once again 1.0 cm proximal to the dentate line. Once this was accomplished, the distal pulled through bowel was resected utilizing electrocautery and passed off the table as specimen. We then completed our second layer of the anastomosis at the level of the previous resection utilizing interrupted absorbable sutures from mucosa to mucosa.

Upon completion of the procedure, a debriefing checklist was completed to share information critical to the postoperative care of the patient. The patient tolerated the procedure well, *was extubated in the operating room*, and was transported to the postanesthesia care unit in stable condition thereafter.

37 Duhamel Procedure

Kate Savoie and Brian D. Kenney

Indications and Benefits

- Hirschsprung disease

Risk and Alternatives

- Risks: Bleeding, infection, anastomotic leak, intraabdominal abscess, iatrogenic injury to the ureter, traction injury to the spleen, inappropriate leveling
- Alternatives: Soave procedure, Swenson procedure

Essential Steps

1. Midline laparotomy or trocar placement.
2. Adhesiolysis, if necessary.
3. Take down colostomy or perform leveling biopsies.
4. Mobilize the distal colon to the level of the rectum.
5. Transect the aganglionic colon and send to pathology.
6. Develop the retrorectal space.
7. Incise the rectum proximal to the dentate line.
8. Pass the normoganglionic bowel through enterotomy and into rectum.
9. Secure the colon to the rectum with interrupted sutures.
10. Perform a stapled anastomosis to create a common channel.
11. Close fascia and subcutaneous tissues.

Notes These Variations

- A transabdominal stapling technique to create the common channel has been described.

Template Operative Dictation

Preoperative Diagnosis Hirschsprung disease

Posteroperative Diagnosis Same as preoperative diagnosis

Findings Same as postoperative diagnosis

Anesthesia General

Specimen Colon

K. Savoie (✉)
Nationwide Children's Hospital, Department of Pediatric Surgery, Columbus, OH, USA
e-mail: Kate.savoie@nationwidechildrens.org

B. D. Kenney
Pediatric Intensive Care Unit, Nationwide Children's Hospital, Department of Pediatric Surgery, Columbus, OH, USA

D. J. Papandria et al. (eds.), *Operative Dictations in Pediatric Surgery*,
https://doi.org/10.1007/978-3-030-24212-1_37

Drains {Drains}

Implants {Implants}

Estimated Blood Loss ____

Indications This is *a/an ___-day/week/month/year-old male/female* with Hirschsprung disease. He/she was deemed to be a suitable candidate for a Duhamel pull-through procedure.

Procedure in Detail Following satisfactory induction of anesthesia, the patient was placed in a lithotomy position and appropriately padded. Timeouts were performed using both preinduction and pre-incision safety checklists with participation of all present in the operative suite. These confirmed the correct patient, procedure, operative site, and additional critical information prior to the start of the procedure. The abdomen and rectum were then prepped and draped in the usual sterile fashion including the use of an iodine-impregnated incision drape.

[Choose One]

If an open approach was performed: A *left paramedian incision with a curvilinear transition to a transverse suprapubic incision/ midline incision* was made and carried down through the subcutaneous tissues using electrocautery to expose the peritoneum.

If a minimally invasive approach was performed: *An incision was made at the umbilicus and a/an __-mm port placed. The abdomen was then insufflated, which the patient tolerated well. Two additional ___-mm ports were placed in the left and right abdomen.*

Adhesiolysis was performed and the bowel run in its entirety from the ligament of Treitz to the *leveling colostomy sigmoid colon.*

[Choose One]

If no previous leveling colostomy was performed: A full-thickness biopsy was then taken just above the peritoneal reflection, with an additional biopsy at the suspected transition zone based on the contrast enema/operative inspection. Additional biopsies were taken at 10 cm intervals sequentially until normal ganglions cells were present and the absence of hypertrophic nerves is confirmed. As the transition zone was noted to be in the descending/transverse colon, the phrenicocolic ligament and attachments to the spleen were divided with suture ligatures/cauterization. The mesentery was then sequentially divided proximally to the transition zone, with care to preserve the marginal artery of Drummond and the Arc of Riolan.

If previous leveling colostomy performed: The mobilization of the colostomy was then started by creating an elliptical incision around the stoma. The subcutaneous tissues were dissected away from the intradermal portion of the colon until it was able to be returned to the abdomen.

{Continue dictation}

The aganglionic portion of colon was mobilized distally by taking down the white line of Toldt and releasing the colon from its retroperitoneal attachment, taking care to stay along the colon wall. The colon was mobilized distally to the level of the splaying of the tinea. The rectum was dissected circumferentially down to the mid-rectum and the mesentery divided with sequentially to this level. The rectum was then transected with a/an ___-mm stapler using a/an ___ (color) load. Blunt dissection was then performed to develop the presacral space behind the rectum with care to obtain hemostasis.

The proximal end of the bowel was then brought down into the presacral space. There was adequate length and no undue tension was appreciated.

The Lone Star retractor pins were placed circumferentially. Once the dentate line was identified, the retractor pins were repositioned above this line. Through a transanal approach, the posterior wall of the rectum was then opened 1 cm proximal to the dentate line and this dissection was carried into the retrorectal space. The end of the proximal rectum was then grasped and pulled through this incision until all of the colon was exteriorized up to the transition zone. The anterior half of the colon was incised and secured to the rectal wall with multiple ___-0 *vicryl/ silk* sutures in an interrupted fashion. The mesentery of the colon was then divided. The posterior wall of the colon was divided and similarly secured to the inferior aspect of the rectal wall. The specimen was then passed off to pathology and the proximal margin was verified on frozen section to have ganglion cells.

A/an ___-mm ___ (color) stapler as then used to create a common channel between the posterior rectal wall and the normoganglionic colon. Care was taken to ensure that the all anterior redundancy was removed. The Lone Star pins were then removed and the anastomosis was inspected and felt to be hemostatic.

The abdomen was again inspected and hemostasis ensured. A catheter tipped syringe was then placed into the rectum and the peritoneal cavity was irrigated. The anastomosis was then tested by filling the rectal pouch with air. The irrigation fluid was then removed.

If an open approach was performed: *The fascia was then reapproximated using a/an __-0 vicryl/prolene/ PDS suture in a running/ interrupted/ figure of eight fashion. The subcutaneous tissues were reapproximated with a/an ___-0 vicryl and the skin closed with a/an ___-0 vicryl/ monocryl.*

If a minimally invasive approach was performed: *The trocars were removed under direct visualization to confirm hemostasis. The abdomen was then desufflated and the umbilical port removed. The umbilicus was then closed with a single __-0 vicryl/ prolene/ PDS. The skin was closed at all the port sites with a/an ___-0 vicryl/ monocryl.*

The skin was cleaned and dried and then *dermabond/ steri-strips and gauze* were applied.

If a colostomy reversal was performed: *The fascia at the previous colostomy site was then closed with interrupted/ running/figure of eight ___-0 prolene sutures. The skin was then partially closed with a/an __-0 vicryl, leading a looped vessel loop through the base of the wound to allow for drainage.*

All counts were correct at the end of the case and the attending of record was present and scrubbed for *all/key* portions of the case.

Upon completion of the procedure, a debriefing checklist was completed to share information critical to the postoperative care of the patient. The patient tolerated the procedure well, *was extubated in the operating room*, and was transported to the postanesthesia care unit in stable condition.

Soave-Like Transanal Endorectal Pull-Through

38

Devin R. Halleran, Richard J. Wood, and Marc A. Levitt

Indications and Benefits

- Hirschsprung disease
- Benefits: Removal of diseased distal bowel in a fashion to minimize the risk for injury to the nerves of the pelvis

Risks and Alternatives

- Standard risks (bleeding, infection, need for additional procedures, risks of anesthesia)
- Injury to adjacent structures (anal sphincter, dentate line, prostate, urethra, vagina, nervi erigentes)
- Fecal, urinary, and sexual dysfunction
- Obstruction secondary to retained, re-fused, or rolled-up rectal cuff
- Transition zone pull-through
- Anastomotic stricture
- Twist of pull-through
- Alternatives: Swenson, Duhamel

D. R. Halleran · R. J. Wood · M. A. Levitt (✉)
Nationwide Children's Hospital, Center for Colorectal and Pelvic Reconstruction, Columbus, OH, USA
e-mail: marc.levitt@nationwidechildrens.org

Essential Steps

Combined Abdominal and Transanal Approach

1. Gain laparoscopic or open access to the abdominal cavity.
2. Perform full-thickness biopsy to determine the level of the normal ganglionic bowel.
3. Mobilize the descending and sigmoid colon from its peritoneal attachments.
4. Begin circumferential dissection down into the pelvis right at the bowel wall.
5. When intraabdominal dissection is complete place the patient in a legs up position.
6. Place Lone Star pins to hide dentate line.
7. Placement of circumferential interrupted silk sutures 1.0 cm proximal to dentate line.
8. Using electrocautery, start with submucosal dissection, dissecting the mucosa from the muscular layer, for a distance of approximately 1–2 cm.
9. Incise rectal muscle circumferentially, allowing for the remainder of the dissection to be performed in a full-thickness fashion along the bowel.
10. Pull through the rectum and sigmoid colon to 5 cm above the site of the ganglionic frozen section.
11. Placement of deep layer of sutures circumferentially at the resection margin from mus-

D. J. Papandria et al. (eds.), *Operative Dictations in Pediatric Surgery*,
https://doi.org/10.1007/978-3-030-24212-1_38

cle to colonic serosa, 1 cm proximal to dentate line.
12. Resection of aganglionic segment of rectum and colon.
13. Incision of the muscular cuff posteriorly.
14. Performing of second layer of anastomosis from mucosa to mucosa.

Transanal Approach Only

1. Placement of Lone Star pins to hide the dentate line.
2. Placement of circumferential interrupted silk sutures 1.0 cm proximal to dentate line.
3. Using electrocautery, start with submucosal dissection, dissecting the mucosa from the muscular layer, for a distance of approximately 1–2 cm.
4. Incision of rectal muscle circumferentially, allowing for the remainder of the dissection to be performed in a full-thickness fashion along the bowel.
5. Performing full-thickness biopsy to verify the level of normal ganglionic bowel.
6. Ligation of branches of the sigmoid mesentery transanally.
7. Pull-through of the rectum and sigmoid colon based on the frozen section.
8. Placement of deep layer of sutures circumferentially at the resection margin from muscle to colonic serosa, 1 cm proximal to dentate line.
9. Resection of aganglionic segment of rectum and colon.
10. Incision of the muscular cuff posteriorly.
11. Performance of a second layer of anastomosis from mucosa to mucosa.

Note These Variations

- Note that depending on the length of the segment of aganglionic bowel, an abdominal portion may be needed in addition to the transanal approach.

Template Operative Dictation

Preoperative Diagnosis Hirschsprung disease

Postoperative Diagnosis Same as preoperative diagnosis

Findings Same as postoperative diagnosis

Procedure(s) Performed Soave-like transanal endorectal pull-through

Anesthesia *General*

Specimen Rectal biopsy x __, *sigmoid colon*, and rectum.

Estimated Blood Loss ___

Indications This is a/an ___-*day/week/month/year*-old *male/female* with Hirschsprung disease. *The child underwent previous suction/full-thickness rectal biopsy which showed absence of ganglion cells and hypertrophic nerve cells. The child to this point has been managed with rectal irrigations. The prior contrast enema is compatible with a transition zone at the level of the rectosigmoid.* He/she was deemed to be a suitable candidate for Soave-like transanal endorectal pull-through.

Procedure in Detail Following satisfactory induction of anesthesia, the patient was placed in the *supine/prone* position and appropriately padded. Timeouts were performed using both preinduction and pre-incision safety checklists with participation of all present in the operative suite. These confirmed the correct patient, procedure, operative site, and additional critical information prior to the start of the procedure. *The ostomy (if one is present) was covered.* The child underwent a total body preparation and was then draped in the usual sterile fashion.

[Choose One]

If Laparoscopic abdominal dissection required: The patient was placed in the supine position. An incision was made through the umbilicus and carried down to the umbilical stalk where the fascia was incised, revealing the peritoneum, which was carefully opened so as to avoid causing injury to the underlying abdominal viscera. A *4-mm* port was placed and secured with a *3–0 silk* suture. The abdomen was then insufflated using CO_2. Additional *3-mm* incisions were then made in the *right upper quadrant, right lower quadrant,* and *left upper quadrant* through which we placed our additional ports under direct visualization.

If Open abdominal dissection required: The patient was placed in the supine position. An *infraumbilical/Pfannenstiel* incision was made and carried down to the umbilical stalk where the fascia was incised, revealing the peritoneum, which was carefully opened so as to avoid causing injury to the underlying abdominal viscera.

We identified the sigmoid colon and brought the bowel through our incision, and performed a full-thickness biopsy, which we sent to pathology for frozen section. We began to mobilize the splenic flexure, *which we continued down the white line of Toldt.* At this point, we were informed that our biopsy demonstrated normal ganglion cells with no evidence of hypertrophic nerves. *The sigmoid and distal descending colon was then separated from the left retroperitoneal attachements up to just distal to the splenic flexure. The arcade was preserved proximally to the level of the mid-descending colon.* This level of bowel reached the peritoneal reflection easily. The peritoneal reflection was then opened circumferentially and dissection along the bowel wall carried out to *approximately 2 cm* below the reflection.

We then focused our attention on the transanal portion of the procedure. With the patient still in the supine position, we placed the patient's legs up and examined the anus, which was noted to be in the correct anatomical position. The Lone Star retractor was then brought into the field and initially placed at the level of the mucocutaneous junction. Once this was accomplished, we then further retracted at the level of the dentate line circumferentially, so that the dentate line was no longer visible and therefore could not be damaged during the dissection. We then placed circumferential interrupted silk sutures, approximately 1.0 cm proximal to the dentate line, to provide uniform circumferential tension. We then utilized electrocautery to perform a mucosal incision above the dentate line with care to strip the mucosa from the underlying muscle. This was carried proximally for approximately *1–2 cm,* after which we incised the muscle layer circumferentially and proceed from that point with a full-thickness dissection. We took care throughout the dissection to stay right on the bowel to avoid injury to the pelvic nerves and vessels. Dissection then continued proximally until we met the distal portion of our abdominal dissection. At this point, we were able to enter the peritoneum, and we ligated *any remaining branches of the sigmoid mesentery transanally and we were able to pull through the rectum and sigmoid colon.* We decided to transect the bowel *5 cm* proximal to this to minimize the chance of pulling through a portion of the transition zone. We then incised the muscular cuff at the posterior aspect in an attempt to avoid an obstruction in the future. At this level, we placed a deep layer of sutures circumferentially at the level of the resection margin, from muscle to colonic serosa, which was once again 1.0 cm proximal to the dentate line. Once this was accomplished, the distal pulled through bowel was resected utilizing electrocautery and passed off the table as specimen. We then completed our second layer of the anastomosis at the level of the previous resection utilizing interrupted absorbable sutures from mucosa to mucosa.

If Transanal only: The patient was placed in the *prone* position. The anus was examined and noted to be in the correct anatomical position. The Lone Star retractor was then brought into the field and initially placed at the level of the mucocutaneous junction. Once this was accomplished, we then further retracted at the level of the dentate line circumferentially, so that the dentate line was no longer visible and therefore could not be damaged during the dissection. We then placed circumferential interrupted silk sutures, approximately 1.0 cm proximal to the dentate line, to provide uniform circumferential tension. We then utilized electrocautery to perform a mucosal incision above the dentate line with care to strip the mucosa from the underlying muscle. This was carried proximally for approximately *1 to 2 cm*, after which we incised the muscle layer circumferentially and proceed from that point with a full-thickness dissection. We took care throughout the dissection to stay right on the bowel to avoid injury to the pelvic nerves and vessels. At this point, we pulled the sigmoid colon forth and took a full-thickness biopsy which we sent to pathology. Dissection then continued proximally. Once we were able to enter the peritoneum, we ligated the *branches of the sigmoid mesentery transanally and we were able to pull through the rectum and sigmoid colon.* We were then informed that our prior biopsy contained normal ganglion cells without hypertrophic nerves. We decided to transect the bowel 5 cm proximal to this to minimize the chance of pulling through a portion of the transition zone. We then incised the muscular cuff at the posterior aspect in an attempt to avoid an obstruction in the future. At this level, we placed a deep layer of sutures circumferentially at the level of the resection margin, from muscle to colonic serosa, which was once again 1.0 cm proximal to the dentate line. Once this was accomplished, the distal pulled through bowel was resected utilizing electrocautery and passed off the table as specimen. We then completed our second layer of the anastomosis at the level of the previous resection utilizing interrupted absorbable sutures from mucosa to mucosa.

Upon completion of the procedure, a debriefing checklist was completed to share information critical to the postoperative care of the patient. The patient tolerated the procedure well, *was extubated in the operating room*, and was transported to the postanesthesia care unit in stable condition thereafter.

39 Laparoscopic Colonic Mapping

David Coyle and Karen A. Diefenbach

Indications and Benefits

- Hirschsprung's disease confirmed by rectal biopsy where the level of the transition zone has not been previously identified or where a transition zone proximal to the splenic flexure is suspected.
- Hirschsprung's disease confirmed by rectal biopsy where imaging suggests a recto-sigmoid transition zone, but there is poor decompression of the proximal colon despite washouts
- Benefits: Accurate localization of the transition zone prior to attempting a transanal approach for a pull-through procedure

Risks and Alternatives

- Standard risks (bleeding, infection, need for additional procedures, risks of anesthesia).
- Injury to adjacent structures (small bowel, spleen).
- Leak from enterotomy repair.
- False positive/negative biopsy, inadequate biopsy specimen.

D. Coyle (✉)
Nationwide Children's Hospital, Division of Pediatric Surgery, Columbus, OH, USA
e-mail: David.coyle@nationwidechildrens.org

K. A. Diefenbach (✉)
Nationwide Children's Hospital, Columbus, OH, USA
e-mail: Karen.Diefenbach@nationwidechildrens.org

- Alternatives: A transanal approach for pull-through surgery with frozen section leveling biopsies performed as the colon is delivered with open or laparoscopic assistance to mobilize the colon as required.

Essential Steps

Open Colonic Mapping

1. While seromuscular biopsies allow assessment of the myenteric plexus and avoid the risk of spillage of colonic contents, full-thickness biopsies additionally facilitate histological assessment of the submucosal plexus where nerve trunk hypertrophy can be observed.
2. Ensure that biopsies are taken proximal to a grossly visible transition zone. Where none is obvious, then the sigmoid colon, splenic flexure, and transverse colon can be biopsied next.
3. A biopsy of the terminal ileum is indicated if histopathological inspection of a frozen section biopsy proximal to the transverse colon is not normal. *Do not* biopsy the appendix, as this is not a reliable indicator of involvement of the right colon and may lead to unnecessary resection of a valuable portion of the colon.
4. Ensure that information regarding both the presence of ganglion cells *and* nerve size in the biopsy specimens is obtained before completion of the procedure.

D. J. Papandria et al. (eds.), *Operative Dictations in Pediatric Surgery*,
https://doi.org/10.1007/978-3-030-24212-1_39

Laparoscopic Colonic Mapping

1. The minimally invasive approach follows the same principles as the open operation.
2. Primary access is through a transverse umbilical incision, through which the colon above the transition zone to be biopsied is exteriorized with assistance from a single working port, usually in the right lower quadrant to best approach the left and transverse colon. However, if extensive/total colonic mapping is indicated, additional laparoscopic ports and intracorporeal biopsies are useful. These port sites can continue to be used if it is decided to proceed directly to a pull-through operation.

Note These Variations

- In some patients, for example, those in whom Hirschsprung's disease first presented with cecal perforation, an ileostomy may already be present and needs to be avoided in placement of a working port.
- If intraoperative frozen section analysis of the colonic biopsies indicates abnormal innervation at or proximal to the splenic flexure, a diverting ileostomy should be performed and pull-through surgery delayed pending permanent section histology and to allow growth and maturation of colonic blood supply, specifically, the right marginal artery.

Template Operative Dictation for Colonic Mapping

Preoperative Diagnosis Hirschsprung's disease

Postoperative Diagnosis Same as preoperative diagnosis

Findings Biopsy at ___ colon: Positive for ganglion cells

Transition point seen at ___ *colon/splenic flexure/hepatic flexure*

Ileostomy sized to Hegar size ___

Procedure(s) Performed *Laparoscopic* Colonic Mapping for Hirschsprung's disease

Anesthesia General Anesthesia

Specimen(s) *Full-thickness/seromuscular* colonic biopsies taken at ___ (include all levels).

Drains None

Implants None

Estimated Blood Loss Minimal

Indications This is a/an ___*-day/week/month/year*-old *male/female* with biopsy-confirmed Hirschsprung's disease. *He/she* was deemed to be a suitable candidate for laparoscopic colonic mapping.

Procedure in Detail Following satisfactory induction of anesthesia, the patient was placed in supine position and appropriately padded. Timeouts were performed using both preinduction and preincision safety checklists with participation of all present in the operative suite. These confirmed the correct patient, procedure, operative site, and additional critical information prior to the start of the procedure. The patient was placed in the supine position and was prepped and draped in the standard surgical fashion.

[Choose One]

For open approach: The abdominal cavity was entered through an *upper/lower* abdominal *transverse/oblique/midline* incision.

For laparoscopic approach: A/an ___-mm incision was made at the level of the umbilicus and the peritoneal cavity entered. A/an ___*-mm port/Veress needle* was placed through this incision and the abdomen insufflated to a pressure of ___ mmHg. A second ___-mm port was placed under direct vision in the right lower quadrant.

{Continue dictation}

[Choose One]

If transition zone noted: The colon was inspected and a suspected transition zone noted in the *sig-*

moid/descending/distal transverse colon. This part of the colon was mobilized and a biopsy site was chosen proximal to the suspected transition zone.

If no transition zone noted: The colon was inspected and no transition zone was noted. Therefore, the first biopsy was taken in the sigmoid colon.

{Continue dictation}

A/an __-cm *seromuscular/full-thickness* biopsy transverse elliptical biopsy was excised using sharp dissection from the antimesenteric border of colon and handed off the operating table to go for frozen section histological inspection. The defect was closed in *one/two* layers using ___-0 Vicryl suture. Each biopsy was evaluated for the presence of ganglion cells and normal nerve trunks. This procedure was repeated until *a normal appearing biopsy was identified/ the entire colon and the terminal ileum had been biopsied.*

If performing a diverting ileostomy at this procedure:

{Continue dictation}

As a result of *extensive/total colonic involvement/failure to thrive/the need to wait for final pathologic evaluation of the specimens*, the decision was made to proceed with diverting ileostomy. The terminal ileum was identified and a site at least 10 cm proximal to ileocecal valve was chosen to bring up as an ileostomy. This segment of bowel was divided using *a(n) EndoGIA stapler/GIA stapler/___* and the distal limb was tacked to the proximal small bowel approximately 8 cm proximal to the staple line. *An incision was made in the right lower quadrant/the right lower quadrant port site was extended* to allow formation of the ileostomy and the proximal ileum was brought up through this incision. The ileum was tacked to the fascia with interrupted ___-0 Vicryl sutures.

[Choose One]

If open: The incision was then closed using *interrupted/running ___-0 Vicryl/PDS/___* suture(s) to close fascia and a running subcuticular ___-0 ___ suture to close the skin.

If laparoscopic: The abdomen was then deflated and the ports removed. The fascia at the umbilical incision was closed using ___-0 Vicryl. *The fascia at the other port site(s) was closed using ___-0 Vicryl suture.* The skin at all incisions was closed using a ___-0 Monocryl subcuticular suture.

{Continue dictation}

If doing an ileostomy: The staple line was then resected from the end ileostomy and it was then matured in the standard Brooke fashion using *___-0 Vicryl sutures.* Enough redundancy was allowed to give an approximately 1 cm area of Brooking above our skin level. A stoma bag appliance was placed over the stoma.

Dressings were placed. The sponge and instrument count was correct at the end of the case. Upon completion of the procedure, a debriefing checklist was completed to share information critical to the postoperative care of the patient. The patient tolerated the procedure well, *was extubated in the operating room*, and was transported to the postanesthesia care unit in stable condition thereafter.

Laparoscopic Leveling Colostomy for Colonic Aganglionosis

40

David Coyle and Karen A. Diefenbach

Indications and Benefits

- Confirmed or suspected Hirschsprung-associated enterocolitis not responsive to non-operative measures or severe/life-threatening enterocolitis as a first presentation of Hirschsprung's disease.
- Confirmed Hirschsprung's disease with excessively distended colon despite rectal irrigations and thus not suitable for primary pull-through.
- Benefits: Provides a safe way to decompress the colon without the added morbidity of an ileostomy; Once the patient is appropriately leveled colon brought up for the colostomy is all that needs to be pulled through for the colo-anal anastomosis.

Risks and Alternatives

- Standard risks (bleeding, infection, need for additional procedures, risks of anesthesia)
- Injury to adjacent structures (spleen, liver, small bowel, ureter)
- Colostomy retraction or prolapse
- Parastomal hernia
- Maturation of colostomy in aganglionic or transition zone bowel.
- Alternatives: Diverting ileostomy

Essential Steps

Access

1. A supraumbilical transverse laparotomy should provide access to the entire colon in an infant, which is the typical age range for this procedure to be performed if performing it open.
2. Dilated colon can add difficulty in this operation when performed as a minimally invasive procedure. If possible, one of the working ports should be placed at the site of the future colostomy, which may be determined on initial inspection for the location of the transition zone.

Biopsy and Choice of Colostomy Site

1. Biopsies may be full thickness or seromuscular. Seromuscular biopsies preclude visualization of the submucosal nerve plexus where hypertrophic nerve trunks may be observed but limit contamination, which may be of particular benefit when performing the biopsies intra-corporeally.

D. Coyle (✉)
Nationwide Children's Hospital, Division of Pediatric Surgery, Columbus, OH, USA
e-mail: David.coyle@nationwidechildrens.org

K. A. Diefenbach (✉)
Nationwide Children's Hospital, Columbus, OH, USA
e-mail: Karen.Diefenbach@nationwidechildrens.org

D. J. Papandria et al. (eds.), *Operative Dictations in Pediatric Surgery*,
https://doi.org/10.1007/978-3-030-24212-1_40

2. The colostomy is brought up at the site of biopsy with confirmed presence of ganglion cells. It is important that the colostomy is well tacked to the fascia to reduce the risk of prolapse in dilated bowel, especially if it is transverse colon.

Note These Variations

- In patients in whom leveling biopsy frozen section analysis is abnormal proximal to the splenic flexure, consideration should always be given to mapping the remaining colon and carrying out a diverting ileostomy, as correct interpretation of frozen section biopsies at this level can be challenging and so further decision-making is often best served by waiting on permanent section histology.

Template Operative Dictation (Open)

Preoperative Diagnosis [Choose one] *Hirschsprung's disease/Hirschsprung-associated enterocolitis*

Postoperative Diagnosis Same as preoperative diagnosis

Findings Same as postoperative diagnosis

Procedure(s) Performed Laparoscopic leveling colostomy for colonic aganglionosis

Anesthesia General anesthesia

Specimen ___ colonic biopsies taken from ___ (list all sites).

Drains None

Implants None

Estimated Blood Loss ___ mL

Indications This is a/an ___*-day/week/month/year*-old *male/female* with *Hirschsprung's disease/Severe Hirschsprung-associated enterocolitis/suspected severe Hirschsprung-associated enterocolitis*. Due to the *colonic dilatation not responsive to rectal irrigations/severe Hirschsprung-associated enterocolitis not responsive to nonoperative therapy*, he/she was deemed to be a suitable candidate for laparoscopic leveling colostomy for colonic aganglionosis.

Procedure in Detail Following satisfactory induction of anesthesia, the patient was placed in supine position and appropriately padded. Timeouts were performed using both preinduction and preincision safety checklists with participation of all present in the operative suite. These confirmed the correct patient, procedure, operative site, and additional critical information prior to the start of the procedure. The abdomen was then prepped and draped in the usual sterile fashion.

A/an ___-cm transverse incision was placed in the left *upper/lower* quadrant. The incision was deepened to fascia and through to peritoneum using electrocautery for hemostasis. The peritoneum was entered and opened the full length of the incision. The visible transition zone was identified at the level of the *sigmoid/descending/transverse/ascending colon* and a/an ___-mm *seromuscular/full-thickness* biopsy was excised sharply from the antimesenteric border of colon and handed off the operating table to go for frozen section histological inspection. The defect was closed in *one/two* layers using ___-0 ___ suture. An additional biopsy was taken proximal to the dilated segment just above the transition zone and closed in the same manner. This procedure was repeated until the frozen section histology demonstrated the presence of ganglion cells in the absence of hypertrophic nerve trunks. The biopsy site first identified as meeting these criteria was selected to be brought out as a leveling colostomy.

[Choose One]
If divided colostomy: The bowel was divided at this biopsy site using a/an ___ stapler load and the

proximal end brought up *at the medial/lateral end of the incision/through a separate ___-cm incision placed in the right/left upper/lower quadrant*. This segment was tacked to the fascia of the anterior abdominal wall. The distal segment was tacked to the side wall of the proximal segment for ease in dissection at the next staged operation. The remaining laparotomy wound was then closed in layers using ___-0 ____ sutures to close fascia and ___-0 ___ sutures to close the skin. The stapler line was then resected and the stoma matured using interrupted ___-0 ___ sutures.

If loop colostomy: The bowel at this biopsy site was brought up *at the medial/lateral end of the incision/through a separate ___ cm incision placed in the right/left upper/lower quadrant* and secured to the fascia using interrupted ___-0 ___ sutures. The remaining laparotomy wound was then closed in layers using ___-0 ____ sutures to close fascia and ___-0 ___ sutures to close the skin. The colostomy loop was opened using *cautery/sharp scissors* along its antimesenteric border. A loop colostomy was matured in the Brooke style using ___-0 ___ sutures with sufficient redundancy to allow a 1 cm area of Brooking above the level of the skin. *The distal limb of the colostomy was partially closed using a 3–0 prolene/nylon purse-string suture to limit distal spillover of fecal content.* A stoma bag appliance was placed over the stoma *and wounds were dressed with ___.*

The sponge and instrument count was correct at the end of the case. Upon completion of the procedure, a debriefing checklist was completed to share information critical to the postoperative care of the patient. The patient tolerated the procedure well, *was extubated in the operating room,* and was transported to the postanesthesia care unit in stable condition thereafter.

Template Operative Dictation (Laparoscopic)

Preoperative Diagnosis [**Choose one**] *Hirschsprung's disease/Hirschsprung-associated enterocolitis*

Postoperative Diagnosis Same as preoperative diagnosis

Findings Same as postoperative diagnosis

Procedure(s) Performed Laparoscopic leveling colostomy for colonic aganglionosis

Anesthesia General anesthesia

Specimen ___ colonic biopsies taken from ___ (list all sites).

Drains None

Implants None

Estimated Blood Loss ___ mL

Indications This is a/an ___*-day/week/month/year*-old *male/female* with *Hirschsprung's disease/Severe Hirschsprung-associated enterocolitis/Suspected severe Hirschsprung-associated enterocolitis*. Due to the *colonic dilatation not responsive to rectal irrigations/severe Hirschsprung-associated enterocolitis not responsive to nonoperative therapy*, he/she was deemed to be a suitable candidate for laparoscopic leveling colostomy for colonic aganglionosis.

Procedure in Detail Following satisfactory induction of anesthesia, the patient was placed in supine position and appropriately padded. Timeouts were performed using both preinduction and preincision safety checklists with participation of all present in the operative suite. These confirmed the correct patient, procedure, operative site, and additional critical information prior to the start of the procedure. The abdomen was then prepped and draped in the usual sterile fashion.

A ___ port was placed at the level of the umbilicus being careful to avoid the umbilical vessels. The peritoneum was safely entered and the abdomen was insufflated to a pressure of ___ mmHg. Two additional ports were placed, one in the right lower quadrant and one in the left upper quadrant. The visible transition zone was identified at the level of the *sigmoid/descending/transverse/ ascending colon* and a/an ___-mm *seromuscular/ full-thickness* biopsy was excised sharply from the antimesenteric border of colon and handed off the operating table to go for frozen section histological inspection. The defect was closed in *one/two* layers using ___-0 ___ suture. An additional biopsy was taken proximal to the dilated segment just above the transition zone and closed in the same manner. This procedure was repeated until the frozen section histology demonstrated the presence of ganglion cells in the absence of hypertrophic nerve trunks. The biopsy site first identified as meeting these criteria was selected to be brought out as a leveling colostomy. A/an ___-cm incision was made at the site selected for the stoma and extended into the peritoneal cavity and the biopsy site was brought up through this incision.

[Choose One]

If divided colostomy: The bowel was divided at this biopsy site using a ___ stapler load. The distal bowel was tacked to the proximal bowel at least 5 cm proximal to the staple line. The proximal end was brought up through this incision and was tacked to the fascia of the anterior abdominal wall. The ports were removed and the fascia at each incision was closed using ___-0 ___ sutures and ___-0 ___ sutures to close the skin. The stapler line was then resected and the stoma was matured using interrupted ___-0 ___ sutures.

If loop colostomy: The bowel at this biopsy site was secured to the fascia using interrupted ___-0 ___sutures. The ports were removed and the fascia at each incision was closed using ___-0 ___ sutures and ___-0 ___ sutures to close the skin. The colostomy loop was opened using *cautery/ sharp scissors* along its antimesenteric border. A loop colostomy was matured in the Brooke style using ___-0 ___ sutures with sufficient redundancy to allow a 1 cm area of Brooking above the level of the skin. *The distal limb of the colostomy was partially closed using a 3–0 prolene/nylon purse-string suture to limit distal spillover of fecal content.* A stoma bag appliance was placed over the stoma *and wounds were dressed with* ___.

The sponge and instrument count was correct at the end of the case. Upon completion of the procedure, a debriefing checklist was completed to share information critical to the postoperative care of the patient. The patient tolerated the procedure well, *was extubated in the operating room*, and was transported to the postanesthesia care unit in stable condition thereafter.

Posterior Sagittal Anorectoplasty: Male

41

Rebecca M. Rentea, Richard J. Wood, and Marc A. Levitt

Indications and Benefits

- Indication: Anorectal malformation
- Benefits: Creation of adequately sized anus, separation of distal rectum from urinary tract (congenital fistula) and anatomic optimization for future continence

Risks and Alternatives

- Standard risks (bleeding, infection, need for additional procedures, risks of anesthesia)
- Rectal injury
- Stenosis/stricture of rectum
- Retention of remnant of original fistula
- Injury to urethra
- Injury to prostate
- Injury to bladder, bladder neck
- Injury to surrounding structures, that is, ureter, seminal vesicles, vas deferens
- Mislocation of anus
- Breakdown of posterior sagittal incision
- Rectourethral fistula (recurrent, acquired, or persistent fistula)
- Alternatives: colostomy with mucous fistula

Essential Steps

1. Identification of fistula
2. Stimulation of muscle complex-mark anterior and posterior limits
3. Posterior sagittal incision
4. Separate fistula/rectum from urethra, prostate, bladder neck
5. Stimulate muscle complex again to determine site of anoplasty
6. Anoplasty

Subsection 2

1. Subsection Step 1
2. Subsection Step 2

Note These Variations

- Laparoscopic mobilization of fistula inserting into bladder, bladder neck, or high into prostate

R. M. Rentea (✉)
Children's Mercy, University of Missouri -Kansas City, Department of Pediatric Surgery, Kansas City, MO, USA
e-mail: rrentea@cmh.edu

R. J. Wood · M. A. Levitt
Nationwide Children's Hospital, Center for Colorectal and Pelvic Reconstruction, Columbus, OH, USA

D. J. Papandria et al. (eds.), *Operative Dictations in Pediatric Surgery*, https://doi.org/10.1007/978-3-030-24212-1_41

Operative Dictation

Preoperative Diagnosis Anorectal malformation

Postoperative Diagnosis Same as preoperative diagnosis

Findings Same as postoperative diagnosis

Procedure(s) Performed Posterior sagittal anorectoplasty (including laparoscopic ligation of __fistula)

Anesthesia *General*

Indications This is a/an ___-day/week/month/year-old male with anorectal malformation. He was/was not previously diverted with a colostomy/mucous fistula and following high pressure distal colostogram demonstrating a ____-fistula, was deemed to be a suitable candidate for posterior sagittal anorectoplasty (including laparoscopic ligation of __fistula).

Procedure in Detail Following satisfactory induction of anesthesia, the patient was placed in the supine position and appropriately padded. Timeouts were performed using both preinduction and preincision safety checklists with participation of all present in the operative suite. These confirmed the correct patient, procedure, operative site, and additional critical information prior to the start of the procedure.

A Coude Foley catheter was passed into the bladder. The perineum (and lower abdomen if appropriate) was then prepped and draped in the usual sterile fashion.

[Choose One]

If Perineal Fistula: Inspection of the perineum revealed the distal rectum ending as a tiny hole anterior to the sphincter mechanism, consistent with a rectoperineal fistula. The patient was placed in the prone position to begin the repair. Multiple silk sutures were placed in the mucocutaneous junction of the fistula.

If no Fistula or Recto Urethral Fistula at Bulbar or Low Prostatic Level: Inspection of the perineum revealed no fistula, and distal colostogram confirmed this. The patient was placed supine on the operating room table. A posterior midline incision was created, staying perfectly in the midline, and divided the skin, subcutaneous tissue, parasagittal fibers, and muscle complex. The bulge of the rectal wall was encountered in the midline in the area of the bulbar urethra. The posterior rectal wall was opened and multiple silk stitches were placed in it to provide ease in obtaining circumferential mobilization. There was no rectourethral fistula. The lateral rectal walls were mobilized laterally and then anteriorly, taking great care to shave the rectum off of the posterior urethra which lies below. The rectum was mobilized until it reached the perineum.

A posterior sagittal incision was then made through the skin and subcutaneous tissues. The sphincter mechanism was easily delineated a pink ellipse in the skin and we went directly through this, delineating the entire posterior wall of the rectum, noting a whitish fascia surrounding it. Dissection was performed laterally to define the lateral plane and then began to come circumferentially around the sutures. The rectum was then lifted superiorly and the common wall between the rectum and urethra were dissected. The rectum was completely separated from the posterior wall of the urethra until the areolar tissue was reached defining the two separate walls. Dissection of the attachments to the rectum was performed to gain adequate length of rectum to allow the anoplasty to reach the perineum without tension. There was approximately 1–2 cm of fistula distal to the normal rectal tissue. The perineal body was closed utilizing multiple layers of long-term absorbable sutures up to the anterior limit of the sphincter mechanism. Tension was then placed on the rectum and Vicryl sutures were used to tack the rectum to the posterior edge of the muscle complex all the way to the level of the levator up to the level of the skin. The reconstruction of the posterior sagittal incision was performed by reapproximating the ischiorectal fat and parasagittal fibers. The skin was closed with interrupted Vicryl sutures. The anoplasty was performed utilizing multiple interrupted Vicryl sutures. A __# Hegar dilator was able to pass straight and easily into the rectum. The rectum was healthy and viable at the anoplasty and inverted nicely after cutting of the sutures.

Preoperative high pressure distal colostogram revealed a rectoprostatic/rectobulbar/rectobladder neck fistula. [Only for high prostatic or bladder neck]. (The patient then underwent a total body preparation so that we could enter the abdomen easily if necessary.) A Foley catheter was passed into the bladder. The operation was begun in the prone position for the posterior sagittal approach.

[Choose One]

If Prostatic Fistula: We began the operation in prone position for the posterior sagittal approach, with careful padding. We made a pure midline posterior sagittal incision, staying perfectly in the midline, and divided the skin, subcutaneous tissue, parasagittal fibers, and muscle complex, all the way down until we identified the coccyx and the area just beneath it and we began to look for the rectum. We placed silk sutures in this area to mobilize this tissue forward until we were able to visualize what appeared like rectal tissue. We then placed silk sutures in this and divided it in the midline. We then placed multiple silk stitches for mobilization in the rectal wall. We then identified, inferior to this, the rectourethral fistula at the prostatic level, placing a lacrimal duct probe in it. We placed silk sutures proximal to this fistula, and then carefully dissected the rectal wall off of the posterior urethra, taking special care to define the lateral walls first before beginning the anterior dissection. We then began a circumferential mobilization of the rectum taking all attachments and dissecting within the white fascia that envelopes the rectum, preserving the intramural blood supply. We mobilized the rectum until it reached the perineum.

There was approximately 1–2 cm of fistula distal to the normal rectal tissue. The perineal body was closed utilizing multiple layers of long-term absorbable sutures. The skin was closed with interrupted sutures at the skin level up to the anterior limit of the sphincter mechanism. Tension was then placed on the rectum and Vicryl sutures were used to tack the rectum to the posterior edge of the muscle complex all the way to the level of the levator and up to the level of the skin. The reconstruction of the posterior sagittal incision was performed by reapproximating the ischiorectal fat and parasagittal fibers. The skin was closed with interrupted Vicryl sutures. The anoplasty was performed utilizing multiple interrupted Vicryl sutures with excision of the very distal fistulous tissue. The very distal fistulous tissue was excised. A __# Hegar dilator was able to pass straight and easily into the rectum. The rectum was healthy and viable at the anoplasty and inverted nicely after cutting of the sutures.

If Rectobulbar Fistula: We made a pure midline posterior sagittal incision, staying perfectly in the midline, and divided the skin, subcutaneous tissue, parasagittal fibers, and muscle complex. Visible in the center of the incision was the posterior rectal wall. We identified the true rectal wall into which we placed multiple silk stitches for mobilization. We then identified interior to this, after the posterior rectal wall was opened, the rectourethral fistula at the bulbar urethral level. We mobilized the rectum, first with dissection along the lateral wall, and then medially dissecting it off the posterior urethra. We took the attached bands, keeping the rectal wall intact and thus preserving its intramural blood supply. We continued this mobilization until the rectum reached the perineum.

There was approximately 1–2 cm of fistula distal to the normal rectal tissue. The perineal body was closed utilizing multiple layers of long-term absorbable sutures. The skin was closed with interrupted sutures at the skin level up to the anterior limit of the sphincter mechanism. Tension was then placed on the rectum and Vicryl sutures were used to tack the rectum to the posterior edge of the muscle complex all the way to the level of the levators and up to the level of the skin. The reconstruction of the posterior sagittal incision was performed by reapproximating the ischiorectal fat and parasagittal fibers. The skin was closed with interrupted 400 Vicryl sutures. The anoplasty was performed utilizing multiple interrupted Vicryl sutures. A __# Hegar dilator was able to pass straight and easily into the rectum. The rectum was healthy and viable at the anoplasty and inverted nicely after cutting of the sutures.

If Rectobladder Neck: The patient is placed supine. Laparoscopically or through a lower midline laparotomy was performed to find the distal rectum which was connected to the bladder neck. We successfully mobilized it. This required extensive delicate dissection of the small blood vessels to the distal rectum, relying on its intramural blood supply, and we were able to get the rectum to reach. We needed to (or did not need to) take down the mucous fistula. We were able to delineate the rectum's insertion into the bladder neck. We stayed intimately next to the rectum for our dissection, identified the vas deferens and preserved them and continued our dissection down until the rectum ended in essentially a point at the bladder neck. Here, we placed a single PDS Endoloop to take care of the fistula, and thus ad a mobile piece of rectum, its blood supply dependent on the inferior mesenteric artery (IMA). We opened via a small perineal incision remaining in supine position with legs up staying perfectly in the midline. The sphincter mechanism in such patients is often quite anterior and near the base of the scrotum. We palpated through the small perineal incision behind the pubis and anterior to the sacrum, defining the pathway through which the rectum would be passed. We then grasped the rectum and pulled it through and it reached for our anoplasty without difficulty.

There was approximately 1–2 cm of fistula distal to the normal rectal tissue. Tension was then placed on the rectum and Vicryl sutures were used to tack the rectum to the posterior edge of the muscle complex through the small perineal incision. The anoplasty was performed utilizing multiple interrupted Vicryl sutures. A __#Hegar dilator was able to pass straight and easily into the rectum. The rectum was healthy and viable at the anoplasty and inverted nicely after cutting of the sutures. The few millimeters of posterior sagittal incision was closed with interrupted Vicryl.

Upon completion of the procedure, a debriefing checklist was completed to share information critical to the postoperative care of the patient. The patient tolerated the procedure well, was extubated in the operating room, and was transported to the postanesthesia care unit in stable condition thereafter.

Posterior Sagittal Anorectoplasty: Female

42

Rebecca M. Rentea, Richard J. Wood, and Marc A. Levitt

Indications and Benefits

- Anorectal malformation
- Benefits: creation of perineal body, adequately sized anus, anatomic optimization for future continence

Risks and Alternatives

- Standard risks (bleeding, infection, need for additional procedures, and risks of anesthesia)
- Rectal injury
- Stenosis/stricture of rectum
- Injury to vagina
- Injury to surrounding structures
- Mislocation of anus
- Breakdown of perineal body
- Rectovaginal fistula
- Wound dehiscence
- Alternatives: Colostomy with mucous fistula

Essential Steps

1. Identification of fistula
2. Stimulation of muscle complex – mark anterior and posterior limits
3. Place sutures circumferentially at mucocutaneous junction of fistula
4. Posterior sagittal incision
5. Separate fistula/rectum from vagina
6. Stimulate sphincter complex again to determine site of anoplasty
7. Reconstruction of perineal body
8. Anoplasty

Note These Variations

- Use of laparoscopy/abdominal approach for rectovaginal fistulas

Operative Dictation

Preoperative Diagnosis Anorectal malformation

Findings Same as postoperative diagnosis

R. M. Rentea (✉)
Children's Mercy, University of Missouri -Kansas City, Department of Pediatric Surgery, Kansas City, MO, USA
e-mail: rrentea@cmh.edu

R. J. Wood · M. A. Levitt
Nationwide Children's Hospital, Center for Colorectal and Pelvic Reconstruction, Columbus, OH, USA

D. J. Papandria et al. (eds.), *Operative Dictations in Pediatric Surgery*,
https://doi.org/10.1007/978-3-030-24212-1_42

Procedure(s) Performed Posterior sagittal anorectoplasty – female

Anesthesia *General*

Indications This is a/an ___-day/week/month/year-old female with an anorectal malformation specifically *[anorectal malformation defect]*. She was deemed to be a suitable candidate for posterior sagittal anorectoplasty – female.

Procedure in Detail Following satisfactory induction of anesthesia, the patient was placed in prone position and appropriately padded. Timeouts were performed using both preinduction and preincision safety checklists with participation of all present in the operative suite. These confirmed the correct patient, procedure, operative site, and additional critical information prior to the start of the procedure. A Foley catheter was passed into the bladder. The perineum was then prepped and draped in the usual sterile fashion.

Inspection of the perineum revealed the urethra and vagina to be normal. (*A cystoscope was utilized to delineate the urethra, which was normal. She also had a normal bladder neck that contracted well, with normal bladder mucosa). Passage of the scope into the introitus demonstrated a normal vaginal lumen, no vaginal septum, and a normal appearing single cervix.* Prior to the administration of paralytic anesthetic agent, a muscle stimulator was utilized to delineate the sphincter mechanism. The anterior and posterior limits of the sphincter mechanism were then marked.

[Choose One]

If Rectovesibular Defect: Inspection of the perineum revealed the distal rectum to be in the vestibule. After completion of the cystoscopy, the patient was placed in the prone position to begin the repair. Multiple silk sutures were placed at the mucocutaneous junction of the rectum, which was in the vestibule of the vagina.

If Rectoperineal: Inspection of the perineum revealed the distal rectum ending as a tiny hole at the anterior aspect of the sphincter mechanism, consistent with a rectoperineal fistula. The patient was placed in the prone position to begin the repair. Multiple silk sutures were placed in the mucocutaneous junction of the fistula.

If no Fistula Defect: Inspection of the perineum revealed no fistula. The urethra and vagina were normal. The patient was placed in the prone position to begin the repair. The bulge of the rectal wall was encountered in the area of the posterior vagina. We opened the posterior rectal wall and placed multiple silk stitches in it for mobilization. We continued to open the posterior rectal wall in its midline moving anteriorly. Multiple silk sutures were placed across the most anterior rectal wall. There was no rectovaginal fistula. The lateral rectal walls were mobilized anteriorly taking care to shave the rectum off the posterior vagina.

If Rectovaginal: Inspection of the perineum revealed a rectovaginal fistula – the urethra was visible anterior, and the vagina had a septum (or no septum) through which the rectovaginal fistula was visible. A circumferential body prep from her nipples to toes was performed in the usual sterile fashion. We began the operation prone with a long posterior sagittal incision staying within the midline. This incision was carried down perfectly in the midline splitting the parasagittal fibers, ischiorectal fat, muscle complex, and levators. This dissection was carried down until the *single vagina or two hemivaginas* were visualized.

If Two Hemivaginas: The two hemivaginas were both opened up posteriorly and the septum was resected.

Since the vagina shared a common wall with the urethra, this was not dissected. A single vaginal orifice was created utilizing interrupted Vicryl sutures. If rectum reached from below, the operation proceeded like for a vestibular fistula. If rectovaginal fistula is higher, then the patient was then placed in the supine on the operating room table and a diagnostic laparoscopy was performed. Utilizing hook cautery and blunt dissection, the rectovaginal fistula was isolated and divided at its insertion into the vagina. The rectum was then carefully mobilized until it could be brought down into the muscle complex (which had been previously stimulated and marked) under direct laparoscopic visualization. The colonic/rectal orientation was again confirmed laparoscopically and the ports were removed, and port sites closed. The sphincter complex was stimulated and incised enough to pull-through the rectum under direct visualization and performed the anoplasty.

If no Laparoscopy was Performed: A posterior sagittal incision was then made through the skin and subcutaneous tissues.

The sphincter mechanism was easily delineated with a pink ellipse and we went directly through this, delineating the entire posterior wall of the rectum, noting a whitish fascia surrounding it. Dissection was performed laterally to define the lateral plane and then began to come circumferentially around the sutures. The rectum was then lifted superiorly and the common wall between the rectum and vagina was dissected. The rectum was completely separated from the posterior wall of the vagina until a typical areolar tissue reached which defines the two separate walls. Dissection of the attachments to the rectum was performed to gain adequate length of rectum to allow the anoplasty to reach the perineum without tension. There was approximately 1–2 cm of fistula distal to the normal rectal tissue. The perineal body was closed utilizing multiple layers of long-term absorbable sutures. The skin was closed with interrupted sutures at the skin level up to the anterior limit of the sphincter mechanism. Tension was then placed on the rectum and Vicryl sutures were used to tack the rectum to the posterior edge of the muscle complex all the way to the level of the levators and up to the level of the skin. The reconstruction of the posterior sagittal incision was performed by reapproximating the ischiorectal fat and parasagittal fibers. The skin was closed with interrupted Vicryl sutures. The anoplasty was performed utilizing multiple interrupted Vicryl sutures. A __# Hagar dilator was able to pass straight and easily into the rectum. The rectum was healthy and viable at the anoplasty, and inverted nicely after cutting of the sutures.

Upon completion of the procedure, a debriefing checklist was completed to share information critical to the postoperative care of the patient. The patient tolerated the procedure well, *was extubated in the operating room*, and was transported to the postanesthesia care unit in stable condition thereafter.

Cloacal Reconstruction with Total Urogenital Mobilization

43

Rebecca M. Rentea, Richard J. Wood,
and Marc A. Levitt

Indications and Benefits

- Indication: Cloaca
- Benefits: Separation of colorectal and urogenital tract

Risks and Alternatives

- Standard risks (bleeding, infection, need for additional procedures, and risks of anesthesia).
- Injury to adjacent structures rectum, vagina, urethra.
- Urethrovaginal fistula.
- Persistent urogenital sinus.
- Remnant of original fistula.
- Length of native vagina inadequate to reach perineum.
- Vaginal stenosis.

R. M. Rentea (✉)
Children's Mercy, University of Missouri -Kansas City, Department of Pediatric Surgery, Kansas City, MO, USA
e-mail: rrentea@cmh.edu

R. J. Wood · M. A. Levitt (✉)
Nationwide Children's Hospital, Center for Colorectal and Pelvic Reconstruction, Columbus, OH, USA
e-mail: Richard.wood@nationwidechildrens.org; marc.levitt@nationwidechildrens.org

Essential Steps

Insert Subsection Titles in Bold Italic as Needed (or omit for simple procedures)

1. Definition of cloacal anatomy by endoscopy and cloacagram
2. Posterior sagittal approach
3. Mobilization of the rectum and separation of it from the posterior vagina
4. Mobilization of the urogenital complex as a unit including incising of the suspensory ligaments of the urethra
5. Urethroplasty
6. Introitoplasty
7. Rectoplasty
8. Closure of the posterior sagittal incision

Operative Dictation

Preoperative Diagnosis Cloaca

Postoperative Diagnosis Same as preoperative diagnosis

Findings Same as postoperative diagnosis

Procedure(s) Performed Cloacal reconstruction

Indications This is a/an ___-*day/week/month/year*-old female with *long/short* channel cloaca.

D. J. Papandria et al. (eds.), *Operative Dictations in Pediatric Surgery*,
https://doi.org/10.1007/978-3-030-24212-1_43

She was deemed to be a suitable candidate for cloacal reconstruction.

Procedure in Detail Following satisfactory induction of anesthesia, the patient was placed in the supine position and appropriately padded. Timeouts were performed using both preinduction and preincision safety checklists with participation of all present in the operative suite. These confirmed the correct patient, procedure, operative site, and additional critical information prior to the start of the procedure. A total body prep was performed in the usual sterile fashion.

The perineum was carefully inspected noting an anorectal malformation with a single perineal orifice, describing a cloacal malformation. Utilizing electrical stimulation, a well-defined sphincter mechanism, also represented by a pinkish ellipse where the sphincter belonged, was visualized and marked. The patient was placed prone. A long posterior sagittal incision was performed staying within the midline. The posterior sagittal incision was carried down in the midline-splitting the parasagittal fibers, muscle complex, and levator muscles. This incision was opened down to the level of the perineum, including the entire common channel. The orifice of the rectum was clearly identified. Multiple silk sutures were placed to provide uniform traction to the rectum. The rectum was dissected to define the lateral plane. Dissection was continued anteriorly, carefully separating the rectum from the posterior wall of the vagina being sure to keep the vaginal and rectal walls intact. Dissection was continued until the vagina and rectum were distinct and separate structures and the typical areolar plane between them was reached. During the dissection the thickness of both vaginal wall as well as rectal wall was checked utilizing a lacrimal duct probe. The rectum then required some further mobilization by removing some of its attached fascia until it reached the perineum comfortably and without tension for the planned anoplasty.

Total Urogenital Mobilization (TUM): The rectum was then lifted out and retracted superiorly, out of the field so that attention could be directed toward the total urogenital mobilization. Traction sutures were placed completely around the urogenital tract anteriorly approximately 5 mm posterior to the clitoris, and around the entire vagina. The urethra was then easily visualized and was cannulated with a Foley catheter. Circumferentially, mobilization was then performed around the urogenital tract utilizing the silk sutures for continuous traction. The anterior suspensory ligaments to the urethra were divided which allowed good mobilization. The vagina was evaluated to see if it would reach the perineum, and this required further mobilization along the lateral aspect of the vagina. This was performed carefully to preserve the blood supply to the vagina. The common channel was then split in the midline. Multiple fine 5-0 Vicryl sutures were then utilized to reapproximate the urethra down to the perineum as well as the now splayed common channel laterally on both sides to recreate the labia minora. The vagina was brought down, again utilizing 5-0 Vicryl sutures to the introitus circumferentially. Posteriorly, the sites of the marked sphincter complex were visualized, and the muscle stimulator was utilized to define the anterior limit of the sphincter. The perineal body was recreated utilizing 4-0 Vicryl sutures to bring soft tissue and muscle as well as the skin together posteriorly. The vagina was well perfused and fit nicely without tension within the labial folds of the introitus.

The sphincter complex was marked, again using visual identification of the sphincter complex as well as electrical stimulation marking the posterior and anterior limits. The levator muscles were closed with several sutures so that the muscles complex lay on either side of the rectum. Gentle tension on the rectum with sutures placed from the posterior edge of the muscle complex to the back wall of the rectum resulted in the rectum lying perfectly within the sphincter mechanism. The completed closure of the posterior sagittal incision was performed up to the skin in layers. The anoplasty was completed with long-term absorbable sutures after trimming off approximately the distal 3 mm of the rectum. The anoplasty was performed under slight tension so that after the sutures were cut, the anus retracted slightly without evidence of prolapse. The posterior sagittal incision closure was performed with interrupted 5-0 Vicryl sutures.

Upon completion of the procedure, a debriefing checklist was completed to share information critical to the postoperative care of the patient. The patient tolerated the procedure well, *was extubated in the operating room*, and was transported to the post anesthesia care unit in stable condition thereafter.

Anal Stricturoplasty

44

Devin R. Halleran, Richard J. Wood, and Marc A. Levitt

Indications and Benefits

- Skin-level stricture after posterior sagittal anorectoplasty in patients with imperforate anus/anorectal malformations
- Some cases of congenital anal stenosis
- Approach only for skin-level, think (1–3 mm) stricture or stenosis
- Benefits: Return of anal opening to age-appropriate size with minimal dissection, not requiring a diversion

Risks and Alternatives

- Standard risks (bleeding, infection, need for additional procedures, risks of anesthesia)
- Injury to adjacent structures (external anal sphincter)
- Re-stricturing
- Alternatives: Dilation

D. R. Halleran · R. J. Wood · M. A. Levitt (✉)
Nationwide Children's Hospital, Center for Colorectal and Pelvic Reconstruction, Columbus, OH, USA
e-mail: devin.halleran@nationwidechildrens.org; Richard.wood@nationwidechildrens.org; marc.levitt@nationwidechildrens.org

Essential Steps

1. Prior to starting the procedure, measure the size of the anal opening using a Hegar dilator.
2. Place four traction sutures in the anal skin at the 2, 4, 8, and 10 o'clock positions.
3. Apply slight tension in opposing directions to two sutures and radially incise the skin between the two sutures until the stricture releases.
4. Suture the rectal mucosa to the skin longitudinally with absorbable sutures.
5. Repeat steps 3 and 4 for all quadrants, incising at the 12, 3, 6 and 9 o'clock positions.
6. At the completion of the procedure, measure the anal opening using a Hegar dilator to ensure the size is appropriate for the age of the patient.
7. This technique can usually double the circumference (e.g., Hegar 8 to Hegar 16).

Template Operative Dictation

Preoperative Diagnosis *Skin-level anal stricture after posterior sagittal anorectoplasty/congenital anal stenosis.*

Postoperative Diagnosis Same as preoperative diagnosis

Findings Same as postoperative diagnosis

D. J. Papandria et al. (eds.), *Operative Dictations in Pediatric Surgery*,
https://doi.org/10.1007/978-3-030-24212-1_44

Procedure(s) Performed Anal stricturoplasty

Anesthesia *General*

Estimated Blood Loss ___

Indications This is a/an ___-*day/week/month/year*-old *male/female* with a *skin-level anal stricture after posterior sagittal anorectoplasty/congenital anal stenosis*. He/she was deemed to be a suitable candidate for anal stricturoplasty.

Procedure in Detail Following satisfactory induction of anesthesia, the patient was placed in *supine/prone* position and appropriately padded. Timeouts were performed using both preinduction and preincision safety checklists with participation of all present in the operative suite. These confirmed the correct patient, procedure, operative site, and additional critical information prior to the start of the procedure. The perineum was then prepped and draped in the usual sterile fashion.

Prior to starting the procedure, the anus was inspected and found to accommodate a size __ Hegar. Silk traction sutures were then placed in the anal skin at the 2, 4, 8, and 10 o'clock positions and each grasped with a mosquito clamp. Taking two of the stitches and applying traction in opposite directions, radial incisions were made using electrocautery into the skin between the two suture and some of the anal mucosa until the stricture released. The rectal mucosa was then sutured to the skin in a longitudinal fashion with *4-0 Vicryl*. This was repeated in all four quadrants incising at the 12, 3, 6, and 9 o'clock positions. The anus was again inspected and noted to accept a size __ Hegar after the procedure. There were no complications. All counts were correct at the end of the case.

Upon completion of the procedure, a debriefing checklist was completed to share information critical to the postoperative care of the patient. The patient tolerated the procedure well, *was extubated in the operating room*, and was transported to the postanesthesia care unit in stable condition thereafter.

Vaginoplasty and Vaginal Replacement

45

Alejandra Vilanova-Sánchez, Geri D. Hewitt, and Marc A. Levitt

Indications and Benefits

- Mullerian agenesis (Mayer-Rokitansky-Kuster-Hauser syndrome – MRKH) with failed vaginal dilation
- Distal vaginal atresia with high vagina (vagina does not reach the perineum)
- Patients with anorectal malformations or urogenital sinus with vaginal agenesis
- *Benefits*: Allow normal perineum anatomy, vaginal intercourse, menstrual egress, conception

Risks and Alternatives

- Standard risks: Colo-colostomy or enteroenterostomy anastomotic leak
- Injury to adjacent structures: Injury to the bladder, rectum, gynecologic structures, ureters, colonic, or small bowel mesentery. Inadequate blood supply to neovagina leading to stenosis or acquired atresia
- *Alternatives:*
  - In MRKH, the first-line therapy is serial vaginal dilation of the vaginal dimple (the rate of success of vaginal dimple dilations is close to 90%). An adequate introitus, presence of a vaginal dimple, and persistent dilation increase likelihood of success.
  - In distal vaginal agenesis with normal upper vagina, uterus, and cervix: If the distal vagina is close to the perineum (<3 cm), an anastomosis of the distal vaginal pouch to the perineum could be tried. The distal vagina can be mobilized using a laparoscopic technique. If the distal vaginal pouch is >3 cm from the perineum, a vaginal interposition or any other vaginoplasty technique should be performed to avoid tension on the anastomosis and potential vaginal stricture.
  - Vaginoplasty techniques: McLeod technique with skin flaps, vulvar flaps, Vecchietti technique, rotational flap procedures.

Essential Steps for Vaginal Replacement Using Sigmoid Colon

1. The patient is placed in a lithotomy position with the feet in stirrups.
2. Foley catheter placement.

A. Vilanova-Sánchez
Hospital La Paz, Department of Pediatric Surgery, Madrid, Spain

G. D. Hewitt (✉)
Nationwide Children's Hospital, Department of Surgery, Columbus, OH, USA
e-mail: Geri.Hewitt@osumc.edu

M. A. Levitt
Nationwide Children's Hospital, Center for Colorectal and Pelvic Reconstruction, Columbus, OH, USA
e-mail: marc.levitt@nationwidechildrens.org

D. J. Papandria et al. (eds.), *Operative Dictations in Pediatric Surgery*,
https://doi.org/10.1007/978-3-030-24212-1_45

3. A midline laparotomy is performed from umbilicus to the pubis symphysis.
4. The pelvis is inspected for the presence of ovaries, Fallopian tubes, and uterus.
5. Colonic arcade examination. The inferior mesenteric artery (IMA) and left colic arteries are identified. The sigmoid arcade and marginal artery are identified.
6. A 10–15-cm sigmoid colon segment is isolated with a selected blood supply.
7. The selected bowel is divided (proximal and distal) with a 60 mm stapler.
8. Bowel continuity is restored by an end-to-end colonic anastomosis.
9. *The stapler lines are removed from both ends and oversewn with absorbable suture at proximal end unless it is anastomosed to proximal vagina.*
10. *If distal vaginal atresia: Pelvic dissection of the upper vaginal until the vaginal pouch was identified. Anastomosis of the sigmoid segment from the vaginal pouch to the proximal neovagina.*
11. Elevate legs further to gain better access to the perineum by flexing thighs toward abdomen.
12. *If MRKH: Incision through the vaginal dimple and blunt dissection to create a tunnel between the urethra and the rectum until peritoneal cavity is reached.*
13. *If distal vaginal agenesis with normal upper vagina and uterus: Incision between the urethra and the anus. Blunt dissection in front of the rectum until the peritoneal cavity is reached.*
14. The neovagina is then brought to the perineum through the tunnel previously created in a isoperistaltic manner.
15. Perineal anastomosis with 4/0 interrupted absorbable stitches to the perineum (introitus).
16. Abdominal closure.

Note These Variations

- The neovagina could be done with sigmoid colon, descending colon, or small bowel. For all the options, a careful selection of the blood supply to the graft must be done.
- Depending on the length of mesentery, the isolated segment is usually brought down to the perineum in an isoperistaltic fashion.
- Laparoscopy has been described for this operation, but is technically challenging to do the staple line removal, suturing for anastomosis or suture line repair.

Template Operative Dictation

Preoperative Diagnosis Vaginal agenesis

Postoperative Diagnosis Same as preoperative diagnosis

Findings *Complete/partial vaginal agenesis.* Normal ovaries

Procedure Performed Sigmoid vaginoplasty

Anesthesia *General*

Estimated Blood Loss ____ mL

Indications This is a/an ___*-day/week/month/year*-old *female* with Mullerian agenesis. She was deemed to be a suitable candidate for vaginal interposition.

Procedure in Detail Following satisfactory induction of anesthesia, the patient was placed in dorsal lithotomy position and appropriately padded. Timeouts were performed using both preinduction and preincision safety checklists with participation of all present in the operative suite. These confirmed the correct patient, procedure, operative site, and additional critical information prior to the start of the procedure. The abdomen and the perineum was then prepped and draped in the usual sterile fashion. A Foley catheter was inserted in the bladder in the sterile field. We performed a midline laparotomy from the umbilicus to 2 cm above the pubic symphysis. We opened in the midline by layers, and entered the peritoneal cavity. The peritoneal cavity was inspected and a normally rotated bowel was noted. We then inspected the colonic mesentery. The inferior mesenteric artery and its branches, the left colic artery and its branch to the sigmoid, and the superior hemorrhoidal artery were carefully identified. A segment of sigmoid colon approximately 10 cm long is selected that is perfused by a sigmoid branch parallel to the bowel. The sigmoid section to be used as neovagina was dissected proximally and distally, making sure that the vascular arcade was left intact. The colon is transected with a 60 mm GIA stapler at the proximal and distal parts. We continued with the end-to-end colocolonic anastomosis using absorbable 4-0 interrupted stitches. The mesenteric defect was closed without disruption of blood supply with interrupted 4/0 absorbable stitches.

[Choose One:]

If Mullerian structures are not present (complete vaginal agenesis with no uterus): *She had Mullerian agenesis with no midline structure or fallopian tubes identified. Both stapler lines were removed from the neovagina. The proximal end of the neovagina was then closed in two layers, with 4/0 interrupted absorbable suture. We then paid attention to the perineum. We further elevated the patient's legs. A blind vaginal dimple was identified posterior to a normal urethral meatus. The vaginal dimple was incised vertically and a blunt dissection with electrocautery was started taking care to not injure the urethra or the rectum. The peritoneal cavity was entered. We inserted a Babcock forceps through the perineum up to abdominal cavity. The assistant surgeon who was on the abdominal field presented the selected piece for neovagina. The distal end of the neovagina was grasped and was then pulled through the pelvis down to the perineum in an isoperistaltic manner ensuring its vascular pedicle remained in the correct orientation. The proximal neovagina was fixed to the posterior bladder in the midline using absorbable 4/0 interrupted sutures.*

If Mullerian structures are present (distal vaginal agenesis): A normal uterus and upper vagina were identified. We began the dissection of the posterior uterus, taking care of the blood supply. We continued the dissection of the upper vagina until the distal limit of the vaginal pouch was found. It was detached from its attachments to the pelvis. A lumen was confirmed. The staple line of the proximal edge of the neovagina was resected. We approximated the vaginal replacement to the distal portion of the upper vaginal pouch to perform the proximal anastomosis. No tension was noted. The end-to-end colo-vaginal anastomosis was performed with 4/0 interrupted stitches. We then paid attention to the perineum. We further elevated the patient's legs. No vaginal opening or dimple was identified. The urethra and the anus were noted to be in the correct place. At the intended site of the introitus, a vertical incision was made with electrocautery. A blunt dissection between the urethra and the rectum was performed until the peritoneal cavity was entered. We identified the distal pouch of the vagina anastomosed to the neovagina. The distal end of the neovagina was grasped from the perineum and was then pulled down through tunnel dissected previously. The pedicle was pulled through in an isoperistaltic manner ensuring that its vascular pedicle remained in the correct orientation, without twist or tension.

We checked that the pedicle was not under tension and the neovagina was well vascularized. An introitoplasty was then performed using 4-0 interrupted absorbable stitches to secure the distal sigmoid colonic mucosa to the new introital skin. Hemostasis was ensured in the pelvis. The colocolonic anastomosis looked well perfused. We closed the muscular and fascia layer with interrupted stitches. Subcutaneous and subcuticular layers were closed with interrupted 4/0 stitches. Upon completion of the procedure, a debriefing checklist was completed to share information critical to the postoperative care of the patient. The patient tolerated the procedure well, *was extubated in the operating room*, and was transported to the postanesthesia care unit in stable condition.

46 Augmentation Enterocystoplasty

Christina B. Ching

Indications

- Reduction of bladder storage pressure
- Increased urinary volume storage
- Preservation of upper urinary tract health
- Urinary continence

Benefits

- Continence
- Protection of urinary upper tract

Risks/Complications

- Intraoperative/Immediate postoperative
  - Injury to adjacent structures
  - Urine leak
  - Urine fistula
  - Urinary tract infection
  - Mucus production– clogging tubes
  - Tube dislodgement/malfunctioning
  - Electrolyte abnormalities
  - Bowel leak
  - Bowel obstruction
  - Bowel fistula
  - Wound infection
- Long term
  - Urinary incontinence
  - Urinary tract infection
  - Bladder stones
  - Mucus production – increasing risk of bladder stones and urinary tract infection
  - Bladder rupture
  - Electrolyte abnormalities and vitamin B12 deficiency
  - Bowel obstruction
  - Malignant transformation

Alternatives

- Clean intermittent catheterization with pharmacologic treatment
  - Anticholinergic/beta-3 adrenergic receptor agonist medication
  - Intravesical Botulinum Type-A toxin injection
- Indwelling catheter (urethral or suprapubic)
- Incontinent diversion
- Autoaugmentation

Essential/Critical Steps

1. Abdominal incision
2. Bladder mobilization and adequate bivalving

C. B. Ching (✉)
Nationwide Children's Hospital, Department of Pediatric Urology, Columbus, OH, USA
e-mail: Christina.Ching@nationwidechildrens.org

D. J. Papandria et al. (eds.), *Operative Dictations in Pediatric Surgery*,
https://doi.org/10.1007/978-3-030-24212-1_46

3. Bowel identification and harvesting of bowel segment for augmentation with good blood supply and at least 15 cm proximal to terminal ileum
4. Reestablishment of bowel continuity
5. Preparation of bowel segment for augmentation
6. Bowel to bladder anastomosis
7. Check bowel to bladder anastomosis for leaks
8. Postoperative drainage of bladder
9. Close the abdomen

Needed Equipment

- Retractor (Bookwalter, Denis-Browne)
- Stapler
- Foley catheters

Note These Variations

- Usually done with catheterizable channel.
- May be done with bladder neck procedure.
- Minimal invasive technique is possible.
- Various bowel segments can be used such as stomach, jejunum, ileum, and colon. Ileum and sigmoid colon are most common.

Template Operative Dictation

Preoperative Diagnosis Neurogenic bladder, urinary incontinence, and hydronephrosis

Postoperative Diagnosis Same

Findings Small, trabeculated, fibrotic bladder; normal bowel

Procedure (s) Performed Augmentation enterocystoplasty, open suprapubic tube placement.

Anesthesia General +/− *epidural*

Specimen None

Drains __F suprapubic tube, __F *urethral Foley and/or catheterizable channel Foley, Jackson-Pratt pelvic drain, nasogastric tube.*

Estimated Blood Loss ____ ml

Indications This is a/an ___-year-old *male/female* with *neurogenic bladder, urinary incontinence, and hydronephrosis*. Preoperative urodynamics showed signs of *a poorly compliant and small capacity bladder*. Prior bladder management included ______. *He/she* was deemed to be a suitable candidate for augmentation enterocystoplasty.

Procedure in Detail The patient was brought back to the operating room by anesthesia and placed in supine position and appropriately padded. ***If the child is older:*** *Pneumatic compression stockings were applied to the extremities prior to anesthetic induction.* Timeouts were performed using both preinduction and preincision safety checklists with participation of all present in the operative suite. These confirmed the correct patient, procedure, operative site, and additional critical information prior to the start of the procedure. After adequate induction of anesthesia and endotracheal intubation, *an epidural and a nasogastric tube were placed*. With the patient in the supine position, the abdomen was then prepped and draped in the usual sterile fashion. Preoperative antibiotics were given. A ___F transurethral catheter was inserted under sterile conditions on the table. Urine was collected and sent for culture to facilitate postoperative antibiotic management.

An *infraumbilical midline/Pfannenstiel* incision was made. Dissection proceeded through the subcutaneous tissue down to the rectus fascia. The rectus fascia was cleared of subcutaneous tissue and then opened longitudinally in the midline. The rectus muscles were split in the midline; the supravesical space was developed; and the bladder was exposed. The bladder was distended with saline through the sterile transurethral Foley in order to facilitate blunt dissection of the space of Retzius. The bladder was freed anteriorly down to the pubic symphysis and laterally from the pelvic side walls. The *Bookwalter/Denis-Browne retractor* was then placed to facilitate visualization.

If Performing Bladder Neck Reconstruction: *The bladder neck was identified and bladder neck procedure was performed.*

The peritoneum was then identified and opened sharply. The *ileum/sigmoid* was inspected to find an area that would reach the bladder easily and supplied by a nice vascular pedicle. ***If performing ileal augmentation:*** *The area of ileum being identified was at least 15 cm proximal to the terminal ileum/ileocecal junction.* The segment of bowel is marked with superficial silk sutures on either end. Abdominal sponges were then placed to pack the bowel away.

The bladder is then opened in a bivalve manner. This was done in the *transverse/sagittal* plane. ***If performing a catheterizable channel such as appendicovesicostomy:*** *This was done as an inverted "U" incision on the anterior wall of the bladder to enable some of the anterior wall to fold backwards to elongate the posterior wall of the bladder for the catheterizable channel to reach the umbilicus/right lower quadrant and provide an adequate tunnel for catheterizable channel placement in the bladder.* The bladder was opened with a wide mouth to prevent an hourglass configuration or waist between the bladder and augmentation.

The sponges packing the bowel away were then readjusted to enable the previously selected bowel segment to be included in the incision.

[Choose One:]

If an ileal augmentation is chosen: The ileal bowel segment initially identified was confirmed to be at least 15 cm proximal to terminal ileum/ileocecal junction. 20–25 cm of ileum proximal to that was then measured for use in augmentation. The bowels segment was checked one last time for a good vascular pedicle. The selected loop of bowel was then taken out of continuity with the rest of the bowel via blue intestinal load linear cutter stapler incision on either side. The bowel continuity was reestablished with a side-to-side stapled anastomosis using a linear cutter and transverse anastomosis staplers. The butt end was oversewn and thus reinforced with imbricating/Lembert sutures of 4-0 *Vicryl/silk*. The mesentery defect was closed carefully with superficial interrupted 4-0 Vicryl sutures so as not to catch any major mesentery blood supply or cause bleeding.

If a sigmoid augmentation is chosen: The sigmoid section was identified as being a redundant loop in close proximity to the bladder and about 20 cm long. The bowel segment was checked one last time for a good vascular pedicle. The selected loop of bowel was then taken out of continuity with the rest of the bowel via blue intestinal load linear cutter stapler incision on either side. The bowel continuity was reestablished with hand sewn end-to-end bowel anastomosis using interrupted 2-0 *Vicryl/silk*. The mesentery defect was closed carefully with superficial interrupted 4-0 sutures so as not to catch any major mesentery blood supply or cause bleeding.

Towels were then placed on either side of the isolated bowel segment to collect any bowel spillage. One end of the staple line was sharply removed and the segment irrigated with warm antibiotic saline solution. The staple line on the opposite side was then sharply removed. The bowel segment was then detubularized by opening the bowel on the antimesenteric border. The bowel was reconfigured, in *an/a "U"/"S"* shape configuration with 2-0 Vicryl sutures bringing the bowel walls together.

If performing catheterizable channel* via *appendicovesicostomy: *The catheterizable channel was then harvested, prepared, and performed at this time.*

The most mobile segment of bowel was then identified to come down anteriorly over the bladder. The bowel segment was anastomosed to the bladder with running but intermittently locking 2-0 Vicryl suture in a full-thickness layer from the posterior wall of the bladder and working laterally. Prior to closing the anterior wall and completing the augmentation, a ___F suprapubic tube was brought out of the native bladder. A 3-0 Vicryl purse string suture was placed around the SPT where it was brought through the bladder wall. The tube was then brought out the left lower abdomen. The balloon was minimally inflated just to be sure it did not get pulled out but to avoid being in the way or inadvertently being popped during the final stages of the bladder/bowel closure. A __F catheter was also left in the *urethra/catheterizable channel* with the balloon also minimally inflated. The anterior wall of the bowel to bladder anastomosis was then completed with full-thickness running 2-0 Vicryl. The bladder was then irrigated with antibiotic saline to ensure patency and test the anastomosis for leaks. Leaks were repaired with interrupted figure-of-eight 3-0 Vicryl suture. The SPT/Foley balloons were then filled with the rest of the water. Tubes were secured to the skin with 0 silk sutures.

At the end of the case, the pelvis was irrigated and evaluated for hemostasis. *A Jackson-Pratt drain was placed to exit the right lower quadrant and secured to the skin.* When adequate hemostasis was ensured, the fascia was closed with *running/interrupted 2-0/0* Vicryl. The incision was irrigated. Scarpas fascia was then closed with interrupted 4-0 Vicryl. Skin was closed with running *5-0 Monocryl/Vicryl/staples*. A dressing *of skin glue/mastisol with adhesive tape and sponges was*/were then placed.

At the end of the case, all sponge and needle and instrument counts were correct. All tubes were placed to gravity drainage.

Upon completion of the procedure, a debriefing checklist was completed to share information critical to the postoperative care of the patient. The patient tolerated the procedure well, *was extubated in the operating room*, and was transported to the anesthesia post-operative care unit in stable condition thereafter.

Urinary Conduit

47

Molly E. Fuchs and Daniel G. Dajusta

Indications

- Neurogenic bladder with noncompliance with catheterization regimen
- Deterioration of renal function with a continent urinary diversion
- Patients' desire to have urinary diversion that does not require catheterization
- Prior bladder perforation because of trauma or noncompliance

Essential Steps

1. Low midline incision.
2. Mobilize peritoneum off of the bladder anteriorly and laterally.
3. Identify the ileocecal valve and measure 15 cm proximal to the ileocecal valve.
4. Identify a section of ileum (no closer than 15 cm to the ileocecal valve) that is mobile enough to reach the bladder.
5. Isolate 15–20 cm of ileum with GIA stapler out of this mobile section of intestine.
6. Reanastomose the intestine in a standard side-to-side fashion stapled anastomosis.
7. Close the mesenteric defect.
8. Excise the staple line off the isolated portion of ileum and irrigate the intestine with saline.
9. An inverted U incision is made on the anterior superior portion of the bladder to accommodate the spatulated intestine.
10. Anastomose the ilium to the bladder with interrupted Vicryl suture.
11. Reinforce the anastomosis of the ilium to the bladder with interrupted Vicryl sutures through the detrusor and the serosa of the bowel.
12. Place a large Foley through the ileum and into the bladder and inflate the bladder with sterile water (ensure that the balloon is in the bladder and not in the ileum.
13. Identify an area on the abdomen appropriate for the stoma (ideally marked by enterostomal nurses prior to the beginning of surgery).
14. Bring the distal end of the bowel up through the skin and mature the stoma in a brooked fashion.
15. Irrigate the peritoneum with copious amounts of sterile saline.
16. Close the abdomen in standard fashion.
17. Place enterostomal appliance on the urinary stoma with Foley in the stoma bag.
18. A urethra foley or suprapubic tube should be left in place as a secondary mode of drainage during healing to keep the bladder empty.

M. E. Fuchs (✉) · D. G. Dajusta
Nationwide Children's Hospital, Department of Pediatric Urology, Columbus, OH, USA
e-mail: molly.fuchs@nationwidechildrens.org; Daniel.dajusta@nationwidechildrens.org

D. J. Papandria et al. (eds.), *Operative Dictations in Pediatric Surgery*,
https://doi.org/10.1007/978-3-030-24212-1_47

Note These Variations

- Colon can be utilized for the urinary conduit if deemed appropriate
- The length of bowel necessary for the conduit varies based on the patient's body habitus and body wall thickness
- Urinary conduit can be performed with a minimally invasive technique, typically robotic assisted. Port placement is as follows: 12-mm camera port at the umbilicus, 8-mm robotic ports placed 8–10 cm lateral in a line across the abdomen and an additional 8-mm port in the right lower quadrant, 1–2 cm superior and medial to the anterior superior iliac spine. A 12-mm assistant port is also typically necessary in the left upper quadrant for retraction and stapler use

Complications

- Injury to the surrounding structures (bowel or vasculature)
- Stomal stenosis
- Stomal prolapse
- Poor drainage of urine from the incontinent stoma

Template Operative Dictation

Preoperative Diagnosis Neurogenic bladder

Postoperative Diagnosis Same

Procedure *Ileovesicostomy/Colovesicostomy*, and reanastomosis of bowel

Indications This is a/an ____-year-old *male/female* with *myelomeningocele/anorectal malformation/neurogenic bladder* whose bladder has been managed with clean intermittent catheterization but because of *poor compliance with catheterization program and renal insufficiency/prior bladder perforation/patient* preference, we discussed options and the patient and family have opted for an incontinent urinary diversion. After discussion of the surgical options, risks, benefits, and alternatives of ileovesicostomy procedure, the family agreed to proceed with surgery.

Procedure in Detail After informed consent was attained, the patient was brought to the operating room and placed on the operating room table in the supine position. General endotracheal anesthesia was induced and all of the patient's pressure points were padded appropriately. An operative time out was performed to confirm patient identification and procedure to be performed. The patient was prepped and draped in the normal sterile fashion with chlorhexidine. A Foley catheter was placed in the bladder per the urethra on the sterile field and the balloon inflated with sterile water.

A low midline incision was made extending from just inferior to the umbilicus down to the pubic symphysis. Dissection was carried down to the level of the fascia and the abdomen was entered in the midline distally, paying special attention to split the rectus muscle in the midline. Upon entering the space of Retzius, the peritoneum was carefully dissected off the anterior and lateral portions of the bladder, freeing the bladder from its peritoneal attachments. With the bladder adequately freed, the peritoneum was then entered and a *Bookwalter/Denis-Browne* retractor was placed in the incision and we identified the terminal ileum and cecum.

[Choose One:]
Ileovesicostomy: A 20-cm portion of ileum that was freely mobile was identified and we measured to ensure that it was greater than 15 cm proximal to the ileocecal valve. A robust vascular arcade was clearly visualized supplying this portion of the ileum so the mesentery was carefully dissected off the bowel, and the LigaSure™ was used to isolate the section of ileum. A GIA 60 stapler was used to transect the ileum. The ileum was then reanastomosed in the standard side-to-side fashion using a stapler technique. The two staple lines were then excised off the isolated piece of ileum. The bowel was then irrigated out clear with an asepto syringe.

Colovesicostomy: The redundant sigmoid colon was identified and a 20-cm section of colon with a generous vascular pedicle was marked out with silk stay sutures to mark the proximal and distal margins of the bowel resection. A robust vascular arcade was clearly visualized supplying this portion of the colon so the mesentery was carefully dissected off the bowel, and the LigaSure™ was used to isolate the section of colon. A GIA 60 stapler was used to transect the colon. The colon was then reanastomosed in the standard side to side fashion using a stapler technique. The two staple lines were then excised off the isolated piece of colon. The bowel was then irrigated out clear with an asepto syringe.

The bladder was then opened using an inverted U shaped incision at the anterior superior portion of the bladder using electrocautery. The bladder was opened and the Foley catheter was visualized in the urethra. The opening was widely patent and the proximal portion of the bowel was then anastomosed to the bladder, starting with the posterior portion of the anastomosis. This was performed with interrupted, absorbable sutures and once the bowel was anastomosed circumferentially, reinforcing sutures were place as a second layer through the serosa of the bowel to the detrusor muscle circumferentially. A large bore Foley (22 Fr) was passed through the conduit to ensure that the anastomosis was widely patent where it communicated with the bladder.

The previously marked stoma site on the abdomen was then identified and a circumferential skin incision was made by grabbing the skin with a Kocher clamp and we dissected out the fat down to the level of the fascia. A cruciate incision was made in the fascia and stretched the fascial opening to accommodate the conduit. The distal end of the bowel was then brought up through the fascia and the stoma was created and brooked in the standard fashion. A large bore Foley (22 Fr – 24 Fr) was placed through the conduit and into the bladder. The balloon was filled and we ensured that the balloon was all the way in the bladder by feeling the balloon manually before closing the abdomen.

The abdominal cavity was copiously irrigated with sterile saline and the retractor was removed. The fascia was closed with interrupted 0 Vicryl sutures in a figure of eight fashion. The subcutaneous tissue closed with 4-0 Vicryl and the skin closed with 5-0 Monocryl subcuticular stitch. Steri-Strips were placed on the incision and Telfa, and Medi-pore tapes were placed on the incision as a dressing. A stoma appliance was placed on the stoma with the Foley draining into the urostomy bag.

Sponge and needle counts were correct ×2 at the end of the procedure. The patient was extubated and taken to the recovery room in stable condition.

Appendicovesicostomy/Mitrofanoff

48

Molly E. Fuchs and Daniel G. Dajusta

Indications

- Neurogenic bladder and inability to catheterize per urethra
- Urethral stricture disease and inability to catheterize per urethra

Essential Steps

1. Low midline incision.
2. Identify terminal ileum and cecum.
3. Evaluate the presence of appendix and size of appendix (if no appendix or appendix <4 cm in length, appendicovesicostomy is not possible and Monti channel is necessary).
4. Mobilize cecum so that appendix can reach bladder without tension on mesentery.
5. Evaluate blood supply to appendix to ensure adequate vasculature after appendectomy.
6. Appendectomy ensuring that vasculature is preserved. Suture ligate appendiceal stump and imbricate the cecum over it.
7. Ensure that appendix can reach the bladder and up to the umbilicus without being on tension or twisting the vascular pedicle.
8. Pass an 8-Fr straight catheter into the appendix to ensure patency.
9. Incise the tip of the appendix in a cruciate fashion to allow both ends of the appendix to be open and allow straight cath to come through.
10. Secure catheter in place with a holding stitch through the appendix and the catheter.
11. Mobilize the bladder anteriorly and laterally so that it can be brought nearly up to the umbilicus.
12. Open the bladder longitudinally on the anterior surface of the bladder, ensuring that the incision does not extend through the dome of the bladder cranially and does not extend through the bladder neck caudally.
13. Make a small cystotomy on the posterior portion of the bladder, just caudal to the dome of the bladder. It may be necessary to dissect the peritoneal reflection off of the posterior portion of the bladder.
14. After creating this cystotomy, carefully create a submucosal tunnel between the detrusor muscle and the bladder mucosa. Make this tunnel in the caudal direction toward the bladder neck. This tunnel should measure 4 cm in length.
15. Once a 4-cm tunnel is created, incise the mucosa at the bottom of the tunnel where the intravesical appendicovesicostomy will be matured.

M. E. Fuchs (✉) · D. G. Dajusta
Nationwide Children's Hospital, Department of Pediatric Urology, Columbus, OH, USA
e-mail: molly.fuchs@nationwidechildrens.org; Daniel.dajusta@nationwidechildrens.org

D. J. Papandria et al. (eds.), *Operative Dictations in Pediatric Surgery*,
https://doi.org/10.1007/978-3-030-24212-1_48

16. Pass the distal end of the appendix through the cystotomy with the catheter in place and through the submucosal tunnel.
17. Secure the appendix to the posterior portion of the distal end of the tunnel with an absorbable suture that incorporates detrusor and mucosa to secure the channel in place.
18. Mature the remainder of the intravesical portion of the stoma with interrupted absorbable suture bringing only the mucosa to the lumen of the appendix.
19. Place an absorbable suture on the outside of the bladder and secure it to the appendix so that it does not slide within the tunnel. Be sure that the vasculature to the appendix is not compromised.
20. Remove the catheter from the appendicovesicostomy and pass it through the channel to be sure that it catheterizes easily.
21. Place an 8-Fr Foley catheter through the appendicovesicostomy and ill the balloon.
22. Close the bladder with absorbable suture.
23. Make an inverted V incision at the base of the umbilicus so that the apex of the V is cranial and the wide base of the flap is caudal.
24. Make an incision in the fascia large enough to accommodate the appendicovesicostomy.
25. Bring the back end of the catheter up through the umbilical incision followed by the proximal end of the appendicovesicostomy.
26. With the appendicovesicostomy up through the umbilical incision, bring the bladder up to the anterior abdominal wall and secure it with an absorbable suture to take tension off the appendicovesicostomy. This can be achieved with 1 or more sutures.
27. Spatulate the appendix on the antimesenteric side and bring the apex of the V flap down to the apex of the spatulation and secure it with absorbable suture.
28. Mature the remainder of the stoma with interrupted absorbable suture.
29. Remove the catheter and attempt catheterization again if desired to ensure that the appendicovesicostomy is catheterized easily.
30. Irrigate the abdominal cavity gently.
31. Close the abdomen in the usual fashion.
32. Secure appendicovesicostomy catheter with drain stitch so that it does not get pulled on or become dislodged prematurely.

Note These Variations

- Pfannenstiel incision may be utilized with a potential limitation being the cecal mobilization can be challenging with this incision, particularly if the patient has had prior surgery and the cecum is not freely mobile.
- The appendicovesicostomy can be tunneled on the bladder anteriorly, particularly if the bladder is not being opened for any other reason during the operation (i.e., simultaneous bladder augmentation) If the appendicovesicostomy is implanted anteriorly, an extravesical tunnel is created by incising the detrusor muscle and closing the detrusor tunnel over the appendix as in a Lich-Gregoir reimplantation technique.
- If the appendix does not easily reach the umbilicus or if there is another reason that the umbilicus is not the optimal position for the skin stoma, the appendicovesicostomy can be brought up to the right lower quadrant and matured in a tension-free fashion.
- Minimally invasive techniques can be utilized for this operation, typically robotic-assisted laparoscopy. In this case, the appendectomy is performed, followed by the critical step of bladder mobilization. The bladder needs to be adequately mobilized from the anterior abdominal wall and stretched up towards the umbilicus and re-secured to the abdominal wall prior ot the appendix being implanted into the bladder. This allows the distance between the umbilicus and the bladder to be minimized. The appendix is then implanted into the posterior portion of the bladder in a Lich-Gregoir fashion. Port placement for robotic variation is as follows: 12-mm camera port at the umbilicus, 8-mm robotic port a hand breadth lateral to the camera port on each side, and an additional 8-mm robotic port in the right lower

quadrant, 1–2 cm medial and superior to the right anterior superior iliac spine.

Complications

- Injury to the surrounding structures (bowel or vasculature)
- Devascularization of the appendix
- Stomal stenosis
- Difficulty catheterizing

Template Operative Dictation

Preoperative Diagnosis Neurogenic bladder and inability to catheterize per urethra

Postoperative Diagnosis Same

Procedure Creation of appendicovesicostomy (Mitrofanoff)

Indications This is a/an ____-year-old *male/female* with *myelomeningocele/anorectal malformation/neurogenic bladder* who is not able to empty *his/her* bladder adequately and requires intermittent catheterization. Catheterization per urethra *has not been successful/is not possible/is very painful and challenging*. After discussion of the surgical options, risks, benefits, and alternatives of appendicovesicostomy procedure, the family has agreed to proceed with surgery.

Procedure After informed consent was attained, the patient was brought to the operating room and placed on the operating room table in the supine position. General endotracheal anesthesia was induced and all of the patient's pressure points were padded appropriately. An operative time out was performed to confirm patient identification and procedure to be performed. The patient was prepped and draped in the normal sterile fashion with chlorhexidine. A Foley catheter was placed in the bladder per the urethra on the sterile field and the balloon inflated with sterile water.

A low midline incision was made extending from just inferior to the umbilicus down to the pubic symphysis. Dissection was carried down to the level of the fascia and the abdomen was entered in the midline distally, paying special attention to split the rectus muscle in the midline. Upon entering the space of Retzius, the peritoneum was carefully dissected off the anterior and lateral portions of the bladder, freeing the bladder from its peritoneal attachments. With the bladder adequately freed, the peritoneum was then entered, and a *Bookwalter/Denis Browne* retractor was placed in the incision and we identified the terminal ileum and cecum. The appendix was identified. The appendix measured ___ cm and was determined to be adequate for appendicovesicostomy. The cecum was adhered to the abdominal side wall and did not allow for the appendix to reach the bladder. The cecum was carefully mobilized off the side wall by incising the white line of Toldt and this freed the cecum up so that it was freely mobile and the appendix reached the bladder. The blood supply to the appendix was adequate and there was a very clear arcade that could be used once the appendix is transected from the cecum. A small window was created in the mesentery at the base of the appendix. A right angle clamp was placed across the base of the appendix and the appendix transected above the clamp. A 2-0 chromic was then used to suture ligate the appendiceal stump. The stump was them imbricated with cecum overlying it with interrupted 2-0 silk sutures. The detached appendix was then evaluated and there was an adequate mesentery with good blood supply remaining.

An 8-Fr straight catheter was then advanced into the open end of the appendix and advanced until it was at the tip of the appendix. A cruciate incision was made at the tip of the appendix overlying the tip of the catheter to allow the catheter to pass all the way through the appendix. A stay suture was placed at the distal end of the appendix and tied loosely. *A small fecalith was pushed out of the distal appendix in the process and it was disposed of.* The 8 Fr straight catheter passed easily through the appendix without any resistance, and it was secured in place with a 4-0 Vicryl suture so that approximately 1 cm was sticking out distally (This securing suture is placed at the proximal end of the appendix and catheter and a 4-cm tail left at the end of the suture and will be used later in the operation to pass the appendix through the umbilicus). The appendix was adequately mobilized from the cecal dissection that it reached the umbilicus and the bladder without too much tension on the vascular pedicle.

[Choose One:]

***Posterior Implantation*:** The bladder was then grasped with two Allis clamps on the anterior surface. A longitudinal incision was made on the bladder in the midline and extended toward the bladder neck but stopped at least 2 cm prior to reaching the bladder neck. A 3-0 chromic suture was placed at the apex of the incision to ensure that it did not extend into the bladder neck. The incision was extended cranially but not as far as the dome of the bladder. The peritoneum was carefully dissected off the posterior portion of the bladder and a small full thickness cystotomy was made at the superior and posterior portion of the bladder. A small hemostat was advanced through the small cystotomy and stretched to accommodate the appendix. The detrusor muscle was then grasped with a hemostat at the small cystotomy and tenotomy scissors were used the carefully create a submucosal tunnel between the detrusor muscle and the bladder mucosa. Care was taken to ensure that the tunnel was 4-cm long and wide enough not to restrict the appendix when it is passed through. Once an adequate tunnel was created, the tenotomy scissors were used to create a hole in the mucosa distally in the tunnel. A right angle was gently passed backwards through the tunnel and out the cystotomy and the distal stay suture on the appendix was grasped and the appendix was gently pulled into the bladder and through the tunnel with the catheter in place. The appendix fit nicely in the tunnel. A 3-0 Vicryl suture was then placed in the posterior portion of the appendix at the distal portion of the tunnel, securing the appendix to the detrusor muscle and the mucosa. The remainder of the intravesical orifice was matured with 4-0 chromic suture bringing the bladder mucosa to the lumen of the appendix. The extravesical portion of the tunnel was then evaluated and with the tunnel on gentle stretch, a 3-0 Vicryl suture was placed through the extravesical detrusor muscle and secured to the appendix to ensure that the appendix did not slide through the tunnel. Once the appendicovesicostomy was secured, the straight catheter was removed and the channel was catheterized without any resistance. An 8-Fr Foley catheter was then advanced into the channel and 3 cc of sterile water was instilled into the balloon. The bladder was then closed in 2 layers of absorbable suture.

***Anterior Implantation*:** The bladder was grasped with a *Babcock/Allis* and brought up to the umbilicus to ensure that it would reach just inferior to the umbilicus. *If more mobilization is required, dissect further laterally and anteriorly.* The anterior wall of the bladder was evaluated and using a marking pen a 4-cm tunnel was marked out. Stay stitches were placed in the anterior wall of the bladder for retraction and a 4-cm incision was made in the detrusor muscle down to the level of the mucosa ensuring that the bladder mucosa was not violated. The dissection was carried down to the mucosa so that the mucosa bulged out when the bladder was filled. The edges of the detrusor trough were elevated up off the mucosa on either side using tenotomy scissors. A small incision was then made in the mucosa in the most caudal portion of the trough. This was widened to approximately the size of the appendiceal lumen. A 3-0 Vicryl suture was placed at the apex of the trough through the detrusor and the mucosa and brought up to the appendix. When it was tied down, the appendix was secured to the base of the trough. The appendix was then matured to the mucosa with the distal tip of the tube in the bladder. Once this was complete, the appendix was laid in the detrusor trough and the detrusor was then closed over the appendix with 4-0 Vicryl interrupted sutures creating a tunnel. Every other suture closing the detrusor over the appendix incorporated a small bite of the outer lumen of the appendix to prevent sliding within the tunnel. Once the tunnel was completely closed, the straight catheter was removed and the appendicovesicostomy was catheterized without any resistance. A 12-Fr Foley catheter was then placed in the channel and 3 cc of sterile water instilled into the balloon.

A small inverted V incision was made at the inferior base of the umbilicus and extended down to the level of the fascia ensuring that the flap was adequately vascularized. A small incision was made in the fascia at the base of the umbilicus and a hemostat was placed in this incision and stretched to accommodate the appendix. A hemostat was then placed from outside to inside through this incision and the back of the Foley and the stay suture on the proximal end of the appendix was grasped and one at a time, brought up through the umbilical incision. With the appendix up through the incision, the bladder was tacked to the anterior abdominal wall with *2-0/3-0* Vicryl sutures relieving any tension on the appendicovesicostomy stoma. Once the bladder was secure, the appendix was spatulated at the skin level on the antimesenteric surface approximately 1 cm. A 4-0 vicryl suture was used to anastomose the tip of the skin v flap down to the apex of the spatulation on the appendix. The remainder of the stoma was then matured with 4-0 Vicryl interrupted sutures.

The abdominal cavity was copiously irrigated with sterile saline and the retractor was removed. The fascia was closed with interrupted 0 Vicryl sutures in a figure of eight fashion. The subcutaneous tissue was closed with 4-0 Vicryl and the skin was closed with 5-0 Monocryl subcuticular stitch. Steri-Strips were placed on the incision and Telfa and Medi-pore tapes were placed on the incision as a dressing. The Mitrofanoff catheter was secured in place with a 2-0 nylon drain stitch. Neosporin ointment was placed on the Mitrofanoff stoma and a drain sponge was placed around the tube with Medi-pore tape around it.

Sponge and needle counts were correct ×2 at the end of the procedure. The patient was extubated and taken to the recovery room in stable condition.

Circumcision

49

Nicholas Beecroft and Daryl J. McLeod

Indications and Benefits

- Family/patient preference (cultural/religious/social).
- Symptomatic or persistent phimosis.
- Recurrent balanitis or balanoposthitis.
- Recurrent paraphimosis.
- Urinary tract infections.
- Lichen sclerosis (balanitis xerotica obliterans).
- Benefits: Reduces the risk of urinary tract infection in first year of life, reduces the risk of sexually transmitted infections, and reduces the risk of penile cancer.

Risks and Alternatives

- Standard risks (bleeding, infection, need for additional procedures, and general/regional anesthesia)
- Injury to adjacent structures (urethra or glans)
- Skin dehiscence
- Excess skin removed
- Persistent redundant foreskin
- Penile concealment/secondary phimosis (cicatrix)
- Meatal stenosis
- Skin bridging/adhesions
- Suture tracks
- Alternatives: Steroid cream or dorsal slit in patients with symptomatic phimosis but who wish to avoid circumcision

Essential Steps

1. Retract the foreskin completely, remove smegma, and manually lyse adhesions prior to surgical preparation(If unable to retract, will need dorsal slit and second preparation in surgical sterile field).
2. Surgical preparation and drape.
3. Monopolar cautery is set at 15 coagulation and 15 cut (authors' preference).
4. Injection of local anesthesia for penile block if no regional block performed (before or after procedure per surgeon preference).
5. Retract the foreskin.
6. Place glans holding suture dorsal to meatus (5-0 Proline on taper needle; authors' preference).
7. If prominent frenulum, lift up and away from penis and using cutting current incise this band, lightly touch any bleeding with coagulation current to achieve hemostasis.

N. Beecroft
The Ohio State University College of Medicine, School of Medicine, Columbus, OH, USA
e-mail: Nicholas.Beecroft@osumc.edu

D. J. McLeod (✉)
Nationwide Children's Hospital, Department of Surgery, Section of Urology, Columbus, OH, USA
e-mail: daryl.mcleod@nationwidechildrens.org

D. J. Papandria et al. (eds.), *Operative Dictations in Pediatric Surgery*,
https://doi.org/10.1007/978-3-030-24212-1_49

8. With penis on full stretch, mark the distal (inner) line of the incision below the glans of the penis leaving a 1–2-cm glans collar.
9. Incise the distal (inner) circumferential incision through skin only with either knife or cutting electrocautery current.
10. Using combination of sharp dissection and/or cutting and coagulation electrocautery current, partially deglove the penis down to the level where proximal incision is expected to be made.
11. With the penis on full stretch, reduce foreskin over the glans taking care not to pull up any ventral scrotal skin onto the shaft and mark the proximal (outer) line of the incision just distal to the impression made by the free edge of the glans collar (If there is concern about scrotal skin at the level of the proximal shaft, the proximal (outer) circumcision incision can be carried more distal on the ventral surface to allow this skin to drop down).
12. Incise the proximal (outer) circumferential incision through skin only with either knife or cutting electrocautery current.
13. Connect the two circumferential incisions and remove the intervening foreskin (If the penis was initially degloved down to the level of the proximal incision, the intervening foreskin can be removed with minimal further dissection).
14. Meticulously evaluate for any bleeding and achieve complete hemostasis with coagulation electrocautery current.
15. Reapproximate the skin edges with interrupted full thickness or running subcuticular 4-0 or 5-0 fast absorbing sutures.
16. Apply wrap dressing or surgical glue (as per surgeons' preference).
17. Remove holding suture.

Note These Variations

- Rather than degloving the penis after the initial incision, both circumferential incisions (inner and outer) may be made followed by carful dissection of the intervening foreskin from the underlying tissue and shaft to allow removal.
- While marking the proximal (outer) incision, if the imprint of the free edge of the collar is not visible, a dorsal and ventral slit can be made to identify the appropriate level prior to excising the redundant foreskin.
- If penile torsion is present, the penis rotation should be corrected after complete degloving and positioned in the appropriate orientation as sutures are placed. More severe levels of penile torsion (>90 degrees) may require an absorbable anchoring suture proximally at the dorsal midline. (Knowledge of penile neurovascular anatomy is required to safely perform this step.)
- If moderate-to-severe tethering of the scrotum to penile shaft skin is noted, a formal scrotoplasty may be required to avoid a poor surgical outcome.
- If there is a prominent pubic fat pad where the penis becomes concealed when off traction, an absorbable anchoring suture proximally at the dorsal midline may be necessary to avoid healing complications. (Knowledge of penile neurovascular anatomy is required to safely perform this step.)
- Varying degrees of penile chordee with or without hypospadias require additional surgical maneuvers not covered in this chapter.

Template Operative Dictation (Open)

Preoperative Diagnosis Intact foreskin/phimosis

Postoperative Diagnosis Same as preoperative diagnosis

Findings Intact foreskin/phimosis

Procedure(s) Performed Circumcision

Anesthesia General/local

Specimen Foreskin (no need to send as specimen unless concern for abnormal pathology or institutional policy)

Estimated Blood Loss Minimal

Indications This is a/an ___-*day/week/month/year*-old male with an intact foreskin. The family did request circumcision.

Procedure in Detail Following satisfactory induction of general anesthesia, the patient was placed in the supine position on the operating room bed and appropriately padded. A surgical timeout was performed to identify the patient and confirm the procedure. The foreskin was manually retracted clearing preputial adhesions and smegma. The penis and pubic area was then prepped and draped in the typical sterile fashion. In the surgical field, a local penile block was performed, the foreskin was retracted, and a 5-0 Proline holding suture was then placed in the glans dorsal to the meatus. With the penis on stretch using the holding suture, the frenulum was incised with electrocautery and the base coagulated for hemostasis. A 1–2-cm glans collar was marked and incised with electrocautery on cutting current, taking care to only cut the skin layer and avoid any injury to deeper tissues. The penis was then partially degloved using electrocautery. Again with the penis on full stretch, the foreskin was reduced over the glans and the proximal incision was marked just distal to the imprint of the free edge of the glans collar. The proximal circumferential incision was made using electrocautery on cutting current. A longitudinal incision connecting the two circumferential incisions was made and the intervening foreskin was removed. Hemostasis was achieved with electrocautery. The two skin edges were reapproximated using interrupted 5-0 chromic sutures. A medium tegaderm was cut to size, and then placed as a wrap dressing allong the entire length of the penis. The holding suture was removed. The patient tolerated the procedure well, was extubated in the operating room, and was transported to the post anesthesia care unit in stable condition.

Orchiopexy (Open and MIS Approaches)

50

Christopher Jaeger and Seth A. Alpert

Indications and Benefits

- Absence of spontaneous testicular descent by 6 months of age (corrected for gestational age)
- In prepubertal boys with palpable, undescended testes
- In prepubertal boys with nonpalpable testes
- In cases of acute or intermittent testicular torsion
- Benefits: Testicular cancer prevention/screening, preservation of fertility and psychological

Risks and Alternatives

- Standard surgical risks (bleeding, infection, need for additional procedures, and risks of anesthesia)
- Injury to adjacent structures (testicle, epididymis, ilioinguinal nerve, spermatic cord vessels, and vas deferens)
- Testicular retraction, persistent cryptorchidism, testicular atrophy, postoperative hernia, and testis torsion
- Alternatives: Approach (open or laparoscopic) and/or orchiectomy

Essential Steps

Inguinal Orchiopexy

1. Identification and exposure of the external ring.
2. Opening of the external oblique fascia.
3. Identification and mobilization of the testicle off the gubernaculum and dissection of the cremasteric muscle fibers.
4. Isolation and preservation of the ilioinguinal nerve.
5. Dissecting off the patent processus vaginalis/hernia sac from the cord structures and high suture ligation of the sac.
6. Additional proximal mobilization of the cord structures as needed.
7. Delivery of testis from inguinal region to scrotum.
8. Creation of subdartos pouch for testis.
9. Pexy/fixation of testis to dartos fascia of the hemiscrotum.

Laparoscopic Orchiopexy

1. Infraumbilical or transumbilical incision.
2. Establishment of pneumoperitoneum and identification of testicle or absence of the same.

C. Jaeger (✉)
The Ohio State University Wexner Medical Center, Department of Urology, Columbus, OH, USA
e-mail: Christopher.jaeger@osumc.edu

S. A. Alpert
Nationwide Children's Hospital and The Ohio State University Wexner Medical Center, Section of Urology, Columbus, OH, USA
e-mail: seth.alpert@nationwidechildrens.org

D. J. Papandria et al. (eds.), *Operative Dictations in Pediatric Surgery*,
https://doi.org/10.1007/978-3-030-24212-1_50

3. Release of gubernacular attachments.
4. Mobilization of the cord structures, including spermatic cord vessels and vas deferens.
5. Dissection of peritoneal tissues off the cord structures until the testis is able to reach contralateral internal inguinal ring without significant tension.
6. Pass laparoscopic instrument antegrade from abdominal port adjacent to inferior epigastric vessels and into scrotum.
7. Creation of subdartos pouch and passing a laparoscopic port retrograde into the peritoneal cavity under direct vision through which a second instrument can be utilized to grasp testicle.
8. Pull testicle through the new tract and into appropriate scrotal position.
9. Pexy/fixation of testicle to dartos fascia of the hemiscrotum.
10. Release pneumoperitoneum, remove ports under vision, and close all incisions.

Scrotal Orchiopexy

1. Transverse hemiscrotal or midline scrotal incision.
2. Locate testicle and perform detorsion in cases of testis torsion.
3. Dissect off gubernacular attachments and cremasteric fibers.
4. Dissect the vasal and vascular pedicle proximally by releasing surrounding attachments.
5. Identify any hernia sac, if present, dissect off cord structures, and ligate sac as needed.
6. Creation of subdartos pouch.
7. Pexy/fixation of testicle to dartos fascia of the hemiscrotum.

Note These Variations

- Inguinal orchiopexy
- Laparoscopic orchiopexy
- Scrotal orchiopexy

Template Operative Dictation (Inguinal Orchiopexy)

Preoperative Diagnosis Undescended testicle

Postoperative Diagnosis Same as preoperative diagnosis

Findings Same as postoperative diagnosis

Procedure(s) Performed (Left/right/bilateral) Inguinal orchiopexy

Anesthesia General/regional +/− local

Specimen +/− Inguinal hernia sac

Drains None

Implants None

Estimated Blood Loss ___

Indications This is a/an ___*-day/week/month/year*-old *male* with a palpable undescended testicle. He was deemed to be a suitable candidate for inguinal orchiopexy. The risks and benefits of surgery were discussed with the parents/guardians at length and they agreed to proceed.

Procedure in Detail The patient was correctly identified in the preoperative area and brought to the operating room for surgery. Following satisfactory induction of anesthesia, the patient was placed in supine position and appropriately padded. Timeouts were performed using both preinduction and preincision safety checklists with participation of all present in the operative suite. These confirmed the correct patient, procedure, operative site, and additional critical information prior to the start of the procedure. The lower abdomen and genitalia were then prepped and draped in the usual sterile fashion.

A 1–1.5 in. incision was made in the groin overlying the inguinal canal, and the tissues were dissected down to the external oblique fascia. The external ring was identified and the fascia was opened up to the level of the internal ring.

The ilioinguinal nerve was identified and carefully preserved throughout the entire dissection. The testis was found distal to the external ring *(or within the canal)* and dissected off the gubernaculum. The cremasteric muscle fibers were then dissected both medially and laterally up to the level of the internal inguinal ring *(In cases of a peeping testicle, the gubernaculum is used as a guide to locate the testis at the level of the internal inguinal ring.).* At this point in time, a hernia sac was located along the anteromedial surface of the cord and this was then carefully separated from the spermatic cord vessels and vas deferens with care not to injure the spermatic cord structures. The hernia sac was then isolated, cross clamped, divided, and then high suture ligated. This now allowed for adequate length on the spermatic cord for the testicle to reach the ipsilateral hemiscrotum without any tension. A finger was then inserted through the inguinal incision and placed superficial to the pubic tubercle and in the hemiscrotum, and a transverse hemiscrotal incision was performed. A subdartos pouch was created and a tonsil clamp placed in contact with the fingertip in the hemiscrotum, which was then guided back through the inguinal incision. At this point, the cord structures were confirmed to be orthotopic with the spermatic vessels anterior to the vas deferens. The inferior aspect of the testicle was grasped gently with the clamp and brought straight down to the ipsilateral hemiscrotum in an orthotopic manner. The testis was tacked to the dartos fascia within the scrotum using *(monofilament or braided; permanent or absorbable suture per surgeon preference)* suture, and the testis was replaced back into the scrotum.

The dartos muscle and scrotal incision were closed with absorbable suture. Hemostasis was excellent. An ilioinguinal block was then performed *(if regional anesthesia was not performed).* The inguinal incision was then closed in multiple layers with absorbable suture with great care taken not to injure or entrap the ilioinguinal nerve during fascial closure. Dermabond *(or dressing of choice)* was applied to the incisions.

Upon completion of the procedure, a debriefing checklist was completed to share information critical to the postoperative care of the patient. The patient tolerated the procedure well, *was extubated in the operating room,* and was transported to the postanesthesia care unit in stable condition.

Template Operative Dictation (Laparoscopic Orchiopexy)

Preoperative Diagnosis Nonpalpable testis

Postoperative Diagnosis Same as preoperative diagnosis

Findings Same as postoperative diagnosis

Procedure(s) Performed Laparoscopic orchiopexy

Anesthesia *General* plus local or regional

Specimen None

Drains None

Implants None

Estimated Blood Loss ___

Indications This is a/an ___*-day/week/month/year*-old *male* with nonpalpable testis. He was deemed to be a suitable candidate for laparoscopic orchiopexy. The risks and benefits of surgery were discussed with the parents/guardians at length and they agreed to proceed.

Procedure in Detail The patient was correctly identified in the preoperative area and brought to the operating room for surgery. Following satisfactory induction of anesthesia, the patient was placed in supine position and appropriately padded. Timeouts were performed using both preinduction and preincision safety checklists with participation of all present in the operative suite. These confirmed the correct patient, procedure, operative site, and additional critical information prior to the start of the procedure. The lower abdomen and genitalia were then prepped and draped in the usual sterile fashion.

The bladder was drained completely using a catheter. An infraumbilical *(or transumbilical incision)* was made and the anterior rectus fascia was identified. Using a Veress needle technique *(or Hasson technique per surgeon preference)*, the abdomen was insufflated to create a pneumoperitoneum and a 5-mm Versa step laparoscopy port was placed in the abdomen through the incision. The laparoscope was placed through the port and diagnostic laparoscopy was then performed.

We looked at the ipsilateral internal ring and found the testicle sitting proximal to the entrance of the ring. We then proceeded to place two additional 3-mm *(or 5-mm)* laparoscopic ports on either side of the abdomen lateral to and at the level of the umbilicus under direct vision.

The testicle was grasped with a Maryland grasper and the attachments to the gubernaculum within the inguinal canal were carefully dissected to free the testicle from the inguinal canal. During this time, the vas deferens was carefully observed and the presence of a long looping vas was noted *(if present)*. Once the gubernacular attachments were freed with preservation of the vas, a triangular shaped peritoneal flap was created with the medial aspect being medial to the vas and the lateral aspect being lateral to the gonadal blood vessels. The blood vessels were dissected as far proximally as possible. The vas was dissected all the way close to the posterior aspect of the bladder with care to free the peritoneal flap from the ipsilateral ureter without injuring it. After the dissection was completed, the testicle reached the contralateral internal ring without tension.

The bladder was once again emptied *(if needed)* and a small ipsilateral transverse hemiscrotal incision was made. A laparoscopic Maryland grasper was passed through the ipsilateral working port, medially to the inferior epigastric vessels and lateral to the obliterated umbilical ligament into the groin and out through the scrotal incision. A 5-mm *(or 12-mm, per preference)* laparoscopic port was passed retrograde into the abdomen over the Maryland grasper and the port placed into the peritoneal cavity. Through this port, the testicle was grasped inferiorly and brought down into the scrotum. (*The abdomen can be desufflated at this point if needed to assist with the testis reaching the scrotum.)*

[Choose One:]

If testicle did not reach the scrotum: (1) The insufflation was maintained/restarted and the peritoneum overlying the vessels was removed and the cord further skeletonized. At this point, the testis had enough length to reach the scrotum. (2) The testis was still on tension and instead of skeletonizing the cord further, we proceeded with transection of the gonadal vessels to perform a Fowler-Stephens procedure. The peritoneal attachments along the vas deferens were maintained and the spermatic vessels were cleaned off. A 5-mm laparoscopic clip applier was used and two clips were placed proximally and one distally along the vessels. The vessels were transected in between the clips and further dissection distally was done to unfurl the remaining cord structures between the testis and vas deferens, which gave enough length for the testicle to reach the dependent portion of the scrotum.

If/when testicle did reach the scrotum: A subdartos pouch was created and the testicle was stitched to the bottom of the dartos pouch without significant tension using a __-0 silk *(or Prolene)* suture. The dartos fascia overlying the incision was closed with a running *(or interrupted)* __-0 absorbable suture and the skin reapproximated with absorbable stitches.

All ports were removed under direct vision, the CO_2 gas was completely evacuated, and the fascia and skin were closed with absorbable suture. Dermabond *(or dressing of choice)* was used to cover the incisions as skin dressings. Upon completion of the procedure, a debriefing checklist was completed to share information critical to the postoperative care of the patient. The patient tolerated the procedure well, *was extubated in the operating room*, and was transported to the post anesthesia care unit in stable condition thereafter.

Template Operative Dictation (Scrotal Orchiopexy)

Preoperative Diagnosis Undescended testicle

Postoperative Diagnosis Same as preoperative diagnosis

Findings Same as postoperative diagnosis

Procedure(s) Performed Scrotal orchiopexy

Anesthesia General/regional +/– local

Specimen None

Estimated Blood Loss ___

Indications This is a/an ___*-day/week/month/year-*old *male* with a palpable undescended testis. He was deemed to be a suitable candidate for scrotal orchiopexy. The risks and benefits of surgery were discussed with the parents/guardians at length and they agreed to proceed.

Procedure in Detail The patient was correctly identified in the preoperative area and brought to the operating room for surgery. Following satisfactory induction of anesthesia, the patient was placed in supine position and appropriately padded. Timeouts were performed using both preinduction and preincision safety checklists with participation of all present in the operative suite. These confirmed the correct patient, procedure, operative site, and additional critical information prior to the start of the procedure.

We made a transverse *(or midline scrotal incision if procedure is bilateral or done in the setting of testis torsion)* incision in the midscrotum overlying the palpable ipsilateral testis. We bluntly mobilized through the subcutaneous tissue. We identified the testis and placed a hemostat on the tunica of the testis and brought this out into the field. We dissected off the gubernacular attachments as well as the cremasteric fibers both medially and laterally all the way up to the external ring. *(The testis was detorsed into the orthotopic orientation (if the procedure is being done for testis torsion).)* We then carefully freed the testicle of investing tissue down to the vasal and vascular pedicle. The tunica vaginalis was opened and the testis was examined.

If there is evidence of a patent processus vaginalis: A hernia sac was noted along the anteromedial aspect of the cord structures. This was carefully dissected off the spermatic cord vessels and vas deferens. The sac was then isolated, cross-clamped, and then high-suture ligated at the level of the external ring.

Enough length was gained in order to bring the testis in a dependent location in the scrotum. A subdartos pouch was created and the testis was fixed in the scrotum with __-0 silk *(or Prolene)* suture(s). The testis was then placed back into the scrotum and we then closed the scrotal skin with absorbable suture. Dermabond *(or dressing of choice)* was used to cover the incision.

Upon completion of the procedure, a debriefing checklist was completed to share information critical to the postoperative care of the patient. The patient tolerated the procedure well, *was extubated in the operating room*, and was transported to the post anesthesia care unit in stable condition thereafter.

Fowler-Stephens Procedure

51

Kyle J. Van Arendonk and Dai H. Chung

Indications and Benefits

- Indication: High/intraabdominal undescended testis that does not spontaneously descend by 6 months of age and cannot be brought into the scrotum at initial operation without undue tension
- Benefits: Tension-free placement of the testis into the scrotum while avoiding testicular atrophy, allowing for future testicular examinations/surveillance (little to no effect on testicular function/fertility, however)

Risks and Alternatives

- Standard risks (bleeding, infection, need for additional procedures, risks of anesthesia)
- Injury to adjacent structures (vas deferens, testicle, femoral vessels, trocar/Veress needle injury to bowel or bladder)
- Testicular ischemia/atrophy
- Recurrent cryptorchidism
- Alternatives: Single-stage orchiopexy if adequate length exists to allow tension-free placement of the testis into the scrotum with one operation

Essential Steps

First Stage

1. Identification of the vas deferens and testicle
2. Assessment of distance between the testicle and internal inguinal ring and thereby advisability of completing a single-stage procedure
3. Minimal dissection near the testicle with high ligation of the testicular vessels

Second Stage

1. Re-identification of the testis and assessment of perfusion/viability
2. Division of testicular peritoneal attachments
3. Assessment of adequate length to achieve orchiopexy
4. Creation of a dartos pouch and completion of orchiopexy

K. J. Van Arendonk (✉)
Children's Hospital of Wisconsin, Department of Surgery, Milwaukee, WI, USA
e-mail: kvanarendonk@chw.org

D. H. Chung
Children's Medical Center Dallas, Department of Surgery, Dallas, TX, USA
e-mail: Dai.Chung@UTSouthwestern.edu

D. J. Papandria et al. (eds.), *Operative Dictations in Pediatric Surgery*,
https://doi.org/10.1007/978-3-030-24212-1_51

Note These Variations

- Open versus laparoscopic.
- Initial access to the peritoneal cavity (Veress or Hasson) for laparoscopic technique.
- Various trocar types and sizes.
- Electrocautery or clips for division of testicular vessels.
- Some describe a single-stage Fowler-Stephens procedure, but most consider it a two-stage operation with 3–6 months between stages to allow for adequate development of collateral perfusion to the testicle.
- Some prefer orchiopexy with no fixation sutures between the tunica albuginea and dartos to avoid potential damage to the testicle.

Template Operative Dictation (Open, First Stage)

Preoperative Diagnosis High/intra-abdominal undescended *left/right* testis

Postoperative Diagnosis Same as preoperative diagnosis

Findings Same as postoperative diagnosis

Procedure(s) Performed Fowler-Stephens procedure

Anesthesia General anesthesia with *ilioinguinal nerve block/local anesthesia/caudal block.*

Specimen None

Drains None

Implants None

Estimated Blood Loss ___ mL

Indications This is a/an ___*-month/year*-old male with a high undescended testis. He was observed for ___ months without achieving testicular descent into the scrotum. He was thus deemed to be a suitable candidate for Fowler-Stephens procedure to achieve orchiopexy.

Procedure in Detail Following satisfactory induction of anesthesia, the patient was positioned supine with proper padding and support *including a small blue towel bump*. Timeouts were performed using both preinduction and preincision safety checklists with participation of all present in the operative suite. These confirmed the correct patient, procedure, operative site, and additional critical information prior to the start of the procedure. Inguinal and genital areas were prepped and draped in the usual sterile fashion. *Left/right* testis was not palpable in the scrotum or inguinal canal. *Left/right* testis was palpable in the normal scrotal position. *Left/right* inguinal skin incision was made obliquely along the skin crease using a scalpel. Subcutaneous and Scarpa's fascia dissection was performed sharply using Metzenbaum scissors. The external inguinal ring was identified, and the external oblique aponeurosis was incised using a knife and Metzenbaum scissors. The ilioinguinal nerve was identified and preserved. The inner layer of the external oblique aponeurosis was mobilized bluntly to dissect free the inguinal canal. *Left/right* testis of normal size and caliber was found near the *left/right* internal inguinal ring. Due to the very proximal position of the undescended *left/right* testis, the decision was made to proceed with a two-stage Fowler-Stephens orchiopexy. Minimal dissection around the *left/right* testis was performed, staying well wide of the testis. The vas deferens was identified and carefully dissected away from the cord structures. The vascular pedicle was isolated well away from the testis and ligated using ___-0 *silk/Vicryl* ties and transected using Metzenbaum scissors. After hemostasis was confirmed, the external oblique aponeurosis was approximated using a *continuous/interrupted* ___-0 Vicryl stitch. Scarpa's fascia was approximated with ___-0 Vicryl stitch. Skin edges were approximated with a running ___-0 subcuticular *Vicryl/Monocryl* stitch. *Topical skin adhesive/steri-strips and a sterile dressing* were applied. No complications were noted. Sponge and needle counts were correct. Upon completion of the procedure, a debriefing checklist was completed to share information critical to the postoperative care of the patient. The patient tolerated the procedure well, *was extubated in the operating room*, and was transported to the postanesthesia care unit in stable condition.

Template Operative Dictation (Open, Second Stage)

Preoperative Diagnosis High/intraabdominal undescended *left/right* testis.

Postoperative Diagnosis Same as preoperative diagnosis

Findings Same as postoperative diagnosis

Procedure(s) Performed Fowler-Stephens procedure

Anesthesia General anesthesia with *ilioinguinal nerve block/local anesthesia/caudal block*

Specimen None

Drains None

Implants None

Estimated Blood Loss ___ mL

Indications This is a/an ___-*month/year*-old male with a high undescended testis. He was observed for ___ months without achieving testicular descent into the scrotum. He was thus deemed to be a suitable candidate for Fowler-Stephens procedure to achieve orchiopexy. He underwent the first-stage procedure ___ months ago and now presents for the second-stage procedure.

Procedure in Detail Following satisfactory induction of anesthesia, the patient was positioned supine with proper padding and support *including a small blue towel bump*. Timeouts were performed using both preinduction and preincision safety checklists with participation of all present in the operative suite. These confirmed the correct patient, procedure, operative site, and additional critical information prior to the start of the procedure. Inguinal and genital areas were prepped and draped in the usual sterile fashion. *Left/right* inguinal skin incision was made obliquely along the skin crease using a scalpel. Subcutaneous and Scarpa's fascia dissection was performed sharply using Metzenbaum scissors. The external inguinal ring was identified and the external oblique aponeurosis was incised using a knife and Metzenbaum scissors. The ilioinguinal nerve was identified and preserved. The inner layer of the external oblique aponeurosis was mobilized bluntly to dissect free the inguinal canal. *Left/right* testis of normal size and caliber was identified in the inguinal canal. Testis and cord structures were mobilized, and the cremaster fibers were dissected. A patent processus vaginalis consistent with a hernia sac was clamped and dissected away from the vas deferens up to the internal inguinal ring. This dissection was continued further to ensure an adequate length of vas deferens for orchiopexy. The hernia sac was suture ligated using two ___-0 *silk/Vicryl* stitches and excised distally. After further mobilization, the *left/right* testicle appeared to reach down to the scrotum without significant tension. A finger was introduced through the incision and blunt dissection was performed to reach the mid-scrotum. While applying gentle traction to stretch the scrotal skin, a *left/right* transverse scrotal incision was made using a scalpel. Subcutaneous dissection was performed to create a dartos pouch. A small incision was made in the subdartos fascia using electrocautery. A Mayo clamp was then introduced into the inguinal region and the *left/right* testicle was pulled down into the dartos pouch. Proper orientation of the cord structures was confirmed. ___-0 Vicryl stitches were placed from the edge of dartos to the tunica albuginea to secure the testis in the dartos pouch. The scrotal skin incision was approximated using interrupted ___-0 chromic stitches. After hemostasis was confirmed, the external oblique aponeurosis was approximated using a *continuous/interrupted* ___-0 Vicryl stitch. Scarpa's fascia was approximated with ___-0 Vicryl stitch. Skin edges were approximated with a running ___-0 subcuticular *Vicryl/Monocryl* stitch. *Topical skin adhesive/ steri-strips and a sterile dressing* were applied. No complications were noted. Sponge and needle counts were correct. Upon completion of the procedure, a debriefing checklist was completed to share information critical to the postoperative care of the patient. The patient tolerated the procedure well, *was extubated in the operating room*, and was transported to the postanesthesia care unit in stable condition.

Template Operative Dictation (Laparoscopic, First Stage)

Preoperative Diagnosis High/intraabdominal undescended *left/right* testis

Postoperative Diagnosis Same as preoperative diagnosis

Findings Same as Postoperative Diagnosis

Procedure(s) Performed Laparoscopic Fowler-Stephens procedure

Anesthesia General

Specimen None

Drains None

Implants None.

Estimated Blood Loss ___ mL

Indications This is a/an ___-*month/year* old male with a high undescended testis. He was observed for ___ months without achieving testicular descent into the scrotum. He was thus deemed to be a suitable candidate for a laparoscopic Fowler-Stephens procedure to achieve orchiopexy.

Procedure in Detail Following satisfactory induction of anesthesia, the patient was positioned supine with proper padding. The bladder was decompressed with a Crede maneuver. Timeouts were performed using both preinduction and preincision safety checklists with participation of all present in the operative suite. These confirmed the correct patient, procedure, operative site, and additional critical information prior to the start of the procedure. Inguinal, genital, and abdominal areas were prepped and draped in the usual sterile fashion. *Left/right* testis was not palpable in the scrotum or inguinal canal. *Left/right* testis was palpable in the normal scrotal position. *The infraumbilical area was infiltrated with 0.25% Marcaine.* A small curvilinear incision was made.

[Choose One:]

For Veress Needle: *After picking up the anterior abdominal wall with towel clips, a Veress needle was advanced into the abdominal cavity, which was insufflated with carbon dioxide up to ___ mm Hg pressure. The Veress needle was replaced with a 5-mm trocar, and a laparoscope was introduced.*

For Hasson Technique: *The fascia was elevated and incised. The peritoneum was incised, and a 5-mm trocar was inserted into the peritoneal cavity under direct visualization. The abdomen was insufflated with carbon dioxide up to ___ mm Hg, and a laparoscope was introduced.*

Left lower quadrant and suprapubic *3-mm reusable Storz trocars* were placed in the standard fashion. Patient was positioned in Trendelenburg. Intraabdominal *left/right* testis was noted near the *left/right* internal inguinal ring. The decision was made to proceed with the first of a two-stage Fowler-Stephens orchiopexy. The vas deferens was identified and preserved. Minimal wide blunt dissection was performed to isolate the testicular vascular pedicle. Electrocautery was used to transect the testicular vessels well away from the testis. Hemostasis was confirmed, and all laparoscopic instruments were removed. The infraumbilical fascia was approximated using a ___-0 Vicryl stitch. All skin incisions were approximated using *interrupted/running* ___-0 *Vicryl/Monocryl* subcuticular sutures. *Topical skin adhesive/steri-strips and sterile dressings* were applied. No complications were noted. Sponge and needle counts were correct. Upon completion of the procedure, a debriefing checklist was completed to share information critical to the postoperative care of the patient. The patient tolerated the procedure well, *was extubated in the operating room*, and was transported to the postanesthesia care unit in stable condition.

Template Operative Dictation (Laparoscopic, Second Stage)

Preoperative Diagnosis High/intraabdominal undescended *left/right* testis

Postoperative Diagnosis Same as preoperative diagnosis

Findings Same as postoperative diagnosis

Procedure(s) Performed Laparoscopic Fowler-Stephens procedure

Anesthesia General

Specimen None

Drains None

Implants None

Estimated Blood Loss ___ mL

Indications This is a/an ___-*month/year*-old male with a high undescended testis. He was observed for ___ months without achieving testicular descent into the scrotum. He was thus deemed to be a suitable candidate for Fowler-Stephens procedure to achieve orchiopexy. He underwent the first-stage procedure ___ months ago and now presents for the second-stage procedure.

Procedure in Detail Following satisfactory induction of anesthesia, the patient was positioned supine with proper padding. The bladder was decompressed with a Crede maneuver. Timeouts were performed using both preinduction and preincision safety checklists with participation of all present in the operative suite. These confirmed the correct patient, procedure, operative site, and additional critical information prior to the start of the procedure. Inguinal, genital, and abdominal areas were prepped and draped in the usual sterile fashion. *The infraumbilical area was infiltrated with 0.25% Marcaine.* A small curvilinear incision was made.

[Choose One:]
For Veress needle: *After picking up the anterior abdominal wall with towel clips, a Veress needle was advanced into the abdominal cavity, which was insufflated with carbon dioxide up to ___ mm Hg pressure. The Veress needle was replaced with a 5-mm trocar, and a laparoscope was introduced.*

For Hasson technique: *The fascia was elevated and incised. The peritoneum was incised, and a 5-mm trocar was inserted into the peritoneal cavity under direct visualization. The abdomen was insufflated with carbon dioxide up to ___ mm Hg, and a laparoscope was introduced.*

The patient was positioned in Trendelenburg. The *left/right* inguinal canal region was inspected, and a viable, well-perfused, and normal-sized intraabdominal testis was noted. Left lower quadrant and suprapubic *3-mm reusable metal Storz trocars* were placed in the standard fashion. A laparoscopic grasper was used to grip the tissues around the testis and gently dissect the testis from its gubernacular attachment. A wide dissection was performed to mobilize the testis while carefully preserving the vas deferens. Blunt dissection was performed at the *left/right* lateral aspect of the bladder medial to the umbilical vein remnant ligament. While applying gentle traction to stretch the scrotal skin, a *left/right* transverse scrotal incision was made using a scalpel. Subcutaneous dissection was performed to create a dartos pouch. A Veress needle was placed through the scrotal incision into the abdominal cavity under direct visualization. The Veress needle was replaced with a 5-mm expandable trocar, and a laparoscopic grasper was passed through this trocar into the abdominal cavity. The *left/right* testis was grasped and gently pulled down into the dartos pouch. Proper orientation of the testis in the dartos pouch was confirmed. The testis was then secured in the dartos pouch at four quadrants using multiple interrupted ___-0 Vicryl stitches from the edge of dartos to the tunica albuginea. Scrotal skin edges were approximated using interrupted ___-0 chromic stitches. Hemostasis was confirmed. All laparoscopic instruments and ports were removed under direct visualization. The infraumbilical fascia was approximated using an interrupted ___-0 Vicryl stitch. All skin incisions were approximated using *interrupted/running* ___-0 *Vicryl/Monocryl* subcuticular sutures. *Topical skin adhesive/steri-strips and sterile dressings* were applied. No complications were noted. Sponge and needle counts were correct. Upon completion of the procedure, a debriefing checklist was completed to share information critical to the postoperative care of the patient. The patient tolerated the procedure well, *was extubated in the operating room*, and was transported to the postanesthesia care unit in stable condition.

Radical/Simple Orchiectomy

52

Laura Rausch and Harold N. Lovvorn III

Indications and Benefits

- Testicular neoplasm/cancer
- Paratesticular malignancy
- Testicular torsion
- Benefits: Cancer treatment/diagnosis, removal of necrotic testicle/prevention of sepsis

Risks and Alternatives

- Standard risks (bleeding, infection, need for additional procedures, risks of anesthesia)
- Injury to adjacent structures (Ilioinguinal nerve)
- Infertility
- Changes in hormone levels
- Recurrence of cancer/failure to prevent metastasis
- Alternatives: Observation, testicular enucleation for cancer diagnosis

L. Rausch (✉)
Vanderbilt University Medical Center, Department of General Surgery, Nashville, TN, USA
e-mail: laura.a.rausch@vumc.org

H. N. Lovvorn III
Monroe Carell Jr. Children's Hospital at Vanderbilt, Department of Pediatric Surgery, Nashville, TN, USA
e-mail: harold.lovvorn@Vanderbilt.Edu

Essential Steps

Radical Orchiectomy (Cancer Treatment)

1. Make a skin crease incision 1–2 cm above and parallel to the inguinal ligament, ensuring to follow the line connecting the internal and external rings (analogous to an incision for inguinal herniorrhaphy).
   (a) If the tumor/testicle is too large to pass through this incision, may extend incision toward scrotum.
2. Continue the incision through subcutaneous tissue and the Camper's and Scarpa's fascia.
3. Identify external oblique fibers and external inguinal ring.
4. Incise the external oblique aponeurosis along the direction of its fibers through the external ring.
5. Identify and preserve the ilioinguinal nerve and separate it ensuring that one does not damage it during orchiectomy.
6. Take the two leaves of the external oblique fascia (i.e., aponeurosis) with a hemostat and lift anteriorly to dissect freely the spermatic cord (i.e., the testicular vessels and vas deferens) along its length.
7. Isolate the spermatic cord at the pubic tubercle. Wrap a Penrose drain tightly around it and secure with a hemostat to form a tourniquet.

D. J. Papandria et al. (eds.), *Operative Dictations in Pediatric Surgery*,
https://doi.org/10.1007/978-3-030-24212-1_52

8. Stretch the point of entry of the cord into the scrotum with a finger and retract the testicle to the operative site.
9. Identify the gubernaculum and then clamp, divide, and ligate.
10. Confirm diagnosis with inspection; rarely a frozen section is required.
11. Take the spermatic cord in two portions (a vascular portion and the vas deferens) by double clamping, dividing, and ligating above the tourniquet. The cord must be ligated as close as possible to the internal ring to ensure complete removal of the cord tissue.
12. Remove testicle from operative field and send to pathology.
13. Inspect the wound and scrotum for hemostasis.
14. Close the external oblique fascia and external ring in a running fashion, appose scarpa's fascia in a running fashion, and close the skin.

Simple Orchiectomy (for Benign Disorders)

1. Midline scrotal incision is made through skin, subcutaneous tissue, dartos layer, and the tunica vaginalis.
2. The testicle is then delivered through the scrotal incision.
3. The gubernaculum is identified, divided, and ligated.
4. The spermatic cord is then identified above the testicle, clamped, divided, and ligated.
5. Remove the testicle from the operative field and send to pathology.
6. Observe scrotal sac to ensure hemostasis.
7. Two-layer closure performed with a running or interrupted 3-0 absorbable braided suture. Skin is closed with a running 4-0 absorbable monofilament suture.

Template Operative Dictation (Open)

Preoperative Diagnosis Testicular mass/torsion.

Postoperative Diagnosis Same as preoperative diagnosis

Findings Testicular mass/torsion

Procedure(s) Performed Radical/simple orchiectomy

Anesthesia *General*

Specimen Testicular cord and testicle

Drains None

Implants None

Estimated Blood Loss ___ mL

Indications This patient is a/an ___-*day/week/month/year*-old *male* with testicular mass/torsion. He was deemed to be a suitable candidate for radical/simple orchiectomy

Procedure in Detail Following satisfactory induction of general anesthesia, the patient was placed in supine position, and pressure points were appropriately padded. Timeout was performed using both preinduction and preincision safety checklists with participation of all present in the operative suite. These checklists confirmed the correct patient, procedure, operative site, and additional critical information prior to the start of the procedure. The right lower quadrant/left lower quadrant, right inguinal area/left inguinal area, and genitalia were then prepped and draped in the usual sterile fashion.

[Choose One:]
If radical orchiectomy: A small inguinal incision was made and carried down through the subcutaneous tissue to expose the external oblique aponeurosis. This layer was opened along the length of its fibers to expose the spermatic cord and ilioinguinal nerve. The nerve was carefully dissected and retracted medially to preserve it. The spermatic cord was dissected freely, and a Penrose drain was applied tightly around the cord and looped as a tourniquet. Further dissection of the

spermatic cord through mobilization of the dartos fascia distally was performed to free the testicle. The gubernaculum was identified, dissected, and ligated. After these maneuvers, the testicle was delivered into the operative field. Next, the spermatic cord was dissected to the internal inguinal ring. The cord was then divided in two portions, the vascular portion and the vas deferens, by double clamping, dividing, and ligating with 0 silk ties above the tourniquet abutting the internal ring. The testicle and spermatic cord were then removed and sent to pathology. The proximal cord was then observed for hemostasis, and no active bleeding was identified. The floor of the inguinal canal was also examined for hemostasis, which was confirmed. The ilioinguinal nerve was preserved. The external oblique fascia fascia was then re-approximated using running 3-0 Vicryl suture. The wound was then irrigated with sterile water. The subcutaneous tissue with re-approximated with running 3-0 Vicryl suture. The skin was closed with running 4-0 Monocryl suture and dressed with Dermabond.

If simple orchiectomy: A midline scrotal incision was made through the skin of the raphe/septum, subcutaneous tissue, dartos layer, and then the tunica vaginalis. The testicle was palpated, and the gubernaculum was identified. The gubernaculum was divided and ligated. The testicle was then delivered through the scrotal incision. The spermatic cord was identified above the epididymis and then clamped, divided, and ligated. The testicle was then removed and sent to pathology. The remaining scrotal contents were inspected and noted to be normal. Hemostasis was achieved. A two-layer closure of the scrotal incision was performed with 3-0 absorbable suture. The skin was closed using 4-0 Monocryl suture.

Upon completion of the procedure, a debriefing checklist was completed to share information critical to the postoperative care of the patient. The patient tolerated the procedure well, *was extubated in the operating room*, and was transported to the postanesthesia care unit in stable condition.

53 Incision and Drainage of Bartholin Gland Duct Cyst or Abscess with Word Catheter Placement; Marsupialization of Bartholin Gland Duct Cyst or Abscess

Alejandra Vilanova-Sánchez
and Kate A. McCracken

Indications and Benefits

- Symptomatic Bartholin gland duct cysts (causing pain/pressure that interferes with physical and/or sexual activity)
- Bartholin gland duct abscesses
- Benefits: Drainage of cyst fluid or abscess contents provides relief of symptoms and helps to resolve the infection

Risks and Alternatives

- Standard risks (bleeding, infection, need for additional procedures, risks of anesthesia)
- Injury to adjacent structures – vagina, labia, and urethra
- Recurrent cyst or abscess if I&D site closes
- Alternatives: Consider complete Bartholin gland excision in patients with multiple recurrences

A. Vilanova-Sánchez
Hospital La Paz, Department of Pediatric Surgery, Madrid, Spain

K. A. McCracken (✉)
Nationwide Children's Hospital, Department of Pediatric & Adolescent Gynecology, Columbus, OH, USA
e-mail: kate.mccracken@nationwidechildrens.org

Essential Steps

1. Dorsal lithotomy.
2. Bimanual exam to determine the extent of the cyst/abscess.
3. Vertical incision with an 11 blade through the skin into the cyst/abscess (outside the hymen at the 5 or 7 o'clock position on the vulva along inner surface of the cyst/abscess).
4. Drain the purulent material – obtain a culture.
5. Word catheter into the empty cavity – to remain in place for 4–6 weeks.

If Performing a Marsupialization

1. Follow steps 1–2 above.
2. Skin incision with 10 or 15 blades on the vestibule near the medial edge of the labia minora – do not puncture the underlying cyst wall.
3. Incise cyst wall and suture the cyst wall to its adjacent skin edge using interrupted delayed absorbable suture.

Preoperative Diagnosis Bartholin gland duct *cyst/abscess.*

Postoperative Diagnosis Same as preoperative diagnosis.

D. J. Papandria et al. (eds.), *Operative Dictations in Pediatric Surgery*,
https://doi.org/10.1007/978-3-030-24212-1_53

Findings Same as postoperative diagnosis.

Procedure(s) Performed Incision and drainage of Bartholin gland duct cyst or abscess with word catheter placement; marsupialization of Bartholin gland duct cyst or abscess.

Anesthesia General anesthesia or local anesthesia

Specimen Anaerobic and aerobic culture abscess cultures

Drains Word catheter

Estimated Blood Loss 5 mL

Indications This is a/an ___-year-old female with a Bartholin gland duct *cyst/abscess*. She was deemed to be a suitable candidate for an incision and drainage with placement of Word catheter.

Procedure in Detail Following satisfactory induction of anesthesia, the patient was placed in dorsal lithotomy and appropriately padded. Timeouts were performed using both preinduction and preincision safety checklists with participation of all present in the operative suite. These confirmed the correct patient, procedure, operative site, and additional critical information prior to the start of the procedure. The perineum was then prepped and draped in the usual sterile fashion. Inspection of the external genitalia was performed and then a bimanual examination was performed – which confirmed the presence of the *right/left* Bartholin gland duct *cyst/abscess*.

[Choose One:]

Placement of word catheter: A 1-cm incision was made through the skin and into the *cyst/abscess* using an 11-blade scalpel along the inner surface of the *cyst/abscess* outside and parallel to the hymen. Cultures of the *cyst/abscess* fluid were obtained. The contents of the *cyst/abscess* were evacuated and a hemostat was used the break up any loculations. Irrigation of the *cyst/abscess* cavity was performed. Next, the tip of a Word catheter was inserted within the deflated *cyst/abscess* cavity. A syringe was used to inject 2–3 mL of sterile water through the port of the catheter to inflate the catheter balloon. The balloon was inflated to a diameter that would prohibit the catheter from falling out of the incision. The end of the catheter was then tucked inside the distal vagina.

Marsupialization of a cyst/abscess: A 2–3-cm vertical incision was made on the vestibule near the medial edge of the labia minora and approximately 1 cm lateral and parallel to the hymenal ring using a 10- or 15-blade scalpel. The *cyst/abscess* was then incised and cultures of the *cyst/abscess* fluid were obtained. The contents of the *cyst/abscess* were evacuated and a hemostat was used the break up any loculations. Irrigation of the *cyst/abscess* cavity was performed. Next, Allis clamps were placed on the superior, inferior, medial, and lateral edges of the cyst wall and overlying skin. The edge of the *cyst/abscess* wall was sutured to the adjacent skin edge using interrupted 3-0 delayed absorbable sutures.

Hemostasis was noted. Upon completion of the procedure, a debriefing checklist was completed to share information critical to the postoperative care of the patient. The patient tolerated the procedure well, was extubated in the operating room, and was transported to the postanesthesia care unit in stable condition thereafter.

54 Management of Ovarian, Isolated Fallopian Tube, or Adnexal Torsion (Open and MIS Approaches)

Alejandra Vilanova-Sánchez
and Kate A. McCracken

Indications and Benefits

- Ovarian torsion with or without an underlying ovarian cyst – the cyst should be suitable for resection at the same procedure (no imaging or intraoperative findings suggestive of malignancy).
- Isolated fallopian tube torsion (with or without an underlying paratubal cyst).
- Adnexal torsion – involving both the ovary and the fallopian tube.
- Benefits: Restores normal anatomy to ensure adequate vascular perfusion to the ovary and/or fallopian tube. Cystectomy reduces the risk of recurrent torsion, allows for a pathologic diagnosis of the underlying cyst, and relieves pain attributed to the cyst.

Risks and Alternatives

- Standard risks: Bleeding, infection, injury to surrounding structures (gastrointestinal, genitourinary, vascular, neural), need for blood products, anesthesia complications, unplanned oophorectomy, and/or salpingectomy
- Alternatives: None

Essential Steps

1. Pfannenstiel incision/laparoscopic approach.
2. A Foley catheter is placed in the bladder. Consider using a uterine manipulator (Hulka clamp) if performing laparoscopy – this allows for deviation of the uterus during the case, which aides in traction/counter traction of the adnexa.
3. Identify ovaries, fallopian tubes, and uterus.
4. Identify the point of torsion and which portions of the adnexa (ovary, fallopian tube, or both) are involved.
5. Restore normal anatomy by twisting in the reverse direction of the torsion.
6. Observe for evidence of tissue reperfusion. Err on the side of fertility preserving procedures by conserving the ovary and/or fallopian tube, rather than performing an oophorectomy or salpingectomy.
7. If an underlying ovarian cyst is present and suitable for removal, the ovarian cortex is incised using low wattage current. The ovarian cortex is gently grasped and the underlying cyst is dissected away from the cortex using traction, counter traction, and hydrodissection. This technique preserves

A. Vilanova-Sánchez
Hospital La Paz, Department of Pediatric Surgery, Madrid, Spain

K. A. McCracken (✉)
Nationwide Children's Hospital, Department of Pediatric & Adolescent Gynecology, Columbus, OH, USA
e-mail: kate.mccracken@nationwidechildrens.org

D. J. Papandria et al. (eds.), *Operative Dictations in Pediatric Surgery*,
https://doi.org/10.1007/978-3-030-24212-1_54

the ovarian cortex (for details, please refer to Chap. 68: resection of benign ovarian lesions).

8. If an underlying paratubal cyst is present, the mesosalpinx is incised using low wattage current. The mesosalpinx is gently grasped and the underlying cyst is dissected away from the mesosalpinx using traction, counter traction, and hydrodissection.
9. Place the cyst in a tissue-extracting bag; if it is a simple fluid filled cyst, the cyst may be decompressed, allowing the tissue-extracting bag to be removed through a smaller diameter port.
10. Irrigate the cyst bed and achieve hemostasis. It is not necessary to re-approximate the ovarian cortex or mesosalpinx edges.
11. Ensure that all portions of the adnexa remain in the correct anatomic orientation with adequate vascular perfusion.
12. Remove ports and close the laparotomy/port incisions.

Note These Variations

- If there is no underlying cause (e.g., cyst or mass) for torsion and the utero-ovarian ligament appears elongated, the proximal portion of the ligament may be attached to its most distal portion with a 2-0 nonabsorbable suture to shorten the ligament and reduce the risk of recurrent torsion.
- Err on the side of fertility preserving procedures by conserving the ovary and/or fallopian tube, rather than performing an oophorectomy or salpingectomy.
- If an underlying ovarian cyst is identified, but is not distinct from the ovarian cortex due to inflammation and venous congestion, detorsion should be performed without concurrent cystectomy. A pelvic ultrasound should be performed at a later date to reassess the need for an elective cystectomy.
- If intraoperative concerns/suspicion of malignant process, recommend an intraoperative consultation with a pediatric gynecologist and/or pediatric surgeon with training in oncology prior to proceeding with a cystectomy or oophorectomy. Oncologic staging may be necessary. If an expert team is unavailable, we recommend detorsing the adnexa, obtaining pelvic washings, and taking photos, and then referring the patient to an expert in pediatric gynecologic oncology.

Template Operative Dictation (Open)

Preoperative Diagnosis *Ovarian/fallopian tube/adnexal* torsion

Postoperative Diagnosis *Ovarian/fallopian tube/adnexal* torsion

Findings Torsed *right/left ovary/fallopian tube/ovary and fallopian tube*

Procedures Performed *Ovarian/fallopian tube* detorsion, *right/left ovarian cystectomy*

Anesthesia General

Specimen Right/left *ovarian cyst/paratubal cyst*

Estimated Blood Loss ____mL

Indications This is a/an ___*-day/week/month/year*-old female who presented with *pelvic pain/abdominal tenderness/___*. Given her symptoms, exam, and imaging, there was concern that she may have an adnexal torsion. We recommended proceeding with an emergent exploratory laparotomy, possible detorsion, possible cystectomy, possible oophorectomy, and possible salpingectomy.

Procedure in Detail Following satisfactory induction of anesthesia, the patient was placed in supine position and appropriately padded. Timeouts were performed using both preinduction and preincision safety checklists with participation of all present in the operative suite. These confirmed the correct patient, procedure, operative site, and additional critical information prior to the start of the procedure. A Foley catheter was inserted in the urethra prior to start of the procedure. The abdomen was then prepped and draped in the usual sterile fashion.

A Pfannenstiel skin incision was made with the scalpel and carried through to the underlying layer of fascia with monopolar cautery. The fascia was incised in the midline and extended laterally using Mayo scissors. Kocher clamps were used to elevate the superior aspect of the fascial incision, and the underlying rectus muscles were dissected off bluntly and using Mayo scissors. Attention was then turned to the inferior aspect of the fascial incision, which in a similar fashion was grasped with Kocher clamps, elevated, and the underlying rectus muscles were dissected off bluntly and using Mayo scissors. The rectus muscles were separated in the midline. The peritoneum was bluntly dissected, entered, and extended superiorly and inferiorly with good visualization of the bladder. We identified enlarged edematous *left/right ovary/fallopian tube/ovary and adnexa*. A degree twist of the *left/right ovarian/tubal* pedicle was identified. The torsion was gently reduced, restoring the adnexa to its normal anatomic position. Immediately, the ovary (fallopian tube or both) began to return to its normal color, indicating return of vascular flow. We examined the rest of the pelvis and noted a normal uterus, normal contralateral ovary, and normal contralateral fallopian tube.

[Choose One:]

If no underlying ovarian cyst or mass (or fallopian tube cyst) is identified: *We did not identify a mass or cyst.*

If an underlying ovarian cyst is present and suitable for removal: *The ovarian cortex was incised using low wattage current. The ovarian cortex was gently grasped and the underlying cyst was dissected away from the cortex using traction and counter traction. Hemostasis was achieved. The cyst was sent to pathology. (This technique preserves the ovarian cortex. For details, please refer to* Chap. 68*: resection of benign ovarian lesions).*

If an underlying paratubal cyst is present: *The mesosalpinx was incised using low wattage current. The mesosalpinx was gently grasped and the underlying cyst was dissected away from the mesosalpinx using traction and counter traction. Hemostasis was achieved. The cyst was sent to pathology.*

If an underlying ovarian cyst or mass is identified, but not suitable for cystectomy: *The twisted ovary was found to have an associated ____cm × ____cm ovarian cyst (or mass). The ovary was very edematous, with significant venous congestion and the cyst was not distinct from the ovarian cortex. We elected to defer a cystectomy at this time.*

The pelvis was copiously irrigated. Hemostasis was ensured. The fascia was closed with 0 PDS. The subcutaneous layer was closed with 3-0 (or 4-0) Vicryl. The skin was closed with 4-0 Vicryl. Steri-strips were applied. A sterile dressing was placed over the incision. All counts were correct. Upon completion of the procedure, a debriefing checklist was completed to share information critical to the postoperative care of the patient. The patient tolerated the procedure well, *was extubated in the operating room,* and was transported to the postanesthesia care unit in stable condition thereafter.

Template Operative Dictation (Laparoscopic)

Preoperative Diagnosis *Ovarian/fallopian tube/adnexal* torsion

Postoperative Diagnosis *Ovarian/fallopian tube/adnexal* torsion

Findings Torsed *right/left ovary/fallopian tube/ovary and fallopian tube*

Procedures Performed Laparoscopic *ovarian/fallopian tube* detorsion, *right/left ovarian cystectomy*

Anesthesia General

Specimen Right/left *ovarian cyst/paratubal cyst*

Estimated Blood Loss ____mL

Indications This is a/an ___-*day/week/month/year*-old female who presented with *pelvic pain/abdominal tenderness/___*. Given her symptoms, exam, and imaging, there was concern that she may have an adnexal torsion. We recommended proceeding with an emergent exploratory laparotomy, possible detorsion, possible cystectomy, possible oophorectomy, and possible salpingectomy.

Procedure in Detail Following satisfactory induction of anesthesia, the patient was placed in lithotomy position and appropriately padded. Timeouts were performed using both preinduction and preincision safety checklists with participation of all present in the operative suite. These confirmed the correct patient, procedure, operative site, and additional critical information prior to the start of the procedure. A bimanual exam was performed. The abdomen was then prepped and draped in the usual sterile fashion. A Foley catheter was placed under sterile conditions. A speculum was placed vaginally, and the cervix was visualized. The anterior lip of the cervix was grasped with a single toothed tenaculum. A uterine manipulator was placed easily through the patient's cervix into the uterus. The single toothed tenaculum was removed from the cervix and the speculum was removed from the patient's vagina. Gloves were changed and attention was turned to the patient's abdomen.

The umbilicus was infiltrated with 0.5% lidocaine with epinephrine. A skin incision was made with the scalpel and the subcuticular tissue was dissected down to the fascia. The fascia was grasped with Kocher clamps, tented up, and entered sharply with the scalpel. The underlying peritoneum was entered by blunt dissection. The fascial angles were tagged with 0 Vicryl. Pneumoperitoneum was obtained with CO_2 gas to a pressure of 15 mmHg. The laparoscope was introduced and the pelvis and abdomen were explored with the findings as noted above. 0.5% lidocaine with epinephrine was injected in the right lower quadrant. A 5-mm skin incision was made in the right lower quadrant, with care taken to note the anatomical landmarks of the obliterated umbilical vessel and the inferior epigastric vessels. Under direct visualization, the trocar was advanced into the abdominal cavity without difficulty, lateral to the inferior epigastric vessels. In a similar fashion, another 5-mm incision was made in the left lower quadrant and a trocar was advanced into the abdomen. The torsion was gently reduced, restoring the adnexa to its normal anatomic position. Immediately, the ovary (fallopian tube or both) began to return to its normal color, indicating return of vascular flow. We examined the rest of the pelvis and noted a normal uterus, normal contralateral ovary, and normal contralateral fallopian tube.

[Choose One:]

If no underlying ovarian cyst or mass (or fallopian tube cyst) is identified: *We did not identify a mass or cyst.*

If an underlying ovarian cyst is present and suitable for removal: *The ovarian cortex was incised using low wattage current. The ovarian cortex was gently grasped and the underlying cyst was dissected away from the cortex using traction, counter traction, and hydro-dissection to preserve the ovarian cortex. Hemostasis was achieved. The cyst was sent to pathology. (c.f.,* Chap. 68: *resection of benign ovarian lesions).*

If an underlying paratubal cyst is present: *The mesosalpinx was incised using low wattage current. The mesosalpinx was gently grasped and the underlying cyst was dissected away from the mesosalpinx using traction, counter traction, and hydro-dissection. Hemostasis was achieved. The cyst was sent to pathology.*

If an underlying ovarian cyst or mass is identified, but not suitable for cystectomy: *The twisted ovary was found to have an associated ____cm × ____cm ovarian cyst (or mass). The ovary was very edematous, with significant venous congestion and the cyst was not distinct from the ovarian cortex. We elected to defer a cystectomy at this time.*

At this point, the pelvis was copiously irrigated with warmed saline. The pelvis and abdomen were inspected and hemostasis was assured.

The pneumoperitoneum was decreased and again hemostasis was assured. The right ovary and right fallopian tube appeared well perfused and were in the correct anatomic orientation. The two lower quadrant trocars were removed under direct visualization. The umbilical trocar was removed with the laparoscope. The umbilical fascial incision was closed with 0 Vicryl. Subcuticular closure of the trocar sites was accomplished with 4-0 Vicryl. Steri-strips were applied. A sterile bandage was placed over the umbilical incision. Attention was then turned to the vagina. The uterine manipulator was removed. A speculum exam was performed and the cervix was noted to be hemostatic. The speculum was removed from the patient's vagina. The Foley was then removed.

All counts were correct. Upon completion of the procedure, a debriefing checklist was completed to share information critical to the postoperative care of the patient. The patient tolerated the procedure well, *was extubated in the operating room*, and was transported to the postanesthesia care unit in stable condition thereafter.

55 Staging Laparotomy and Oophorectomy for Malignancy

Sara A. Mansfield and Kate A. McCracken

Indications and Benefits

- Solid ovarian mass with concern for malignancy or biopsy-proven ovarian malignancy in children and adolescents
- Benefits: Pathologic diagnosis, resection of cancer

Risks and Alternatives

- Standard risks: Bleeding, infection, injury to surrounding structures (gastrointestinal, genitourinary, vascular, neural), need for blood products, anesthesia complications, and infertility.
- Alternatives: In general, ovarian cystectomy is reserved for symptomatic patients when conservative management has failed; there is a suspicion of torsion, or a tissue diagnosis is indicated.

S. A. Mansfield
The Ohio State University Wexner Medical Center, Department of General Surgery, Columbus, OH, USA
e-mail: sara.mansfield@osumc.edu

K. A. McCracken (✉)
Nationwide Children's Hospital, Department of Pediatric & Adolescent Gynecology, Columbus, OH, USA
e-mail: kate.mccracken@nationwidechildrens.org

Essential Steps

1. A Foley catheter is placed in the bladder
2. Lower midline laparotomy
3. Collection of ascites or washings upon entering the peritoneal cavity
4. Examination of the peritoneal surfaces and liver with biopsy or excision of any nodules
5. Examination and palpation of lymph nodes in the retroperitoneum with sampling of firm or enlarged nodes
6. Inspection of the omentum with resection of abnormal nodules
7. Inspection and palpation of the opposite ovary with biopsy of any abnormal areas
8. Complete resection of the tumor-containing ovary with sparing of the fallopian tube if not involved
9. Abdominal closure

Note These Variations

- Laparoscopic staging is not recommended in the setting of pediatric ovarian masses. The important components in accurate staging for pediatric ovarian germ cell tumors appear to be ascitic cytology, inspection of the pelvic peritoneum, inspection of the omentum, palpation of retroperitoneal lymph nodes, and delivery of an intact specimen to the pathologist.

D. J. Papandria et al. (eds.), *Operative Dictations in Pediatric Surgery*,
https://doi.org/10.1007/978-3-030-24212-1_55

Template Operative Dictation (Open)

Preoperative Diagnosis *Left/right* ovarian mass

Postoperative Diagnosis *Left/right* ovarian mass

Findings cm × cm *left/right* ovarian mass

Procedures Performed Exploratory laparotomy for staging with pelvic washings and *left/right* oophorectomy

Anesthesia General

Specimen *Left/right* ovary; *(pelvic washings for cytology)*

Estimated Blood Loss ____mL

Indications This is a/an ___ *-year*-old female with a *left/right* ovarian mass. Pre-operative evaluation suggests the mass is likely malignant. Given her symptoms, exam, and imaging–there we recommended proceeding with a staging laparotomy and oophorectomy.

Procedure in Detail Following satisfactory induction of anesthesia, the patient was placed in supine position and appropriately padded. Timeouts were performed using both preinduction and preincision safety checklists with participation of all present in the operative suite. These confirmed the correct patient, procedure, operative site, and additional critical information prior to the start of the procedure. A foley catheter was inserted in the urethra prior to start of the procedure. The abdomen was then prepped and draped in the usual sterile fashion. A lower midline skin incision was made with the scalpel and carried through to the underlying layer of fascia using the Bovie. The fascia was incised in the midline. The peritoneum was bluntly dissected, entered, and extended superiorly and inferiorly with good visualization of the bladder.

We identified the *left/right* ovarian cyst–it was approximately cm × cm. It appeared ___. We examined the rest of the pelvis and noted a normal uterus, *normal contralateral ovary/ (abnormal findings)*, and *normal bilateral fallopian tubes / (abnormal findings). There was clear/hemorrhagic ascites present. This was collected for cytology. Saline irrigation was used to collect pelvic washings for cytology.* The peritoneal surfaces along the entire abdomen were palpated and inspected for signs of disease. *Nodules were identified and biopsied/ resected.* The liver was examined and palpated. *This was smooth without signs of metastatic disease.* The omentum was examined. *There were no adhesions or abnormal masses.* The pelvis and retroperitoneum was palpated. *There were no enlarged or firm lymph nodes.* We then proceeded with a *right/left* oophorectomy. The infundibulopelvic ligament was identified and isolated. The ipsilateral ureter was identified and noted to be remote from the area of the infundibulopelvic ligament to be ligated. *We then clamped and suture ligated the infundibulopelvic ligament. The infundibulopelvic ligament was ligated with endoloops and transected. The infundibulopelvic ligament was divided with bipolar cautery.* The mesosalpinx was dissected free and divided with *suture ligation / bipolar cautery*. The utero-ovarian ligament was then suture ligated/divided with bipolary cautery. The intact ovary was then passed off the field for pathology.

The pelvis was copiously irrigated. The fascia was closed with 0 PDS. The subcutaneous layer was closed with 3-0 (or 4-0) Vicryl. The skin was closed with 4-0 Vicryl. Steri-strips were applied. A sterile dressing was placed over the incision. All counts were correct. Upon completion of the procedure, a debriefing checklist was completed to share information critical to the postoperative care of the patient. The patient tolerated the procedure well, *was extubated in the operating room*, and was transported to the postanesthesia care unit in stable condition thereafter.

56 Ovarian Cystectomy for Benign Ovarian Masses (Open and MIS Approaches)

Alejandra Vilanova-Sánchez and Kate A. McCracken

Indications and Benefits

- Symptomatic ovarian masses in women of reproductive age that do not resolve with conservative management *(and have no imaging or intraoperative findings suggestive of malignancy)*
- Benefits: Cessation of symptoms, reduces the risk of ovarian torsion, allows for a pathologic diagnosis of the underlying mass

Risks and Alternatives

- Standard risks: Bleeding, infection, injury to surrounding structures (gastrointestinal, genitourinary, vascular, neural), need for blood products, anesthesia complications, unplanned oophorectomy, and/or salpingectomy.
- Alternatives: In general, ovarian cystectomy is reserved for symptomatic patients when conservative management has failed; there is a suspicion of torsion, or a tissue diagnosis is indicated.

A. Vilanova-Sánchez
Hospital La Paz, Department of Pediatric Surgery, Madrid, Spain

K. A. McCracken (✉)
Nationwide Children's Hospital, Department of Pediatric & Adolescent Gynecology, Columbus, OH, USA
e-mail: kate.mccracken@nationwidechildrens.org

Essential Steps

1. Pfannenstiel incision/laparoscopic approach.
2. A foley catheter is placed in the bladder. *Consider using a uterine manipulator (Hulka clamp) if performing laparoscopy. This allows for deviation of the uterus during the case, which aides in traction/counter traction of the adnexa.*
3. *For a laparoscopic approach, place a 10–12-mm trocar at the umbilicus to allow the specimen to be removed* via *a tissue extraction bag. Two or three additional 5-mm trocars are placed in the lower quadrants or suprapubic region.*
4. Inspect the pelvic anatomy – ovary containing the cyst, contralateral ovary, bilateral fallopian tubes, uterus, and anterior and posterior cul-de-sacs *(if applicable, collect pelvic washings for cytology by irrigating the pelvis with saline).*
5. Incise the ovarian cortex using low wattage current (avoid the vascular hilum of the ovary).
6. Grasp the ovarian cortex and extend the incision allowing the underlying cyst to be dissected away from the cortex using traction, counter traction, and hydrodissection. This technique preserves the ovarian cortex. Err on the side of fertility preserving procedures by conserving the ovary and/or fallopian tube, rather than performing an oophorectomy or salpingectomy.

D. J. Papandria et al. (eds.), *Operative Dictations in Pediatric Surgery*,
https://doi.org/10.1007/978-3-030-24212-1_56

7. Place the cyst in a tissue-extracting bag; if it is a simple fluid-filled cyst, the cyst may be decompressed, allowing the tissue-extracting bag to be removed through a smaller diameter port.
8. Irrigate the cyst bed and achieve hemostasis. It is not necessary to reapproximate the ovarian cortex.
9. Ensure that all portions of the adnexa remain in the correct anatomic orientation with adequate vascular perfusion.
10. Remove ports and close the laparotomy/port incisions.

Note These Variations

- Unilocular cysts <10 cm are generally benign in the setting of normal tumor markers. It is reasonable to aspirate the cyst fluid laparoscopically to allow the cyst to fit in an extraction bag for specimen removal to reduce the morbidity of an open procedure. Make a small incision in the cyst wall with a laparoscopic scissor or electrocautery, and immediately insert a suction tip to quickly evacuate the cyst fluid.
- If there are intraoperative concerns/suspicion of malignant process, recommend an intraoperative consultation with a pediatric gynecologist and/or pediatric surgeon with training in oncology prior to proceeding with a cystectomy or oophorectomy. Oncologic staging may be necessary. If an expert team is unavailable, we recommend obtaining pelvic washings, taking photos, and then referring the patient to an expert in pediatric gynecologic oncology.

Template Operative Dictation (Open)

Preoperative Diagnosis *Left/right* ovarian mass

Postoperative Diagnosis *Left/right* ovarian mass

Findings cm × cm *left/right* ovarian cyst

Procedures Performed Open *left/right* ovarian cystectomy

Anesthesia General

Specimen *Left/Right* ovarian cyst *(pelvic washings for cytology)*

Estimated Blood Loss ____mL

Indications This is a/an ___*-day/week/month/year*-old female with a *left/right* cystic ovarian mass. Preoperative evaluation suggests that the mass is likely benign. Given her symptoms, exam, and imaging, we recommended proceeding with an open ovarian cystectomy.

Procedure in Detail Following satisfactory induction of anesthesia, the patient was placed in supine position and appropriately padded. Timeouts were performed using both preinduction and preincision safety checklists with participation of all present in the operative suite. These confirmed the correct patient, procedure, operative site, and additional critical information prior to the start of the procedure. A foley catheter was inserted in the urethra prior to start of the procedure. The abdomen was then prepped and draped in the usual sterile fashion. A Pfannenstiel skin incision was made with the scalpel and carried through to the underlying layer of fascia using the Bovie. The fascia was incised in the midline and extended laterally using Mayo scissors. Kocher clamps were used to elevate the superior aspect of the fascial incision, and the underlying rectus muscles were dissected off bluntly and using Mayo scissors. Attention was then turned to the inferior aspect of the fascial incision, which in a similar fashion was grasped with Kocher clamps, elevated, and the underlying rectus muscles were dissected off bluntly and using Mayo scissors. The rectus muscles were separated in the midline. The peritoneum was bluntly dissected, entered, and extended superiorly and inferiorly with good visualization of the bladder. We identified the *left/right* ovarian cyst; it was approximately cm × cm. We examined the rest of the pelvis and noted a normal uterus, normal contralateral ovary, and normal bilateral fallopian tubes. Saline irrigation was used to collect pelvic washings for cytology. The ovarian cortex was incised using low wattage current with care taken to start the incision away from the ovarian vasculature. The ovarian cortex was gently grasped and the incision was extended along the ovarian axis to better expose the underlying cyst. The cyst was dissected away from the cortex using blunt dissection with traction and counter traction. The cyst remained intact. Once the cyst was completely separated from the cortex, it was sent to pathology. The cyst bed was irrigated and hemostasis was ensured. The pelvis was copiously irrigated. The fascia was closed with 0 PDS. The subcutaneous layer was closed with 3-0 (or 4-0) Vicryl. The skin was closed with 4-0 Vicryl. Steri-strips were applied. A sterile dressing was placed over the incision. All counts were correct. Upon completion of the procedure, a debriefing checklist was completed to share information critical to the postoperative care of the patient. The patient tolerated the procedure well, *was extubated in the operating room,* and was transported to the postanesthesia care unit in stable condition thereafter.

Template Operative Dictation (Laparoscopic)

Preoperative Diagnosis *Left/right* ovarian mass

Postoperative Diagnosis *Left/right* ovarian mass

Findings cm × cm *left/right* ovarian cyst

Procedures Performed Laparoscopic *left/right* ovarian cystectomy

Anesthesia General

Specimen *Left/right* ovarian cyst; *(pelvic washings for cytology)*

Estimated Blood Loss ____mL

Indications This is a/an ___-*day/week/month/year*-old female with a *left/right* cystic ovarian mass. Preoperative evaluation suggests that the mass is likely benign. Given her symptoms, exam, and imaging, we recommended proceeding with a laparoscopic ovarian cystectomy.

Procedure in Detail Following satisfactory induction of anesthesia, the patient was placed in lithotomy position and appropriately padded. Timeouts were performed using both preinduction and preincision safety checklists with participation of all present in the operative suite. These confirmed the correct patient, procedure, operative site, and additional critical information prior to the start of the procedure. A bimanual exam was performed. The abdomen was then prepped and draped in the usual sterile fashion. A foley catheter was placed under sterile conditions. A speculum was placed vaginally, and the cervix was visualized. The anterior lip of the cervix was grasped with a single-toothed tenaculum. A uterine manipulator was placed easily through the patient's cervix into the uterus. The single-toothed tenaculum was removed from the cervix and the speculum was removed from the patient's vagina. Gloves were changed and attention was turned to the patient's abdomen. 0.5% lidocaine with epinephrine was injected into the umbilicus. A skin incision was made with the scalpel and the subcuticular tissue was dissected down to the fascia. The fascia was grasped with Kocher clamps, tented up, and entered sharply with the scalpel. The underlying peritoneum was entered by blunt dissection. The fascial angles were tagged with 0-vicryl. A 10–12-mm trocar was inserted and pneumoperitoneum was obtained with CO_2 gas to a pressure of 15 mmHg. The laparoscope was introduced and the pelvis and abdomen were explored with the findings as noted above. 0.5% lidocaine with epinephrine was injected in the right lower quadrant. A 5-mm skin incision was made in the right lower quadrant, with care taken to note the anatomical landmarks of the obliterated umbilical vessel and the inferior epigastric vessels. Under direct visualization, the trocar was advanced into the abdominal cavity without difficulty, lateral to the inferior epigastric vessels. In a similar fashion, another 5 mm incision was made in the left lower quadrant and a trocar was advanced into the abdomen. We identified the *left/right* ovarian cyst; it was approximately cm × cm. We examined the rest of the pelvis and noted a normal uterus, normal contralateral ovary, and normal bilateral fallopian tubes. Saline irrigation was used to collect pelvic washings for cytology. The ovarian cortex was incised using low wattage current with care taken to start the incision away from the ovarian vasculature. The ovarian cortex was gently grasped and the incision was extended along the ovarian axis to better expose the underlying cyst. The cyst was dissected away from the cortex using blunt dissection and hydrodissection with traction and counter traction. The cyst remained intact. Once the cyst was completely separated from the cortex, we inserted an endocatch bag through the 10–12-mm trocar and switched the camera to the *left/right* 5-mm trocar.

[Choose One:]

The cyst was too large to be removed intact through the 10–12-mm umbilical port, so we placed the cyst into the endocatch bag and then made a small incision into the cyst wall and immediately inserted a suction device into the cyst to aspirate the cyst contents and decompress the cyst. No spillage into the peritoneal cavity occurred. The specimen was then removed from the pelvis and sent to pathology, along with the cyst contents.

-- or --

The cyst was placed in an endocatch bag, removed from the pelvis, and sent to pathology.

The cyst bed was irrigated and hemostasis was ensured. At this point, the pelvis was copiously irrigated with warmed saline. The pelvis and abdomen were inspected and hemostasis was assured. The pneumoperitoneum was decreased and again hemostasis was assured. The bilateral ovaries and bilateral fallopian tubes appeared well perfused and were in the correct anatomic orientation. The two lower quadrant trocars were removed under direct visualization. The umbilical trocar was removed with the laparoscope. The umbilical fascial incision was closed with 0-vicryl. Subcuticular closure of the trocar sites was accomplished with 4-0 vicryl. Steri-strips were applied. A sterile bandage was placed over the umbilical incision. Attention was then turned to the vagina. The uterine manipulator was removed. A speculum exam was performed and the cervix was noted to be hemostatic. The speculum was removed from the patient's vagina. The foley was then removed. All counts were correct. Upon completion of the procedure, a debriefing checklist was completed to share information critical to the postoperative care of the patient. The patient tolerated the procedure well, *was extubated in the operating room*, and was transported to the postanesthesia care unit in stable condition thereafter.

Hymenectomy

57

Alejandra Vilanova-Sánchez
and Kate A. McCracken

Indications and Benefits

- Imperforate hymen.
- Septate, microperforate, or cribriform hymen interfering with tampon use and/or penetrative vaginal intercourse.
- Benefits: Removing excess hymenal tissue allows menstrual blood egress, tampon use, and penetrative vaginal intercourse.

Risks

Standard risks:

- Bleeding, infection, injury to surrounding structures (e.g., vaginal mucosa, urethra, rectum), need for additional hymenotomy if the excess hymenal tissue is not removed.
- Caution should be observed if performing this procedure in the outpatient setting where adequate resources may not be readily available for control of hemorrhage.
- Ensure you adequately remove all excess hymenal tissue to reduce the risk of scarring and reobstruction.
- Ensure that you have an imperforate hymen, not distal vaginal atresia – which requires a different surgical approach.

Essential Steps

1. Dorsal lithotomy position.
2. Inspection of the external genitalia.
3. Placement of a Foley catheter.
4. Incision in the middle of the hymen with electrocautery.
5. Blood/mucous drainage with aspiration if present.
6. Elliptical incision of the hymen removing excess hymenal tissue.
7. If necessary for hemostasis and to reapproximate the mucosa, perform interrupted absorbable sutures from the edge of the elliptical incision to the external aspect of the hymen.
8. Inspection of the vaginal introitus.

Note This Variation:

In the case of a septate, microperforate, or cribriform hymen, electrocautery is used to remove excess hymenal tissue. The goals of the procedure

A. Vilanova-Sánchez
Hospital La Paz, Department of Pediatric Surgery, Madrid, Spain

K. A. McCracken (✉)
Nationwide Children's Hospital, Department of Pediatric & Adolescent Gynecology, Columbus, OH, USA
e-mail: kate.mccracken@nationwidechildrens.org

D. J. Papandria et al. (eds.), *Operative Dictations in Pediatric Surgery*, https://doi.org/10.1007/978-3-030-24212-1_57

are the same – adequate introitus for menstrual egress, tampon use, and penetrative vaginal intercourse.

Template Operative Dictation

Preoperative Diagnosis Imperforate hymen

Postoperative Diagnosis Imperforate hymen

Findings Imperforate hymen

Procedure Performed Hymenectomy

Anesthesia General anesthesia

Estimated Blood Loss Minimal

Indications This is a/an ___-*day/week/month/year* -old female with an imperforate (or septate, microperforate, cribriform) hymen and hematometrocolpos (or desire for tampon use/penetrative vaginal intercourse). It was recommended that we proceed with a hymenectomy to remove the excess hymenal tissue. The risks, benefits, and alternatives to the planned procedure were discussed. Written informed consent was obtained prior to the procedure.

Procedure in Detail Following satisfactory induction of anesthesia, the patient was placed in dorsal lithotomy position and appropriately padded. Timeouts were performed using both preinduction and preincision safety checklists with participation of all present in the operative suite. These confirmed the correct patient, procedure, operative site, and additional critical information prior to the start of the procedure. The perineum was then prepped and draped in the usual sterile fashion. An external genital exam was performed, and the patient was noted to have normal labia majora and labia minora, clitoris, urethral meatus, perineal body, and anus. A Foley catheter was then inserted under sterile conditions.

[Choose One:]

If imperforate hymen: A bulging imperforate hymen was noted – it was bulging and had a bluish hue secondary to hematometrocolpos. Using electrocautery, an incision was made in the center of the hymen to allow passage of the suction catheter into the vagina. A large amount (or ___mL) of retained blood was aspirated. We then excised the hymenal tissue with electrocautery in an ellipse. *To avoid reobstruction we placed interrupted stitches from the edge of the elliptical incision to the external limit of the hymen, keeping the introitus widely open (optional).* The vagina was irrigated copiously. The introitus easily accommodated two finger breadths.

If septate hymen: The hymen was septate. The septum was grasped with forceps and using electrocautery, we excised the septum. The introitus then easily accommodated two finger breadths.

If microperforate or cribriform hymen: The hymen was microperforate/cribriform. A Kelly (or hemostat) was placed into the hymenal opening and using electrocautery, the hymen was incised in a vertical fashion. Then the extra hymenal tissue on either side was grasped with forceps and excised in an ellipse. *To avoid reobstruction we placed interrupted stitches from the edge of the elliptical incision to the external limit of the hymen, keeping the introitus widely open (optional).*The introitus easily accommodated two finger breadths.

Hemostasis was noted. The Foley catheter was removed. Upon completion of the procedure, a debriefing checklist was completed to share information critical to the postoperative care of the patient. The patient tolerated the procedure well, *was extubated in the operating room* (if applicable), and was transported to the post anesthesia care unit in stable condition.

Drainage of Tubo-Ovarian Abscess 58

Kate A. McCracken

Indications and Benefits

- Suspected intra-abdominal rupture of a tubo-ovarian abscess (TOA) requires prompt surgical intervention combined with antimicrobial therapy.
- Surgical intervention may also be warranted in cases in which patients do not clinically improve after 48–72 h of antibiotic therapy alone. Failure of treatment is defined as: new onset or persistent fever; persistent or worsening abdominal/pelvic tenderness; enlarging pelvic mass; new onset, persistent, or further elevated white blood cell count; signs of sepsis.
- Surgical intervention may be warranted in cases in which minimally invasive interventional radiology drainage techniques are not possible or available.
- Of note, antibiotic therapy is the mainstay of therapy before, during, and after any abscess drainage procedure.
- Benefits: Treatment of tubo-ovarian abscess, prevention of progressive infection.

K. A. McCracken (✉)
Nationwide Children's Hospital, Department of Pediatric & Adolescent Gynecology, Columbus, OH, USA
e-mail: kate.mccracken@nationwidechildrens.org

Risks and Alternatives

- Standard risks: Bleeding, infection, injury to surrounding structures (gastrointestinal, genitourinary, vascular, neural), need for blood products, anesthesia complications, unplanned hysterectomy, oophorectomy, or salpingectomy.
- Alternatives: Minimally invasive abscess drainage via interventional radiology techniques.

Essential Steps

1. Pfannenstiel incision/laparoscopic approach
2. A Foley catheter is placed in the bladder. *Consider using a uterine manipulator (Hulka clamp) if performing laparoscopy – this allows for deviation of the uterus during the course of the procedure, which aids in traction/counter traction of the adnexa.*
3. Identify ovaries, fallopian tubes, and uterus.
4. Identify the tubo-ovarian abscess and involved pelvic structures.
5. Using the suction-irrigator, copiously irrigate and suction all purulent fluid in the pelvis
6. Blunt dissection and/or electrocautery dissection are (is) used to break up all loculated fluid collections.
7. *7. A salpingostomy incision into the involved fallopian tube may be necessary to completely drain the pyosalpinx.*

D. J. Papandria et al. (eds.), *Operative Dictations in Pediatric Surgery*,
https://doi.org/10.1007/978-3-030-24212-1_58

8. Ensure hemostasis and copiously irrigate again.
9. Remove ports and close the laparotomy/port incisions.

Template Operative Dictation (Open)

Preoperative Diagnosis Tubo-ovarian abscess

Postoperative Diagnosis Tubo-ovarian abscess

Findings *Right/left* tubo-ovarian abscess

Procedures Performed Open drainage of a *right/left* tubo-ovarian abscess

Anesthesia General

Specimen Anaerobic and aerobic cultures of abscess fluid

Estimated Blood Loss ____mL

Indications This is a/an ___-*year*-old female who presented with _________. Given her symptoms, exam, and imaging – there was concern that she may a patient with tubo-ovarian abscess. She was started on appropriate antibiotic therapy, however, she clinically did not improve *(or worsened)*. We recommended proceeding with an exploratory laparotomy and drainage of the tubo-ovarian abscess.

Procedure in Detail Following satisfactory induction of anesthesia, the patient was placed in supine position and appropriately padded. Timeouts were performed using both preinduction and preincision safety checklists with participation of all present in the operative suite. These confirmed the correct patient, procedure, operative site and additional critical information prior to the start of the procedure. A Foley catheter was inserted in the urethra prior to start of the procedure. The abdomen was then prepped and draped in the usual sterile fashion.

A Pfannenstiel skin incision was made with the scalpel and carried through to the underlying layer of fascia using the Bovie. The fascia was incised in the midline and extended laterally using Mayo scissors. Kocher clamps were used to elevate the superior aspect of the fascial incision, and the underlying rectus muscles were dissected off bluntly and using Mayo scissors. Attention was then turned to the inferior aspect of the fascial incision, which in a similar fashion was grasped with Kocher clamps, elevated, and the underlying rectus muscles were dissected off bluntly and using Mayo scissors. The rectus muscles were separated in the midline. The peritoneum was bluntly dissected, entered, and extended superiorly and inferiorly with good visualization of the bladder. We identified the *right/left)* tubo-ovarian abscess.

If Gross Pus Identified: There was a copious amount of purulent fluid in the pelvis. There were significant pelvic adhesions secondary to the infection.

We examined the rest of the pelvis and noted a normal uterus, normal contralateral ovary, and normal contralateral fallopian tube. Using blunt dissection, the loculated abscess was broken up and the purulent fluid was sent for culture. The pelvis was copiously irrigated and all purulent fluid was removed. *(Using electrocautery, a longitudinal incision was made in the involved fallopian tube – this allowed the pyosalpinx to be*

The pelvis was copiously irrigated. Hemostasis was ensured. The fascia was closed with 0 PDS. The subcutaneous layer was closed with *3–0* Vicryl. The skin was closed with *4–0* Vicryl. *Steri-strips* were applied. A sterile dressing was placed over the incision. All counts were correct. Upon completion of the procedure, a debriefing checklist was completed to share information critical to the postoperative care of the patient. The patient tolerated the procedure well, *was extubated in the operating room* and was transported to the post anesthesia care unit in stable condition thereafter.

Template Operative Dictation (Laparoscopic)

Preoperative Diagnosis Tubo-ovarian abscess

Postoperative Diagnosis Tubo-ovarian abscess

Findings (Right/left) Tubo-ovarian abscess

Procedures Performed Open drainage of a (right/left) tubo-ovarian abscess

Anesthesia General

Specimen Anaerboic and aerobic cultures of abscess fluid

Estimated Blood Loss ____mL

Indications This is a/an ___-*year*-old female who presented with _________. Given her symptoms, exam, and imaging, there was concern that she may a patient with tubo-ovarian abscess. She was started on appropriate antibiotic therapy; however, she clinically did not improve *(or worsened)*. We recommended proceeding with a diagnostic laparoscopy and drainage of the tubo-ovarian abscess.

Procedure in Detail Following satisfactory induction of anesthesia, the patient was placed in lithotomy position and appropriately padded. Timeouts were performed using both preinduction and preincision safety checklists with participation of all present in the operative suite. These confirmed the correct patient, procedure, operative site, and additional critical information prior to the start of the procedure. A bimanual exam was performed. The abdomen was then prepped and draped in the usual sterile fashion. A Foley catheter was placed under sterile conditions. A speculum was placed vaginally, and the cervix was visualized. The anterior lip of the cervix was grasped with a single toothed tenaculum. A uterine manipulator was placed easily through the patient's cervix into the uterus. The single toothed tenaculum was removed from the cervix, and the speculum was removed from the patient's vagina. Gloves were changed and attention was turned to the patient's abdomen. A dose of 0.5% lidocaine with epinephrine was injected into the umbilicus. A skin incision was made with the scalpel, and the subcuticular tissue was dissected down to the fascia. The fascia was grasped with Kocher clamps, tented up, and entered sharply with the scalpel. The underlying peritoneum was entered by blunt dissection. The fascial angles were tagged with 0-Vicryl. Pneumoperitoneum was obtained with $CO2$ gas to a pressure of 15 mmHg. The laparoscope was introduced and the pelvis and abdomen were explored with the findings as noted above. A dose of 0.5% lidocaine with epinephrine was injected in the right lower quadrant. A 5-mm skin incision was made in the right lower quadrant, with care taken to note the anatomical landmarks of the obliterated umbilical vessel and the inferior epigastric vessels. Under direct visualization, the trocar was advanced into the abdominal cavity without difficulty, lateral to the inferior epigastric vessels. In a similar fashion, another 5-mm incision was made in the left lower quadrant and a trocar was advanced into the abdomen. We identified the (right/left) tubo-ovarian abscess. *(There was a copious amount of purulent fluid in the pelvis. There were significant pelvic adhesions secondary to the infection.)* We examined the rest of the pelvis and noted a normal uterus, normal contralateral ovary, and normal contralateral fallopian tube.

Using blunt dissection, the loculated abscess was broken up, and the purulent fluid was sent for culture. The pelvis was copiously irrigated, and all purulent fluid was removed. *(Using electrocautery, a longitudinal incision was made in the involved fallopian tube – this allowed the pyosalpinx to be completely cleared of all purulent material).*

The pelvis was copiously irrigated. The pelvis and abdomen were inspected and hemostasis was assured. The pneumoperitoneum was decreased and again hemostasis was assured. The two lower quadrant trocars were removed under direct visualization. The umbilical trocar was removed with the laparoscope. The umbilical fascial incision was closed with 0-Vicryl. Subcuticular closure of the trocar sites was accomplished with 4–0 Vicryl. Steri-strips were applied. A sterile bandage was placed over the umbilical incision. Attention was then turned to the vagina. The uterine manipulator was removed. A speculum exam was performed, and the cervix was noted to be hemostatic. The speculum was removed from the patient's vagina. The Foley was then removed. All counts were correct. Upon completion of the procedure, a debriefing checklist was completed to share information critical to the postoperative care of the patient. The patient tolerated the procedure well, *was extubated in the operating room*, and was transported to the post anesthesia care unit in stable condition thereafter.

59 Surgical Management of an Ectopic Pregnancy Via Laparoscopic Salpingectomy or Laparoscopic Salpingostomy

Kate A. McCracken

Indications and Benefits

- Surgical management of an ectopic pregnancy – in some cases, salpingostomy is desired to preserve future fertility. However, cases of tubal rupture, tubal damage, or bleeding may preclude the option to retain the fallopian tube, and a salpingectomy is indicated.
- Benefits: Management of an ectopic pregnancy – which if untreated, may lead to rupture of the fallopian tube, hemorrhage with products of conception, and death.

Risks and Alternatives

- Standard risks: Bleeding, infection, injury to surrounding structures (gastrointestinal, genitourinary, vascular, neural), need for blood products, anesthesia complications, unplanned oophorectomy, and/or salpingectomy.
- Alternatives: In some cases, medical management of an ectopic pregnancy with methotrexate is acceptable.

K. A. McCracken (✉)
Nationwide Children's Hospital, Department of Pediatric & Adolescent Gynecology, Columbus, OH, USA
e-mail: kate.mccracken@nationwidechildrens.org

Essential Steps

1. Patient is placed in dorsal lithotomy position.
2. A Foley catheter is placed in the bladder. *Consider using a uterine manipulator (Hulka clamp) – this allows for deviation of the uterus during the case, which aids in traction/counter traction of the adnexa.*
3. Identify the ectopic pregnancy. Inspect the fallopian tubes, ovaries, and uterus.
4. Lift the affected fallopian tube and perform either a salpingostomy with removal of all ectopic pregnancy tissues or perform a salpingectomy with complete removal of the fallopian tube containing the ectopic pregnancy.
5. Place the specimen in a tissue extracting bag and remove from the pelvis.
6. Ensure hemostasis.
7. Remove ports and close the port incisions.

Template Operative Dictation (Laparoscopic Salpingectomy)

Preoperative Diagnosis *Right/left* ectopic pregnancy

Postoperative Diagnosis *Right/left* ectopic pregnancy

Findings *Right/left* ectopic pregnancy

D. J. Papandria et al. (eds.), *Operative Dictations in Pediatric Surgery*,
https://doi.org/10.1007/978-3-030-24212-1_59

Procedures Performed Laparoscopic *right/left* salpingectomy with removal of ectopic pregnancy

Anesthesia General

Specimen *Right/left* fallopian tube with ectopic pregnancy

Estimated Blood Loss ____mL

Indications This is a/an ___ -*year*-old gravida _________ para ___ female at approximately ___ weeks gestation who presented with vaginal bleeding and abdominal pain. Her quantitative beta-hCG (human chorionic gonadotropin) was ___, and an ultrasound was performed which noted a *right/left* ectopic pregnancy. After a discussion with the patient, we decided to proceed with a laparoscopic procedure to remove the ectopic pregnancy.

Procedure in Detail Following satisfactory induction of anesthesia, the patient was placed in supine position and appropriately padded. Timeouts were performed using both preinduction and preincision safety checklists with participation of all present in the operative suite. These confirmed the correct patient, procedure, operative site, and additional critical information prior to the start of the procedure. A bimanual exam was performed. The abdomen and vagina were then prepped and draped in the usual sterile fashion.

A Foley catheter was placed under sterile conditions. A speculum was placed vaginally, and the cervix was visualized. The anterior lip of the cervix was grasped with a single toothed tenaculum. A uterine manipulator was placed easily through the patient's cervix into the uterus. The single toothed tenaculum was removed from the cervix and the speculum was removed from the patient's vagina. Gloves were changed, and attention was turned to the patient's abdomen.

A dose of 0.5% lidocaine with epinephrine was injected into the umbilicus. A skin incision was made with the scalpel, and the subcuticular tissue was dissected down to the fascia. The fascia was grasped with Kocher clamps, tented up, and entered sharply with the scalpel. The underlying peritoneum was entered by blunt dissection. The fascial angles were tagged with 0-Vicryl. Pneumoperitoneum was obtained with CO_2 gas to a pressure of 15 mmHg. The laparoscope was introduced, and the pelvis and abdomen were explored with the findings as noted above. A dose of 0.5% lidocaine with epinephrine was injected in the right lower quadrant. A 5-mm skin incision was made in the right lower quadrant, with care taken to note the anatomical landmarks of the obliterated umbilical vessel and the inferior epigastric vessels. Under direct visualization, the trocar was advanced into the abdominal cavity without difficulty, lateral to the inferior epigastric vessels. In a similar fashion, another 5-mm incision was made in the left lower quadrant, and a trocar was advanced into the abdomen. The *right/left* fallopian tube containing the ectopic pregnancy was grasped with an atraumatic forceps and using the Ligasure, the mesosalpinx was transected just inferior to the fallopian tube starting from the distal end of the fallopian tube. This process was continued parallel to the fallopian tube and moving toward the uterine cornua. The Ligasure was then placed across the proximal portion of the fallopian tube, and the tube was transected. The fallopian tube containing the ectopic pregnancy was placed in an endocatch bag and the specimen was removed from the abdomen. The pelvis was copiously irrigated. Hemostasis was ensured. The fascia was closed with 0 PDS. The subcutanous layer was closed with 3–0 (or 4–0) Vicryl. The skin was closed with 4–0 Vicryl. Steri-strips were applied. A sterile dressing was placed over the incision.

All counts were correct. Upon completion of the procedure, a debriefing checklist was completed to share information critical to the postoperative care of the patient. The patient tolerated the procedure well, *was extubated in the operating room*, and was transported to the post anesthesia care unit in stable condition thereafter.

Template Operative Dictation (Laparoscopic Salpingostomy)

Preoperative Diagnosis *Right/left* ectopic pregnancy

Postoperative Diagnosis *Right/left* ectopic pregnancy

Findings *Right/left* ectopic pregnancy

Procedures Performed Laparoscopic *right/left* salpingostomy with removal of ectopic pregnancy

Anesthesia General

Specimen *Right/left* ectopic pregnancy

Estimated Blood Loss ____mL

Indications This is a/an ___ -*year*-old gravida ___ para ___ female at approximately ___ weeks gestation who presented with vaginal bleeding and abdominal pain. Her quantitative beta-hCG was ___, and an ultrasound was performed which noted a *right/left* ectopic pregnancy. After a discussion with the patient, we decided to proceed with a laparoscopic procedure to remove the ectopic pregnancy.

Procedure in Detail Following satisfactory induction of anesthesia, the patient was placed in supine position and appropriately padded. Timeouts were performed using both preinduction and preincision safety checklists with participation of all present in the operative suite. These confirmed the correct patient, procedure, operative site, and additional critical information prior to the start of the procedure. A bimanual exam was performed. The abdomen and vagina were then prepped and draped in the usual sterile fashion. A Foley catheter was placed under sterile conditions. A speculum was placed vaginally, and the cervix was visualized. The anterior lip of the cervix was grasped with a single toothed tenaculum. A uterine manipulator was placed easily through the patient's cervix into the uterus. The single-toothed tenaculum was removed from the cervix, and the speculum was removed from the patient's vagina. Gloves were changed, and attention was turned to the patient's abdomen. A dose of 0.5% lidocaine with epinephrine was injected into the umbilicus. A skin incision was made with the scalpel, and the subcuticular tissue was dissected down to the fascia. The fascia was grasped with Kocher clamps, tented up, and entered sharply with the scalpel. The underlying peritoneum was entered by blunt dissection. The fascial angles were tagged with 0-Vicryl. Pneumoperitoneum was obtained with CO_2 gas to a pressure of 15 mmHg. The laparoscope was introduced, and the pelvis and abdomen were explored with the findings as noted above. A dose of 0.5% lidocaine with epinephrine was injected in the right lower quadrant. A 5-mm skin incision was made in the right lower quadrant, with care taken to note the anatomical landmarks of the obliterated umbilical vessel and the inferior epigastric vessels. Under direct visualization, the trocar was advanced into the abdominal cavity without difficulty, lateral to the inferior epigastric vessels. In a similar fashion, another 5-mm incision was made in the left lower quadrant, and a trocar was advanced into the abdomen. The *right/left* fallopian tube containing the ectopic pregnancy was grasped with an atraumatic forceps. A 22-gauge needle inserted through an accessory trocar was used to inject a solution of vasopressin into the mesosalpinx below the ectopic pregnancy. Next using electrocautery, a 1–2-cm longitudinal incision was made in the fallopian tube –the incision was positioned opposite to the mesosalpinx and in the maximally distended portion of the fallopian tube overlying the ectopic pregnancy. Atraumatic forceps was used to hold one edge of the incision while the suction-irrigator tip was placed into the plane between the fallopian tube wall and the ectopic pregnancy. Hydrodissection was performed. Using a combination of hydrodissection and blunt dissection (*alternatively, pregnancy tissue may be extracted with smooth grasping forceps*), the products of conception were removed in their entirety; placed in an endocatch bag and removed from the abdomen *(alternatively small ectopic pregnancies may be removed directly through the trocar without the use of an endocatch bag)*. Hemostasis was achieved using electrocautery. The tubal incision was left open to heal by secondary intention. The pelvis was copiously irrigated. Hemostasis was ensured. The fascia was closed with 0 PDS. The subcutanous layer was closed with 3–0 (or 4–0) Vicryl. The skin was closed with 4–0 Vicryl. Steri-strips were applied. A sterile dressing was placed over the incision. All counts were correct. Upon completion of the procedure, a debriefing checklist was completed to share information critical to the post-operative care of the patient. The patient tolerated the procedure well, *was extubated in the operating room*, and was transported to the postanesthesia care unit in stable condition thereafter.

60 Nephrectomy

Margaret E. Gallagher and Harold N. Lovvorn III

Nephrectomy (Open and Laparoscopic)

Indications and Benefits

- Wilms tumor (nephroblastoma)
- Other renal tumors (e.g., renal cell carcinoma (RCC), clear cell sarcoma of the kidney, rhabdoid tumor of the kidney, congenital mesoblastic nephroma, cystic renal tumor, angiomyolipoma)
- Benefits: Complete removal of disease

Risks and Alternatives

- Standard risks (e.g., bleeding, infection, need for additional procedures, risks of anesthesia)
- Injury to adjacent structures (e.g., aorta, inferior vena cava [IVC], adrenal gland, superior mesenteric artery [SMA])
- Tumor rupture or spillage resulting in subsequent upstaging of a Wilms tumor
- Incomplete resection, residual disease
- Failure to obtain adequate lymph node sampling; failure to perform any lymph node sampling
- Postoperative intussusception
- Alternative: Neoadjuvant chemotherapy and unilateral or bilateral nephron-sparing surgery (NSS); especially useful in bilateral disease or populations at risk to develop multiple metachronous lesions in either kidney (e.g., Wilms tumor predisposition syndromes, such as Beckwith-Wiedemann hemihypertrophy, Denys-Drash, Simpson-Golabi-Behmel, or WAGR [Wilms, aniridia, genitourinary anomalies, mental retardation])

Essential Steps

Open Nephrectomy

1. Position, generally supine, with a soft bump under the appropriate flank.
2. Vary incision depending on size of mass (e.g., upper abdominal transverse, midline, or thoracoabdominal).
3. Explore abdomen for unexpected findings (e.g., rupture or invasion into adjacent organs) and for evidence of metastatic disease, such as to the liver.
4. Medial visceral rotation.
5. Take down lateral attachments of the kidney and begin inferior dissection.
6. Isolate and skeletonize the ureter.
7. Divide ureter at the level of the iliac.
8. Identify and isolate the renal artery and vein(s). Palpate ipsilateral renal vein and

M. E. Gallagher (✉) · H. N. Lovvorn III
Monroe Carell Jr. Children's Hospital at Vanderbilt, Department of Pediatric Surgery, Nashville, TN, USA
e-mail: margaret.gallagher@vumc.org; harold.lovvorn@vumc.org

D. J. Papandria et al. (eds.), *Operative Dictations in Pediatric Surgery*,
https://doi.org/10.1007/978-3-030-24212-1_60

inferior vena cava (IVC) for the presence of tumor extending into these venous structures. Obtain arterial control followed by venous control. If possible, approach hilar vessels to control and divide these structures before aggressive handling of the specimen.
9. Tumor/kidney removal.
10. Complete lymphadenectomy from infrarenal to suprarenal and between the IVC and aorta.
11. Irrigate, ensure hemostasis and close abdominal incision.
12. Consider placing titanium clips at borders of tumor bed to mark radiation field (in the event of tumor spill, bulky lymphadenopathy, or invasion into the retroperitoneum).
13. Central venous catheter placement for adjuvant chemotherapy (unless less than 2 years of age with stage I tumor, favorable histology and weight of tumor <550 gm).

Note These Variations

- Laparoscopic approach, nephroureterectomy
- Unilateral nephron-sparing surgery, open or laparoscopic
- Bilateral nephron-sparing surgery, open or laparoscopic

Template Operative Dictation (Open)

Preoperative Diagnosis Wilms tumor (renal tumor)

Postoperative Diagnosis Wilms tumor (renal tumor)

Findings Same as postoperative diagnosis

Procedure(s) Performed *Right/left* radical nephroureterectomy

Anesthesia General endotracheal

Specimen

1. *Right/left* kidney and ureter
2. Lymph nodes

Drains None

Implants None

Estimated Blood Loss ___

Indications This patient is a/an ___*-month–/year*-old *male/female* who was diagnosed with a *right/left* renal tumor. *He/she* was deemed to be a suitable candidate for nephrectomy and placement of a central venous catheter for chemotherapy.

Procedure in Detail Following satisfactory induction of general anesthesia, the patient was placed in a supine position. A Foley catheter was inserted, and a soft bump was positioned under the *right/left* flank. All pressure points were padded appropriately. Timeouts were performed using both preinduction and preincision safety checklists with participation of all participants present in the operative suite. These physicians and nurses confirmed the correct patient, procedure, operative site, and additional critical information prior to the start of the procedure. The abdomen and flank were then prepped and draped in the usual sterile fashion.

An *upper abdominal transverse/midline/thoracoabdominal* was created over the mass and the abdomen entered. The falciform ligament was divided and a self-retaining *Bookwalter/Thompson* retractor was placed for adequate exposure. Medial visceral rotation was performed of the large intestines *and duodenum*. Gentle retraction of the hollow viscera was achieved with the self-retaining retractor. Operative findings included _______. No extension into the *liver/spleen* was noted, and no evidence of metastases was discovered. The liver was gently retracted cephalad. The attachments along the lateral aspect of the kidney were divided using scissors and electrocautery. Dissection continued along the edge of the lower pole of the kidney and tumor allowing the kidney to be mobilized up and out of the retroperitoneum. Any large retroperitoneal blood vessels to the tumor were identified and ligated between silk ties. The *left/right* renal vein and inferior vena cava (IVC) were palpated for tumor extension. We next identified the ureter, it was skeletonized and traced down to the level of the common iliac vein. The ureter was palpated and there *was/was not* any palpable tumor. The ureter was suture ligated and divided at the level of the iliac. A clip was placed to mark the extension of the ureterectomy. The iliac vein was traced with care cephalad to the inferior vena cava (IVC). The renal artery and vein were then identified and isolated. The artery was identified and ligated between _-0 silk ties and suture ligated with a _-0 silk suture on the aortic side. Once the arterial inflow was controlled, the renal vein was examined, palpated for any tumor extension, and once no tumor burden noted, it was suture ligated in a similar manner to the renal artery. At this point the kidney and tumor were mobilized meticulously from the retroperitoneal bed and removed, taking care to minimize risk of rupture during this manipulation. The specimen was forwarded to pathology. A complete lymphadenectomy or sampling was performed next from infrarenal to suprarenal and between the IVC and aorta. Any lymph nodes identified in the tumor basin were removed and sent as a separate specimen from the kidney/tumor. The abdomen was copiously irrigated with warm saline and hemostasis was assured. Titanium clips were placed at the margins of the tumor bed in the event postoperative radiation is indicated. The colon and small bowel were returned to their normal anatomical position. The self-retaining retractor was released. All sponge, instrument, and needle counts were correct ×2. The abdominal wall was then closed *in layers (if transverse incision)*. A _-0 PDS suture was used for the posterior and anterior rectus layers. 3–0 braided absorbable running suture was used to close Scarpa's, 4–0 braided absorbable deep dermal and 5–0 running monofilament absorbable subcuticular closure was performed. The abdomen was cleaned with a wet and dry gauze and *Dermabond/steri-strips and sterile dressing* was applied. Before awaking the patient from general anesthesia, a tunneled central venous catheter was placed for adjuvant chemotherapy administration (see separate dictation)

Upon completion of the procedure, a debriefing checklist was completed to share information critical to the postoperative care of the patient. The patient tolerated the procedure well, was extubated in the operating room, and was transported to the postanesthesia care unit in stable condition thereafter.

Template Operative Dictation (Laparoscopic)

Preoperative Diagnosis Wilms tumor

Postoperative Diagnosis Same as preoperative diagnosis

Findings Same as postoperative diagnosis

Procedure(s) Performed Laparoscopic nephroureterectomy

Anesthesia General

Specimen
1. *Right/left* kidney
2. Lymph nodes

Drains None

Implants None

Estimated Blood Loss ___

Indications This patient is a/an ___- *month/year*-old *male/female* with a *right/left* renal mass. *He/she* was deemed to be a suitable candidate for nephrectomy *prior to adjuvant chemotherapy/after having received neoadjuvant chemotherapy, which decreased the tumor burden, now allowing for a laparoscopic approach.*

Procedure in Detail Following satisfactory induction of anesthesia, the patient was placed on a beanbag in a modified *right/left* lateral decubitus position with the *right/left* side up approximately 60 degrees. The table was flexed. Timeouts were performed using both preinduction and preincision safety checklists with participation of all present in the operative suite. These confirmed the correctness of patient, procedure, operative site, and additional critical information prior to the start of the procedure. The abdomen and flank were then prepped and draped in the usual sterile fashion.

A 10-mm *infraumbilical/transumbilical* skin incision was created and a 10-mm port was placed using a *Hasson technique/Veress approach*. Pneumoperitoneum was achieved to 15 mmHg. Three additional 5-mm ports were then placed midline of the epigastrium, in the *right/left* lower quadrant, and in the *right/left* flank halfway between the anterior superior iliac spine and the twelfth rib. Medial visceral rotation was performed, mobilizing the colon from the white line of Toldt with the *ultrasonic/thermal energy sealing device*. Dissection then began at the inferior edge of the kidney. Progressing medially the ureter was identified and skeletonized down to the level of the iliac. The ureter was then clipped and divided. The renal artery and vein were next identified and isolated, ensuring enough length to safely clip and divide these vessels. The vein was gently palpated with an atraumatic grasper for the presence of tumor extension. The renal artery was first controlled and divided using *laparoscopic clips/vascular stapler*. Once the artery was divided, attention was directed toward the renal vein which was divided in a similar manner. The remaining renal attachments were taken down with the *ultrasonic/thermal energy sealing device*. Prior to removing the specimen, the lymph node basin was examined and any hilar lymph nodes identified were removed; a thorough lymphadenectomy or sampling was performed from infrarenal to suprarenal and between the inferior vena cava (IVC) and the aorta. The kidney and mass were then placed in a thick specimen bag. The *umbilical/flank port site was upsized/a small Pfannenstiel incision was made* and the specimens removed. The incision size was adequate to allow removal of the mass without any tumor rupture. The renal bed was then examined and hemostasis assured. The ports were removed under direct visualization ensuring no abdominal wall bleeding. Fascia at the umbilical port site was then closed with _-0 braided absorbable suture and all skin incisions closed with a subcuticular _-0 monofilament absorbable suture. *Topical skin glue/Steri-Strips and sterile dressings* were applied. Upon completion of the procedure, a debriefing checklist was completed to share information critical to the postoperative care of the patient. The patient tolerated the procedure well, *was extubated in the operating room*, and was transported to the post anesthesia care unit in stable condition thereafter.

Template Operative Dictation (Laparoscopic Nephron-Sparing Resection of Renal Nodule)

Preoperative Diagnosis Renal mass

Postoperative Diagnosis Same as preoperative diagnosis

Findings Same as postoperative diagnosis

Procedure(s) Performed Laparoscopic nephron-sparing resection of a *left/right* renal nodule

Anesthesia General

Specimen 1. *Right/left* renal mass

Drains __-French *Blake/Jackson-Pratt* drain

Implants None

Estimated Blood Loss ___

Indications This patient is a/an ___-*month/year*-old *male/female* with a *right/left* renal mass. *He/she* has *Beckwith-Wiedemann syndrome/a Wilms tumor predisposition syndrome* and was noted to have a renal mass. *He/She* is now post ___ cycles of chemotherapy and has a persistent nodule measuring ____. *He/She* has been deemed a good candidate for a nephron-sparing operation.

Procedure in Detail Following satisfactory induction of anesthesia, the patient was placed on a beanbag in a modified *right/left* lateral decubitus position with the *right/left* side up approximately 60 degrees. The table was flexed. Timeouts were performed using both preinduction and preincision safety checklists with participation of all team members present in the operative suite. These care providers confirmed the correct patient, procedure, operative site, and additional critical information before the start of the procedure. The abdomen and flank were then prepped and draped in the usual sterile fashion.

A 10-mm *infraumbilical/transumbilical* skin incision was created and a 10-mm port was placed using a *Hasson technique/Veress access*. Pneumoperitoneum was achieved to 15 mmHg. Three additional 5-mm ports were then placed midline of the epigastrium, in the *right/left* lower quadrant, and in the *right/left* flank halfway between the anterior superior iliac spine and the twelfth rib. Medial visceral rotation was performed, mobilizing the colon from the white line of Toldt with the *ultrasonic/thermal energy sealing device*. This maneuver allowed the colon to fall medially. We mobilized the retroperitoneum along the lateral aspect of the kidney up along the peritoneal attachments of the *liver/spleen*. Once we had exposure of the kidney bed we opened Gerota's fascia with the *ultrasonic/thermal energy sealing device*. The hilum was inspected for lymphadenopathy and *none was appreciated/any appreciable lymphadenopathy was sampled*. We continued to mobilize the kidney medially until we could identify the nodule measuring approximately ___ cm. The location matched the patient's preoperative imaging. We saw no other identifiable lesions in the kidney. We then scoured a border along the kidney capsule roughly 5 mm from this nodule using energy. We deepened the rim of renal tissue and proceeded with dissection from the kidney bed. We had no violation of the tumor border. Once the tumor was completely excised it was placed in a laparoscopic specimen bag and removed through the infraumbilical port site. The specimen was brought to pathology and hemostasis verified in the kidney bed. We used *Surgicel®/Tiseel/Fibrillar™* to minimize risk of bleeding and support hemostasis. A __-French *Jackson-Pratt/ Blake* drain was placed along the lateral aspect of the *left/right* upper quadrant to the kidney. We inspected the abdomen for any iatrogenic injury and then removed all ports under direct visualization ensuring absence of abdominal wall bleeding. Fascia at the umbilical port site was then closed with _-0 braided absorbable suture and all skin incisions closed with a subcuticular _-0 monofilament absorbable suture. *Topical skin glue/steri-strips* were applied.

Upon completion of the procedure, a debriefing checklist was completed to share information critical to the postoperative care of the patient. The patient tolerated the procedure well, *was extubated in the operating room*, and was transported to the post anesthesia care unit in stable condition thereafter.

Cholecystectomy

61

Courtney Pisano and Gail E. Besner

Indications and Benefits

- Acute or chronic cholecystitis
- Symptomatic cholelithiasis
- Resolved choledocholithiasis
- Biliary pancreatitis
- Trauma

Risks and Alternatives

- Bleeding, infection, risks of anesthesia
- Injury to the common bile duct or right hepatic duct
- Bile leak
- Abscess
- *Contingent need for conversion from laparoscopic to open cholecystectomy during the progress of the operative procedure*

Essential Steps

Open Cholecystectomy

1. Right subcostal incision.
2. Divide falciform ligament.
3. Inspect the abdomen.
4. Identify the cystic duct and artery.
5. Establish the critical view of safety (make sure the hepatocystic triangle is cleared of fat and fibrous tissue, that the cystic plate is exposed, and that only two structures are seen entering the gallbladder).
6. Ligate and divide cystic duct and cystic artery.
7. Remove gallbladder from the liver bed.
8. *Perform cholangiogram.*
9. Inspect for hemostasis.
10. Close abdomen.

Laparoscopic Cholecystectomy

1. Induce pneumoperitoneum.
2. Inspect abdomen with laparoscope placed through umbilical port.
3. Additional port placement.
4. Grasp the gallbladder fundus and retract it superiorly above the liver.
5. Identify the triangle of Calot.
6. Grasp the infundibulum of the gallbladder, retract laterally.
7. Divide peritoneal attachments.
8. Expose the cystic artery and cystic duct, establishing the critical view of safety (make sure the hepatocystic triangle is cleared of fat and fibrous tissue, that the cystic plate is exposed, and that only two structures are seen entering the gallbladder).

C. Pisano · G. E. Besner (✉)
Nationwide Children's Hospital, Department of Pediatric Surgery, Columbus, OH, USA
e-mail: pisano@nationwidechildrens.org; gail.besner@nationwidechildrens.org

D. J. Papandria et al. (eds.), *Operative Dictations in Pediatric Surgery*,
https://doi.org/10.1007/978-3-030-24212-1_61

9. *Perform cholangiogram.*
10. Take care to identify a point for cystic duct ligation and division sufficiently remote from the common bile duct.
11. Place hemoclips and divide the cystic artery and cystic duct.
12. Dissect the gallbladder from the liver using electrocautery.
13. Check for hemostasis.
14. Removal of the gallbladder per a (dilated) port site alone (if intact) or within an EndoCatch bag (if ruptured).
15. Remove trocars under direct visualization.
16. Closure and dressing.

Robotic Cholecystectomy, Multiport

1. *Administer Indocyanine green (ICG) 4 ml IV at the start of the case in order to use real-time fluorescence imaging guidance.*
2. Abdominal access per umbilical port and diagnostic laparoscopy.
3. Additional port placement.
4. Position the patient and dock the robot prior to deploying instruments.
5. Use an assist port to grasp the gallbladder fundus and retract it superiorly above the liver.
6. Dissect Calot's triangle.
7. Expose the cystic artery and cystic duct, establishing the critical view of safety (make sure the hepatocystic triangle is cleared of fat and fibrous tissue, that the cystic plate is exposed, and that only two structures are seen entering the gallbladder).
8. *Use fluosescence imaging to confirm proper identification of the cystic duct*
9. Ligate and divide the cystic duct and artery.
10. Dissect the gallbladder bed using the heel of the hook.
11. Undock and remove the robot.
12. Removal of the gallbladder per a (dilated) port site alone (if intact) or within an EndoCatch bag (if ruptured).
13. Closure and dressing.

Robotic Cholecystectomy, Single Port

1. *Administer indocyanine green (ICG) 4 ml IV at the start of the case in order to use real-time fluorescence imaging guidance*
2. Abdominal access through a 2.5-cm transumbilical incision.
3. Single-site port deployment and positioning.
4. Position the patient and dock the robot prior to deploying instruments.
5. *Place assist port (5 mm, 10 mm) if needed.*
6. Assist port deployment of a grasper to secure the fundus and pull it up over liver.
7. Dissect Calot's triangle.
8. *Use fluorescence imaging to confirm proper identification of the cystic duct*
9. Ligate and divide the cystic duct and artery.
10. Dissect the gallbladder bed using the heel of the hook.
11. Remove the gallbladder through the port site alone (if intact) or within an EndoCatch bag (if ruptured).
12. Undock and remove the robot.
13. Closure and dressing.

Template Operative Dictation (Open)

Preoperative Diagnosis *Acute/chronic cholecystitis/symptomatic cholelithiasis/choledocholithiasis/biliary pancreatitis*

Postoperative Diagnosis Same as preoperative diagnosis

Findings *Cholelithiasis with/without cholecystitis*

Procedure(s) Performed Cholecystectomy

Anesthesia General anesthesia *with local anesthetic injection (0.25% bupivacaine/0.5% bupivacaine/1% lidocaine/2% lidocaine)*

Specimen Gallbladder to Pathology

Drains None

Implants None

Estimated Blood Loss ___

Indications This is a/an ___*-day/week/month/year*-old *male/female* presented with *right upper quadrant pain/nausea/vomiting/fever/leukocytosis/other*. Diagnostic imaging and workup indicate that the patient has *acute/chronic cholecystitis/choledocholithiasis/symptomatic cholelithiasis/biliary pancreatitis. The patient was not a candidate for laparoscopic cholecystectomy due to __/Laparoscopic cholecystectomy was attempted but converted to open cholecystectomy due to__*. Open cholecystectomy was indicated.

Procedure in Detail The patient was brought to the operating room and placed on the operating table in supine position. Following satisfactory induction of general anesthesia, a time out was completed verifying the patient by two identifiers, the procedure to be performed and the operative site. Appropriate perioperative antibiotics were administered, and the abdomen was prepped and draped in the usual sterile fashion. A subcostal incision was made below the costal margin, extending from the right of xiphoid to the anterior axillary line. Dissection was carried down through the subcutaneous tissues using electrocautery for hemostasis. The fascial layers of the abdomen were divided using electrocautery and the peritoneal cavity was entered. The gallbladder was visualized and traction was placed on the fundus of gallbladder. Using blunt and sharp dissection, the hepatocystic triangle was cleared of fatty and fibrous tissue, and cystic plate was exposed. The cystic duct and artery were identified as the two structures entering the gallbladder.

If cholangiogram: A clip was placed on the cystic duct near the neck of gallbladder. A small incision was made in the cystic duct distal to the clip and a cholangiogram catheter was threaded. A cholangiogram was obtained which showed *absence of filling defects/good bile flow into the duodenum/intact biliary tree/other.*

The cystic duct and artery were ligated using 3–0 silk and then divided. The gallbladder was removed from liver bed using electrocautery to maintain good hemostasis. The gallbladder bed was inspected for bleeding or bile leaks. The peritoneum and the posterior rectus fascia were approximated using *running/interrupted* __. The anterior rectus fascia was approximated using *running/interrupted* __. The subcutaneous fat was closed with _____. The skin was closed using 5–0 Vicryl in subcuticular fashion. The incision was dressed with *Steri-strips/topical skin adhesive.*

All sponge, needle, and instrument counts were correct at the end of the procedure. Upon completion of the procedure, a debriefing checklist was completed to share information critical to the postoperative care of the patient. The patient tolerated the procedure well, *was extubated in the operating room* and was transported to the post anesthesia care unit in stable condition thereafter.

Template Operative Dictation (Laparoscopic)

Preoperative Diagnosis *Acute/chronic cholecystitis/symptomatic cholelithiasis/choledocholithiasis*

Postoperative Diagnosis Same as preoperative diagnosis

Findings *Cholelithiasis with/without cholecystitis*

Procedure(s) Performed Laparoscopic cholecystectomy *with intraoperative cholangiogram*

Anesthesia General anesthesia *with local anesthetic injection (0.25% bupivacaine/0.5% bupivacaine/1% lidocaine/2% lidocaine)*

Specimen Gallbladder to Pathology

Drains None

Implants None

Estimated Blood Loss ___

Indications This is a/an ___ *-day/week/month/year*-old *male/female* presented with *right upper quadrant pain/nausea/vomiting/fevers* and had diagnostic imaging and workup consistent with *cholecystitis/symptomatic cholelithiasis/choledocholithiasis*. The patient was found to be a suitable candidate for laparoscopic cholecystectomy.

Procedure in Detail The patient was brought to the operating room and placed on the operating table in supine position. Following satisfactory induction of general anesthesia, a time out was completed verifying the patient by two identifiers, the procedure to be performed and the operative site. Appropriate perioperative antibiotics were administered, and the abdomen was then prepped and draped in the usual sterile fashion.

A 10-mm incision in the infraumbilical fold was made.

[Choose One:]
For Veress needle: *The fascia was elevated and the Veress needle was inserted. Proper position of the needle was established using aspiration and the saline meniscus test.* Pneumoperitoneum was established using carbon dioxide to a pressure of *12–15 mmHg. A 5 mm/10/12*-mm trocar was then inserted. A 5-mm laparoscope was introduced into the abdomen and the intraperitoneal contents were inspected. No traumatic sequelae of the initial trocar placement were noted.

For Hasson cannula: *Using electrocautery,* dissection was carried down to the level of fascia. The fascia was divided with cautery and *2–0* Vicryl traction sutures were placed on each side of the fascia. The Hasson 10- to 12-mm trocar was then advanced into the abdomen under direct vision and secured to the fascia using the previously placed fascial sutures. A 5-mm laparoscope was introduced into the abdomen and the intraperitoneal contents were inspected. No traumatic sequelae of the initial trocar placement were noted.

Local anesthetic infiltration was used and 5-mm stab incisions were then created for additional trocar sites. Two right subcostal trocars and one epigastric trocar were placed under laparoscopic vision. The right upper quadrant was inspected and *no abnormalities/the following abnormalities were found:* ___. The table was placed into reverse Trendelenburg position with the right side up. A locking atraumatic grasper was introduced into the lateral-most trocar and used to grasp the gallbladder fundus, retracting it superiorly over the dome of the liver.

Using a combination of blunt technique and electrocautery, dissection was then carried out to identify the triangle of Calot, grasping the infundibulum of the gallbladder and retracting it laterally. The peritoneal attachments were divided, exposing the cystic artery and the cystic duct and establishing the critical view of safety.

***If cholangiogram*:** A clip was placed on the cystic duct near the neck of the gallbladder. A small incision was made in the cystic duct distal to the clip, and a cholangiogram catheter was threaded. A cholangiogram was obtained which showed *absence of filling defects/good bile flow into the duodenum/intact biliary tree/other.* Two clips were placed on the retained side and one clip on the specimen side for both artery and duct, followed by sharp transection of each. Care was taken to identify a satisfactory point for cystic duct ligation and division sufficiently remote from the common bile duct.

Dissection was continued with cephalad retraction of the infundibulum and body of the gallbladder. Following mobilization of the gallbladder from its fossa but prior to completing the dissection, the cystic artery and duct stumps were reinspected and clips were found to be in acceptable position, without bleeding or biliary leakage, and the gallbladder fossa was dry. The specimen was then placed in an EndoCatch bag and removed through the umbilical port. The

5-mm trocars were removed under direct laparoscopic vision and hemostasis confirmed at the trocar sites. Following desufflation of the abdomen, the umbilical trocar was removed and site was closed at the fascial level with 2–0 Vicryl in figure-of-eight fashion. The fascia at the 5-mm port sites was closed with interrupted 2–0 Vicryl sutures. The skin at all port sites was closed with 5–0 Vicryl subcuticular sutures. Additional local anesthetic was injected into the port sites as needed. All sites were dressed with Steri-strips/*topic skin adhesive.* A folded 2 × 2 gauze was placed at the umbilical incision. Dressings were secured with TegaDerm.

All sponge, needle and instrument counts were correct at the end of the procedure. Upon completion of the procedure, a debriefing checklist was completed to share information critical to the postoperative care of the patient. The patient tolerated the procedure well, *was extubated in the operating room* and was transported to the post anesthesia care unit in stable condition thereafter.

Template Operative Dictation (Robotic, Multiport)

Preoperative Diagnosis *Acute/chronic cholecystitis/symptomatic cholelithiasis/choledo cholithiasis/biliary pancreatitis*

Postoperative Diagnosis Same as preoperative diagnosis

Findings *Cholelithiasis with/without cholecystitis*

Procedure(s) Performed Robotic multiport cholecystectomy

Anesthesia General anesthesia *with local anesthetic injection (0.25% bupivacaine/0.5% bupivacaine/1% lidocaine/2% lidocaine)*

Specimen Gallbladder to Pathology

Drains None

Implants None

Estimated Blood Loss ___

Indications This is a/an ___ *-day/week/month/year*-old *male/female* presented with *right upper quadrant pain/nausea/vomiting/fever/leukocytosis/other.* Diagnostic imaging and work up indicate patient has *acute/chronic cholecystitis//symptomatic cholelithiasis.* The patient was a candidate for robotic cholecystectomy.

Procedure in Detail The patient was brought to the operating room and placed on the operating table in the supine position. Following satisfactory induction of general anesthesia, a time out was completed verifying the patient by two identifiers, the procedure to be performed and the operative site. Appropriate perioperative antibiotics were administered and an NG tube was then placed to decompress the stomach. Indocyanine green (ICG) 4 ml IV was administered in order to use real-time fluorescence imaging guidance. The abdomen was prepped and draped in a sterile fashion. The robot was positioned to be brought over the patient's right shoulder. A 5-mm port was placed in an umbilical position. Pneumoperitoneum was established using carbon dioxide to a pressure of 12–15 mmHg. Using a 5-mm camera, the abdomen was inspected, and no contraindications to the planned procedure were found. Additional robotic ports were then inserted under direct supervision.

The umbilical port was upsized to a 12-mm laparoscopic port. The table was lowered to clear for the robot. The sterilely draped robot was brought into the field over the patient's right shoulder with the patient in reverse Trendelenburg position with the bed tilted with the right side up. The central column, target anatomy, and camera were aligned. The camera port was docked. The robotic camera was inserted in the 30-degree up position. Additional *two/three* 8-mm robotic ports were placed in the subxiphoid and right subcostal positions and docked. *An additional 5-mm assist port was placed laterally in inferi-*

orly on the right. The camera was turned to the 30-degree down position. A *cautery hook/ Maryland dissector* was placed in for right-handed control and *ProGrasp/Cadiere/ Fenestrated bipolar* foreceps placed for left-handed control. A *laparoscopic 5-mm grasper/ robotic Prograsp foreceps* was deployed the right lateral port and used to grasp the fundus of the gallbladder and retract it over the liver. Calot's triangle was identified and dissected. *Real-time fluorescence was activated to confirm the location of the cystic and common bild ducts.*

Hem-o-lok clips were placed, making sure adequate dissection was done. The cystic duct and artery were then divided using the robotic shears. The gallbladder was dissected off the bed using the heel of the monopolar hook. Meticulous hemostasis was maintained.

An EndoCatch bag was inserted in the umbilical port and the gallbladder placed in the bag and removed. The robot was then undocked and removed from the field. Local anesthetic was injected into the port sites which were closed with *2–0* Vicryl. Steri-strips and Tegaderm dressings were applied.

All needle, sponge and instrument counts were correct at the end of the procedure. Upon completion of the procedure, a debriefing checklist was completed to share information critical to the postoperative care of the patient. The patient tolerated the procedure well, *was extubated in the operating room,* and was transported to the post-anesthesia care unit in stable condition thereafter.

Template Operative Dictation (Robotic, Single Site)

Preoperative Diagnosis *Acute/chronic cholecystitis/symptomatic cholelithiasis/choledocholithiasis/biliary pancreatitis*

Postoperative Diagnosis Same as preoperative diagnosis

Findings *Cholelithiasis with/without cholecystitis*

Procedure(s) Performed Robotic single site cholecystectomy

Anesthesia General anesthesia *with local anesthetic injection (0.25% bupivacaine/0.5% bupivacaine/1% lidocaine/2% lidocaine)*

Specimen Gallbladder to Pathology

Drains None

Implants None

Estimated Blood Loss ___

Indications This is a/an ___ *-day/week/month/ year*-old *male/female* presented with *right upper quadrant pain/nausea/vomiting/fever/leukocytosis/other.* Diagnostic imaging and workup indicate patient has *acute/chronic cholecystitis//symptomatic cholelithiasis.* The patient was a candidate for robotic cholecystectomy.

Procedure in Detail The patient was brought to the operating room and placed on the operating table in supine position. Following satisfactory induction of general anesthesia, a time out was completed verifying the patient by two identifiers, the procedure to be performed and the operative site. Appropriate perioperative antibiotics were administered. Indocyanine green (ICG) 4 ml IV was administered in order to use real-time fluorescence imaging guidance. An NG tube was placed to decompress the stomach. The abdomen was prepped and draped in a sterile fashion.

The umbilicus was everted and a 2.5-cm incision straight through umbilicus was made. The skin was incised using an #11 blade and the subcutaneous fat was divided with electrocautery. The fascia was opened using electrocautery in a vertical direction until the fascial opening easily admitted two fingers to accommodate the single site port. A finger sweep was done to make sure there were no adhesions. The fascia was elevated and the single site port inserted. The abdomen was insufflated (flow at 5, upper pressure limit at 15). The camera port was inserted, the camera inserted in the 30-degree down position, and the abdomen inspected. There were no contraindications to the robotic approach. The patient was placed into reverse Trendelenburg position with the right side slightly elevated. The robot was brought in over the patient's right shoulder. The camera was docked in the 30-degree up position. Cannula 2 was inserted under direct vision and docked. Cannula 1 was the inserted under direct vision and docked. A 5-mm grasper was inserted into the assist port. All port sites were simultaneously burped. The camera was changed to the 30-degree down position.

The crocodile grasper was placed for left-handed control and the cautery hook for right-handed control. The assist port was used to grasp the fundus of gallbladder and pull it up over the liver. Calot's triangle was dissected and the cystic artery and duct identified. *Real-time fluorescence was activated to confirm the location of the cystic and common bile ducts.* Hem-o-lok clips were applied to the cystic duct and artery which were then divided with the robotic shears, leaving two clips on the retained end of the duct and artery. The gallbladder bed was dissected using the heel of the monopolar hook. There were no holes made in the gallbladder, so the grasper that was inserted through the assist port was used to grasp the gallbladder for simultaneous removal with the single site port. The robot was undocked and removed from the field. The single site port and gallbladder were removed. Local anesthetic was injected at the port site. The port site was closed with multiple *2–0* Vicryl figure-of-eight sutures. Steri-strips and 2 × 2/Tegaderm dressings were placed.

All needle, sponge, and instrument counts were correct at the end of the procedure. Upon completion of the procedure, a debriefing checklist was completed to share information critical to the postoperative care of the patient. The patient tolerated the procedure well, *was extubated in the operating room*, and was transported to the postanesthesia care unit in stable condition thereafter.

62 Kasai Portoenterostomy (Open and MIS Approaches)

Stefan Scholz and Lea Wehrli

Indications and Benefits

- Persistent direct hyperbilirubinemia.
- Persistent infantile jaundice with negative medical work-up for alternative.
- Diagnose and treat biliary atresia.
- Benefits: Establish hepatic biliary drainage, improve gastrointestinal absorption for fat-soluble vitamins, and prevent progression of biliary liver cirrhosis.

Risks and Alternatives

- Standard risks (bleeding, infection, need for additional procedures, risks of anesthesia).
- Injury to hepatic arteries or portal vein, small or large bowel.
- Injury to liver at porta hepatis causing bleeding and granulation tissue obstructing bile drainage.
- Anastomotic leak of portoenterostomy (low flow, rare) or jejuno-jejunostomy.
- Postoperative obstruction of Roux limb through adhesions or retrocolonic window.
- Postoperative bowel adhesive obstruction.
- Ascites.
- Ascending cholangitis.
- Deficiency of fat-soluble vitamins.
- Progression of biliary cirrhosis.
- Alternatives: Direct liver transplant after definite diagnosis of biliary atresia by cholangiogram (or ERCP) in cases of advanced liver cirrhosis.

Essential Steps

Cholangiogram

1. Small right subcostal incision to enter the abdomen.
2. Evacuate possible ascites.
3. Retract the liver cranially with malleable retractor and identify gallbladder. Note the size and color of the gallbladder.
4. Place a 5-0 Prolene purse-string suture around the dome of the gallbladder (gallbladder dome may have to be mobilized).
5. Enter the gallbladder with a sharp knife in the center of the purse-string suture, and place a flushed Taut cholangiogram catheter into the

S. Scholz (✉)
University of Pittsburgh School of Medicine, Children's Hospital of Pittsburgh, Department of Pediatric Surgery, Pittsburgh, PA, USA
e-mail: stefan.scholz@chp.edu

L. Wehrli
Children's Hospital of Pittsburgh of UPMC, Department of Pediatric Surgery, Pittsburgh, PA, USA

D. J. Papandria et al. (eds.), *Operative Dictations in Pediatric Surgery*,
https://doi.org/10.1007/978-3-030-24212-1_62

lumen. Note the amount and the color of bile ("white bile?").
6. Tie the purse-string suture around the catheter to obtain a good seal (may add silk tie), and minimize leakage of contrast agent.
7. Place the patient in a good Trendelenburg position.
8. Inject contrast agent with a small syringe into catheter under fluoroscopy guidance (may use flat plate X-ray if quality of fluoroscopy is low).
9. Contrast should flow with minimal resistance into bile system.
10. If distal bile ducts and duodenal outflow is identified but no intrahepatic bile system, compress distal bile duct at the border of the duodenum with a retractor toward the spine to increase outflow pressure.
11. Cholangiogram is complete and normal if contrast reaches the duodenum and the proximal biliary tree within the liver.
12. In cases of biliary atresia, the gallbladder may be minuscule, and there may be only a small amount of "white bile" (mucous). In most cases of biliary atresia, the extrahepatic bile duct has no lumen at all. In about 20% of cases, there is a patent bile duct into the duodenum, but no proximal or intrahepatic bile system can be imaged.
13. If there is a patent bile system, the injection pressure of the contrast, as felt injecting with a small syringe, is minimal. In a patient with Alagille syndrome, the bile system is patent but small in caliber and the pressure may be higher. In case of atretic bile ducts, the injection pressure becomes very high and the contrast may start leaking. High-pressure injections may penetrate into the lymphatic system of the porta hepatis or into the subperitoneal plane, which may be confusing on fluoroscopy.

Laparoscopic Cholangiogram

1. Place a small trocar through the umbilicus, establish pneumoperitoneum and forward the laparoscope.
2. If there is a good-sized gallbladder, the cholangiogram can be performed laparoscopically.
3. Place an additional 3 mm instrument into the right abdomen for liver retraction.
4. Under direct vision, place a Tuohy needle through the abdominal wall, through the liver into the gallbladder to minimize leakage of contrast. Alternatively, the needle (or other catheter) can be placed into the gallbladder dome using a laparoscopic clip.
5. Follow all steps from 7 on for open cholangiogram above.

Kasai Portoenterostomy

1. After definite diagnosis of biliary atresia by means of cholangiogram, extend the right subcostal incision to both sides.
2. Divide the left and right triangular ligaments as well as the falciform ligament to mobilize the liver.
3. With care, rotate the liver anteriorly out of the abdomen using the corners of the incision as retractors behind the right and left hepatic lobes.
4. Mobilize the gallbladder completely, divide the cystic artery, and follow the cystic duct toward the portal vessels.
5. Dissect the peritoneum over the porta hepatis and identify the hepatic artery and its branches.
6. Identify the bile duct remnant and follow this toward the edge of the duodenum. Ligate the bile duct remnant at the border of the duodenum and divide.
7. Follow the bile duct remnant proximally toward the surface of the liver to reach its proximal fibrous cone (if present).
8. Dissect the peritoneum of the fibrous cone anteriorly and laterally to the branches of the hepatic artery. Typically, there are small branches of the hepatic artery entering into the fibrous cone from lateral at its anterolateral border, which can be divided using monopoly or bipolar cautery. Carry this dissection as far lateral as possible to maximize the liver surface covered by the portoenterostomy.

9. Dissect the peritoneum posteriorly behind the bifurcation of the portal vein. Take great care to identify two typical small portal vein branches (one from left and one from right portal vein) entering the posterior aspect of the fibrous cone. Ligate both branches with 6-0 Prolene vs. cautery.
10. Once the complete fibrous cone is dissected on its four borders, laterally to the hepatic arteries and posteriorly behind the portal vein, the biliary remnant is removed from the liver surface. Use small and very sharp scissors for meticulous removal of the scar tissue avoiding any injury to the surface of the liver.
11. Send the biliary remnant to pathology together with a fresh liver wedge biopsy.
12. Place Gelfoam sponge onto the bare hepatic plate and return the liver back into the abdomen.
13. Identify a loop of jejunum about 10 cm distal to the ligament of Treitz, make a window in the mesentery and divide the jejunum with an Endo GIA stapler.
14. Divide the mesentery further to its root and measure a 30–40 cm long Roux loop.
15. Perform a side-to-side jejuno-jejunostomy with a 4-0 PDS running suture directing the stream of enteric contents toward distal.
16. Close the mesenteric gap.
17. Create a window through the retrocolonic mesentery behind the right transverse colon and forward the Roux limp through the window toward the liver.
18. Extrovert the liver from the abdomen again and remove the Gelfoam sponge. Inspect the portal plate for bleeding.
19. Open an antimesenteric enterotomy just proximal to the end of the Roux loop in the appropriate length.
20. Perform an end-to-side portoenterostomy using interrupted 6-0 Maxon sutures maximizing the covered area on the liver surface. The sutures should be placed through the liver well behind the portal bifurcation and just next to the hepatic artery branches on both sides. First, place the back-row sutures. Typically, 8–10 sutures are necessary.
21. Place the liver back into its original position in the abdomen and position the Roux limb into the abdomen and through the transverse colonic mesentery to minimize the chance of kinking and obstruction.
22. Fixate the Roux limb with three sutures into the retrocolonic mesenteric window.
23. Check the orientation of the Roux limb and the jejuno-jejunostomy one last time.
24. Irrigate the abdomen with warm saline.
25. Close the abdominal incision and the skin in multiple layers.

Laparoscopic Kasai Portoenterostomy

1. After definite diagnosis of biliary atresia by means of laparoscopic cholangiogram, place additional three trocars into the right and left abdomen.
2. Retract the liver upwards using either a liver retractor and/or placing a transabdominal suture through the gallbladder remnant.
3. Leaving the gallbladder in place for retraction, divide the cystic artery with hook cautery, and follow the cystic duct toward the portal vessels.
4. Most tissue dissection is performed with hook cautery or careful blunt dissection.
5. Dissect the peritoneum over the porta hepatis and identify the hepatic artery and its branches.
6. Identify the bile duct remnant and follow this toward the edge of the duodenum. Ligate the bile duct remnant at the border of the duodenum and divide.
7. Follow the bile duct remnant proximally toward the surface of the liver to reach its proximal fibrous cone (if present).
8. Dissect the peritoneum of the fibrous cone anteriorly and laterally to the branches of the hepatic artery. Typically, there are small branches of the hepatic artery entering into the fibrous cone from lateral at its anterolateral border, which can be divided using monopoly or bipolar cautery. Carry this dissection as far lateral as possible to

maximize the liver surface covered by the portoenterostomy.

9. Dissect the peritoneum posteriorly behind the bifurcation of the portal vein. Take great care to identify two typical small portal vein branches (one from left and one from right portal vein) entering the posterior aspect of the fibrous cone. Ligate both branches with cautery.
10. Once the complete fibrous cone is dissected on its four borders, laterally to the hepatic arteries and posteriorly behind the portal vein, the biliary remnant is removed from the liver surface. Use very sharp scissors meticulous removal of the scar tissue avoiding any injury to the surface of the liver.
11. Send the biliary remnant to pathology together with a fresh liver wedge biopsy.
12. Place Gelfoam sponge onto the bare hepatic plate.
13. Extent the umbilical incision up- and downwards and exteriorize the small bowel.
14. Identify a loop of jejunum about 10 cm distal to the ligament of Treitz, make a window in the mesentery, and divide the jejunum with an Endo GIA stapler.
15. Divide the mesentery further to its root and measure a 30–40 cm long Roux loop.
16. Perform a side-to-side jejuno-jejunostomy with a 4-0 PDS running suture directing the stream of enteric contents toward distal.
17. Close the mesenteric gap.
18. Place all the bowel back into the abdomen, approximate the umbilical incision and replace the umbilical trocar.
19. Laparoscopically, create a window through the retrocolonic mesentery behind the right transverse colon and forward the Roux limp through the window toward the liver.
20. Remove the Gelfoam sponge. Inspect the portal plate for bleeding.
21. Open an antimesenteric enterotomy just proximal to the end of the Roux loop in the appropriate length.
22. Perform an end-to-side portoenterostomy using interrupted or running 6-0 Maxon sutures maximizing the covered area on the liver surface. The sutures should be placed through the liver well behind the portal bifurcation and just next to the hepatic artery branches on both sides. First, place the back-wall suture.
23. Position the Roux limb into the abdomen and through the transverse colonic mesentery to minimize the chance of kinking and obstruction.
24. Fixate the Roux limb with three sutures into the retrocolonic mesenteric window.
25. Check the orientation of the Roux limb and the jejuno-jejunostomy one last time.
26. Remove the gallbladder and send it to pathology.
27. Irrigate the abdomen with warm saline.
28. Remove all instruments and trocars from the abdomen, close the abdominal incision and the skin in multiple layers.

Note These Variations

- A 5-mm stapler may be utilized to divide the bowel and create the jejuno-jejunostomy and the Roux limb.
- An intraabdominal laparoscopic stapled jejuno-jejunostomy may be performed to create the Roux limb without exteriorization of the intestine.
- The 3 mm laparoscopic bipolar sealer or hook cautery can be used for laparoscopic dissection.

Template Operative Dictation

Preoperative Diagnosis Persistent direct hyperbilirubinemia, possible biliary atresia

Postoperative Diagnosis Biliary atresia

Findings Small gallbladder remnant containing "white bile," atretic biliary system with proximal fibrous cone

Procedures Performed *Laparoscopically assisted/open* cholangiogram, liver wedge biopsy, *laparoscopic/open* cholecystectomy, exploration of extra hepatic bile ducts to rule out biliary atresia, excision of atretic extrahepatic biliary remnant with proximal fibrous cone, jejuno-jejunostomy with creation of 30 cm Roux-en-Y limb, and *laparoscopic/open* Kasai portoenterostomy

Anesthesia General anesthesia

Specimen Gallbladder, liver wedge biopsy, extrahepatic biliary remnant, and fibrous cone

Drains None

Implants None

Estimated Blood Loss Minimal

Indications This ___ *-day/-week/-month*-old *boy/girl* with persistent direct hyperbilirubinemia and jaundice was taken to the operating room for intraoperative cholangiogram to diagnose or rule out biliary atresia.

Procedure in Detail Following satisfactory induction of anesthesia, the patient was placed in supine position and appropriately padded. Timeouts were performed using both pre-induction and pre-incision safety checklists with participation of all present in the operative suite. These confirmed the correct patient, procedure, operative site, instrumentation, and additional critical information prior to the start of the procedure. The abdomen was then prepped and draped in the usual sterile fashion and a broad-spectrum antibiotic was given intravenously.

Cholangiogram

A small right subcostal incision was made to enter the abdomen. This was then carried down to the fascia using electrocautery. The peritoneum was identified and incised to enter the abdominal cavity. *There was a small amount of ascites, which was evacuated. The liver appeared soft and brown with a sharp edge/The liver appeared dark and indurated with a round edge (and a greenish color to it).* The liver was retracted cranially and the gallbladder identified. The gallbladder was very small. A 5-0 Prolene purse-string suture was placed around the dome of the gallbladder after the gallbladder dome was mobilized. The gallbladder was opened with a knife in the center of the purse-string suture and a small amount of white mucous drained. A flushed *Taut* cholangiogram catheter was forwarded into the lumen of the gallbladder and the purse-string suture tied. The patient was placed in a Trendelenburg position.

If laparoscopic cholangiogram*:* An umbilical trocar was placed and pneumoperitoneum established. The peritoneal cavity was inspected for any injuries from abdominal access. The liver appeared soft and brown with a sharp edge/The liver appeared dark and indurated with a round edge (and a greenish color to it). The gallbladder could not be immediately visualized. We then placed a second laparoscopic instrument into the abdomen through a stab incision in the right abdomen. The right lobe of the liver was retracted and the gallbladder identified. (The gallbladder appeared very contracted, and the decision was made to convert to an open procedure.) Under direct vision, a Tuohy needle is introduced through the abdominal wall and directed (transhepatically) into the lumen of the gallbladder.

Under fluoroscopy guidance, a cholangiogram was performed.

The contrast only filled the small gallbladder lumen without progression into the cystic duct and the common bile duct/.The cholangiogram showed a small gallbladder with a patent distal bile duct and outflow into the duodenum. The distal bile duct was compressed at the border of the duodenum onto the spine but a patent proximal extrahepatic and intrahepatic bile system could not be demonstrated.

The cholangiogram was then completed and the parents notified that biliary atresia was confirmed. We then continued with the Kasai procedure.

If cholangiogram negative*:* The cholangiogram showed a patent extra- and intrahepatic bile system with evidence of a normal intrahepatic bile tree and outflow of contrast into the duodenum. *The bile ducts appeared very small and Alagille syndrome should be excluded.* The subcostal incision was closed in a running manner in two layers. *All trocars were removed and the port sites closed.* Scarpa's fascia was approximated and the skin was closed with a subcuticular running stitch. Upon completion of the procedure, a debriefing checklist was completed to share information critical to the postoperative care of the patient. The patient tolerated the procedure well, was extubated in the operating room, and was transported to the postanesthesia care unit in stable condition.

Kasai Portoenterostomy

After confirmation of biliary atresia with the cholangiogram, the right subcostal incision was extended toward lateral and medial. The left and right triangular ligaments were divided to mobilize the liver as well as the falciform ligament. The liver was then rotated out of the abdomen using both corners of the incision as retractors behind the right and left hepatic lobes. The gallbladder was completely mobilized and the cystic artery divided and follow. We then explored the extra hepatic bile system to further confirm the diagnosis of biliary atresia. We carried our dissection along the cystic duct toward the portal vessels. The peritoneum was open at the porta hepatis and the hepatic artery and its branches identified. We then followed the atretic bile duct remnant to the edge of the duodenum. This was ligated at the border of the duodenum and divided. We then dissected the bile duct remnant toward proximal to the surface of the liver until the proximal fibrous cone became visible. We dissected the peritoneum around the fibrous cone anteriorly and laterally all the way to the branches of the hepatic artery. There were two small lateral branches of the hepatic arteries entering into the fibrous cone from lateral, which were divided using monopoly cautery. The dissection was carried as far lateral as possible to maximize the exposed liver surface covered by the portoenterostomy. The peritoneum was then dissected posteriorly behind the bifurcation of the portal vein. Two portal vein branches, one from each portal vein, were seen entering the posterior aspect of the fibrous cone. Both branches were ligated with 6-0 Prolene and cautery. The peritoneal dissection was then completed behind the bifurcation of the portal vein, which was retracted with a vein retractor. The biliary remnant (fibrous cone) was then removed from the liver surface with sharp scissors. Injury to the surface of the liver was avoided and there was minimal bleeding. The biliary remnant was sent to pathology clearly marked for correct orientation. A fresh liver wedge biopsy was then performed at the edge of the liver. Two 4-0 PDS sutures were placed and the wedge was taken with a sharp knife between the two sutures. The liver surface was then cauterized at the cut surface for hemostasis. A small Gelfoam sponge was then placed onto the bare hepatic plate above the portal vein bifurcation and the liver returned back into the abdomen. We then identified a loop of jejunum about 10 cm distal to the ligament of Treitz and made a window in the mesentery. The jejunum was divided with an Endo GIA stapler and the mesentery further divided down to its root. A 30-cm-long jejunal Roux loop was measured. A side-to-side jejuno-jejunostomy was performed with a 4-0 PDS running suture after anti mesenteric enterotomies were opened. The anastomosis was oriented to direct the stream of enteric contents toward the distal small bowel. The mesenteric gap was then closed with interrupted Vicryl sutures. A window was opened through the retrocolonic mesentery to the right of the middle colonic vessels, and the Roux limp was brought through the window toward the liver. The liver was then again extroverted from the abdomen using the skin corners as retractors. The Gelfoam sponge was carefully removed and the portal plate inspected for bleeding. An antimesenteric enterotomy was opened just proximal to the end of the Roux loop. The end-to-side portoenterostomy was then performed using interrupted 6-0 Maxon sutures. The portal plate area on the liver surface covered by the portoenterostomy was maximized behind the portal vein bifurcation and laterally just next to the hepatic artery branches on both sides. The liver back was then placed back into its original position in the abdomen. The Roux limb was then oriented at its optimal position through the transverse colonic mesentery, and the Roux limb was fixated with three sutures into the retrocolonic mesenteric window. The correct positioning and orientation of the Roux limb and the jejuno-jejunostomy were then reconfirmed one last time. The abdomen was irrigated with warm saline.

The subcostal abdominal incision was then closed in a running manner in two layers. Scarpa's fascia was approximated and the skin was closed with a subcuticular running stitch. Upon completion of the procedure, a debriefing checklist was completed to share information critical to the postoperative care of the patient. The patient tolerated the procedure well, was extubated in the operating room, and was transported to the postanesthesia care unit in stable condition.

Laparoscopic Kasai Portoenterostomy

After definite diagnosis of biliary atresia by means of laparoscopic cholangiogram, three additional trocars are placed into the right and left abdomen. The liver was retracted upwards with a liver retractor and a transabdominal suture placed through the gallbladder remnant, which was left in place until the end of the procedure. The cystic artery was divided with hook cautery and followed toward the portal vessels. Careful blunt dissection and hook cautery was used for tissue dissection. The peritoneum over the porta hepatis was opened and the hepatic artery and its branches identified. The bile duct remnant was followed toward the edge of the duodenum and ligated there with a clip. We then followed the bile duct remnant toward the surface of the liver where the fibrous cone was identified. The peritoneum of the fibrous cone was then dissected anteriorly and laterally to the branches of the hepatic artery. The peritoneum was then decided below the fibrous cone behind the bifurcation of the portal vein. The two portal vein branches entering into the fibrous cone were identified and cauterized. The biliary remnant was then removed from the liver surface with sharp scissors without injury to the surface of the liver. A percutaneous liver biopsy was then performed with a biopsy gun. Hemostasis was achieved at the entrance site with cautery. The biliary remnant was sent to pathology together with the fresh liver biopsy. A Gelfoam sponge was placed onto the bare hepatic plate. The umbilical incision was then extended up- and downwards and a neonatal wound retractor placed. The small bowel was exteriorized. A loop of jejunum about 10 cm distal to the ligament of Treitz was identified and a window made into the mesentery. The jejunum was divided with an Endo GIA stapler and the mesentery divided further to its root. A 30-cm-long Roux loop was measured. A side-to-side jejuno-jejunostomy with a 4-0 PDS running suture directing the stream of enteric contents toward distal. A 5 mm Endo-stapler was used to perform a side-to-side jejuno-jejunostomy, and the enterotomy was closed with interrupted Vicryl sutures. The mesenteric gap was closed with Vicryl sutures. The bowel back was the placed back into the abdomen and the wound retractor removed. The umbilical incision was approximated with interrupted sutures and the umbilical trocar placed back into the abdomen. Laparoscopically, a window was made through the retrocolonic mesentery to the right of the middle colic vessels and the Roux limp pass through the window toward the liver. The Gelfoam sponge was the gently removed from the liver surface and the portal plate inspected for any bleeding. An antimesenteric enterotomy just proximal to the end of the Roux loop was then opened with scissors. An end-to-side portoenterostomy was then completed using running 6-0 Maxon sutures for the back row and interrupted sutures for the front row maximizing the covered area on the liver surface. The Roux limb into was then optimally positioned through the transverse colonic mesentery and fixated with three sutures. The orientation of the Roux limb and the jejuno-jejunostomy was reconfirmed one last time. The gallbladder was then removed with hook cautery and sent to pathology. The abdomen was irrigated with warm saline. All instruments and trocars were removed from the abdomen. The fascia of all small abdominal incisions was closed as well as the skin in multiple layers.

A debriefing checklist was completed to share information critical to the postoperative care of the patient. The patient tolerated the procedure well, was extubated in the operating room, and was transported to the postanesthesia care unit in stable condition.

63 Resection of Choledochal Cyst

Amy E. Lawrence and Katherine J. Deans

Indications and Benefits

- Choledochal cyst types I or IV
- Pancreaticobiliary malunion
- Benefits: decreased risk of biliary tract malignancy, decreased risk of pancreatitis and cholangitis

Risks and Alternatives

- Standard risks (bleeding, infection, need for additional procedures, risks of anesthesia)
- Injury to adjacent structures (hepatic artery, portal vein)
- Bile leak
- Biliary strictures
- Intrahepatic stones
- Anastomotic strictures
- Malignancy
- Cirrhosis
- Intrahepatic abscess
- Pancreatitis
- Alternatives: No excision; requires thorough discussion about risks of malignancy

A. E. Lawrence · K. J. Deans (✉)
Nationwide Children's Hospital, Department of Pediatric Surgery, Columbus, OH, USA
e-mail: Katherine.Deans@nationwidechildrens.org

Essential Steps

For Type I, IVa, and IVb Cysts

1. Right subcostal incision.
2. Cholecystectomy.
3. Mobilization of hepatic flexure.
4. Cyst dissection and excision.
5. Wide Kocher maneuver.
6. Hepaticoduodenostomy or Roux-en-Y hepaticojejunostomy
7. If intrahepatic disease is predominantly localized to one lobe, hepatic lobectomy is recommended.
8. Place drain in proximity to anastomosis.
9. Close incision.

Note These Variations

For Type II Cysts

1. Exposure as indicated
2. Complete cyst excision
3. Transverse closure of common bile duct with or without T tube
4. Cholecystectomy

For Type III Cysts

1. ERCP with endoscopic unroofing of choledochocele and sphincterotomy (details not provided in this chapter)
2. Surgical management only in cases where sphincterotomy is difficult to perform or if there is concern for malignancy

D. J. Papandria et al. (eds.), *Operative Dictations in Pediatric Surgery*,
https://doi.org/10.1007/978-3-030-24212-1_63

3. If surgery is indicated:
   (a) Cholecystectomy.
   (b) Via the transected cystic duct, localize the ampulla by passing a Fogarty catheter into the duodenum.
   (c) Extensive Kocher maneuver and intraoperative ultrasound to better identify the anatomy; identify common bile duct and pancreatic duct.
   (d) Transverse duodenotomy in second or third portion of duodenum.
   (e) Intubate pancreatic duct with small Silastic tube.
   (f) Excise intraduodenal biliary cyst.
   (g) Sphincterotomy is performed by suturing duodenal mucosa to bile duct mucosa and pancreatic duct mucosa individually.
   (h) Transverse closure of duodenotomy.

For Type V Cysts

1. If no cirrhosis or malignancy, steps as for Type I or IV with bilateral transhepatic Silastic stents.
2. If progressive liver disease and cirrhosis, consider liver transplantation.

Template Operative Dictation (Open)

Preoperative Diagnosis Type *I/IV* choledochal cyst

Postoperative Diagnosis Same as preoperative diagnosis

Findings Same as postoperative diagnosis

Procedure(s) Performed Resection of choledochal cyst

Anesthesia General anesthesia

Specimen Gallbladder, choledochal cyst

Drains *10 French round Blake drain*

Implants None

Estimated Blood Loss ___

Indications This is a ___ -day/−week/−month/−year-old male/female with a Type I/IV choledochal cyst. He/she was deemed to be a suitable candidate for resection of choledochal cyst.

Procedure in Detail Following satisfactory induction of anesthesia, the patient was placed in the supine position and appropriately padded. Timeouts were performed using both pre-induction and pre-incision safety checklists with participation of all present in the operative suite. These confirmed the correct patient, procedure, operative site and additional critical information prior to the start of the procedure. The abdomen was then prepped and draped in the usual sterile fashion.

A right subcostal incision was made one fingerbreadth below the costal margin in the right upper quadrant. This was carried down through Scarpa's fascia and all muscle layers. The abdomen was entered and the liver was gently retracted superiorly. A Bookwalter retractor was placed.

The gallbladder was dissected off the liver bed starting at the dome. The cystic artery was identified and ligated with the use of ___-0 silk sutures. The cystic duct was then traced down to the level of the common bile duct. The dilation of the common bile duct was identified which extended from **[proximal level]** to **[distal level]**. The choledochal cyst was circumferentially dissected from surrounding structures, starting in the mid-portion of the cyst. A vessel loop was placed securely around the choledochal cyst and dissection was continued both cranially and caudally. An extensive Kocher maneuver was performed to ensure good mobility. Dissection continued toward the duodenum and the head of the pancreas until the transition from dilated cyst to normal ductal size was identified. This dissection was performed very meticulously to ensure that the entire duct was removed without injury to the pancreatic duct. At this point, the cyst was suture ligated and transected.

[If there are concerns about the location of the pancreatic duct:] A ___ cystoscope was introduced through the distal cystic stump to identify the common channel and orifice of the pancreatic duct.

Dissection of the proximal margin was then continued. The cyst was dissected free of the hepatic artery bifurcation and portal vein. The bile duct was transected immediately distal to the bifurcation.

[Choose One:] ***If hepaticoduodenostomy:*** The duodenum was then brought up to the level of the proximal duct and a duodenotomy was created. The hepaticoduodenostomy was fashioned using interrupted ___-0 PDS simple sutures. This was done by putting two corner stitches in for traction and opposition of the cyst and duodenal wall and then a full-thickness single layer anastomosis was performed. The back layer was performed first with the knots on the inside. The anterior layer was performed with knots on the outside.

If Roux-en-Y hepaticojejunostomy: A suitable segment of intestine was mobilized with a Roux-en-Y jejunal limb, approximately 30 cm in length. The anastomosis was created with a retrocolic end-to-side Roux-en-Y hepaticojejunostomy using a single layer of interrupted ___-0 PDS. The bowel was sutured to the mesocolon in three places with interrupted PDS. The distal anastomosis was performed with an end-to-side handsewn anastomosis using interrupted ___-0 PDS.

There was no evidence of leak from the anastomosis. There was no evidence of bleeding. There was no evidence of tension on the hepaticoenteric anastomosis. The Bookwalter retractor was then removed. A ___*-French round channel Blake drain was placed into the RUQ* of the abdomen through a separate stab wound in the right abdomen. The drain was tied in place with a simple ___-0 prolene suture.

The abdominal wound was then closed in layers. Upon completion of the procedure, a debriefing checklist was completed to share information critical to the postoperative care of the patient. The patient tolerated the procedure well, *was extubated in the operating room,* and was transported to the postanesthesia care unit in stable condition thereafter.

Template Operative Dictation (Laparoscopic)

Preoperative Diagnosis Choledochal cyst

Postoperative Diagnosis Same as preoperative diagnosis

Findings Same as postoperative diagnosis

Procedure(s) Performed Laparoscopic resection of choledochal cyst

Anesthesia General

Specimen Gallbladder, choledochal cyst

Drains *None*

Implants None

Estimated Blood Loss ___

Indications This is a__ -day/–week/–month/–year old male/female with a choledochal cyst. He/she was deemed to be a suitable candidate for laparoscopic resection of choledochal cyst.

Procedure in Detail Following satisfactory induction of anesthesia, the patient was placed in the supine position and appropriately padded. Timeouts were performed using both pre-induction and pre-incision safety checklists with participation of all present in the operative suite. These confirmed the correct patient, procedure, operative site and additional critical information prior to the start of the procedure. The abdomen was then prepped and draped in the usual sterile fashion.

A Veress needle was used to enter the abdomen in the infraumbilical region and the abdomen was insufflated to a pressure of 5 mmHg.

This incision was then upsized to a 12 mm trocar. Two more 5 mm trocars were placed on either side of the umbilicus to triangulate the area of the cyst. A large Prolene suture was placed transcutaneously through the falciform ligament and secured extracorporeally to assist in the exposure of the porta hepatis. The cystic artery and duct were identified and isolated. The artery and duct were clipped and divided. The gallbladder was left in the liver bed to assist in traction during dissection. Circumferential dissection of the choledochal cyst began in the midportion of the cyst. The cyst was separated from surrounding structures and divided with electrocautery to facilitate proximal and distal dissection. Distally, dissection continued until the level of the pancreatic tissue where the diameter of the duct was noted to be of normal caliber. The cyst was ligated at that point using an endoloop. Proximally, dissection continued with fine-hook electrocautery. The proximal duct was cut with endoshears just distal to the bifurcation.

An extensive Kocher maneuver was performed to allow easy mobility of the duodenum for preparation of the anastomosis.

[Choose One:]

If hepaticoduodenostomy: At the junction of the first and second part of the duodenum a seromuscular incision was made on the antimesenteric side of the bowel. The submucosa was then opened, and the hepaticoduodenostomy anastomosis was performed using interrupted ___-0 *PDS* sutures. To provide tension-free exposure to the posterior wall, arthroscopy snare needles were inserted through the abdominal wall bilaterally and the corner stitches were grasped and secured extracorporeally at 180 degrees to provide tension and align the anastomosis. Sequential ___-0 *PDS* sutures were placed. After placement of all of the sutures of the posterior row, the sutures were tied using the intracorporeal technique, with the knots internal to the anastomosis. The anterior wall was constructed in a similar fashion with the knots external to the anastomosis. The gallbladder was then dissected from the liver bed and removed through the umbilical port.

If Roux-en-Y hepaticojejunostomy: A suitable segment of intestine was mobilized with a Roux-en-Y jejunal limb, approximately 30–40 cm in length. The anastomosis was created with a retrocolic end-to-side Roux-en-Y hepaticojejunostomy using a single layer of interrupted ___-0 PDS. The bowel was sutured to the mesocolon in three places with interrupted PDS. The distal anastomosis was performed with an end-to-side handsewn anastomosis using interrupted ___-0 PDS.

Port sites were closed in the standard fashion.

Upon completion of the procedure, a debriefing checklist was completed to share information critical to the postoperative care of the patient. The patient tolerated the procedure well, *was extubated in the operating room*, and was transported to the postanesthesia care unit in stable condition thereafter.

Bibliography

Lee H, Hirose S, Bratton B, Farmer D. Initial experience with complex laparoscopic biliary surgery in children: biliary atresia and choledochal cyst. J Pediatr Surg. 2004;39(6):804–7.

Li L, Feng W, Jing-Bo F, Qi-Zhi Y, Gang L, Liu-Ming H, Yu L, Jun J, Ping W. Laparoscopic-assisted total cyst excision of choledochal cyst and Roux-en-Y hepatoenterostomy. J Pediatr Surg. 2004;39(11):1663–6.

Palanivelu C, Rangarajan M, Parthasarathi R, Amar V, Senthilnathan P. Laparoscopic management of choledochal cysts: technique and outcomes—a retrospective study of 35 patients from a tertiary center. J Am Coll Surg. 2008;207(6):839–46.

Santore MT, Deans KJ, Behar BJ, Blinman TA, Adzick NS, Flake AW. Laparoscopic hepaticoduodenostomy versus open hepaticoduodenostomy for reconstruction after resection of choledochal cyst. J Laparoendosc Adv Surg Tech. 2011;21(4):375–8.

Zinner MJ, Ashley SW. Maingot's abdominal operations. New York: McGraw Hill Professional; 2012.

64 Hepatic Resection (Right/Left Hepatectomy; Extended Right/Left Hepatectomy; Wedge Resection)

Justin T. Huntington and Jennifer H. Aldrink

Indications and Benefits

- Hepatoblastoma
- Hepatocellular carcinoma
- Liver metastases
- Benign liver tumors
- Benefits: Potential for cure or local control of tumors

Essential Steps

1. Vascular control and avoidance of major vascular injury
2. Preservation of biliary drainage
3. Complete oncologic resection
4. Appropriate balanced resuscitation with low central venous pressure anesthesia

J. T. Huntington (✉)
Nationwide Children's Hospital, Department of Pediatric Surgery, Columbus, OH, USA
e-mail: Justin.Huntington2@nationwidechildrens.org

J. H. Aldrink
Nationwide Children's Hospital, The Ohio State University College of Medicine, Division of Pediatric Surgery, Department of Surgery, Columbus, OH, USA
e-mail: Jennifer.Aldrink@nationwidechildrens.org

Risks and Alternatives

- Standard risks (bleeding, infection, injury to adjacent structures, need for additional procedures, risks of anesthesia).
- Bile leak, bile duct injury.
- Chyle leak.
- Inadequate resection, positive margins.
- Recurrence.
- Portal hypertension, liver failure.
- Death.
- Alternatives: The preoperative evaluation of the tumor extent (PRETEXT) is used to guide therapeutic decisions for hepatoblastoma in terms of resection, neoadjuvant treatment, or transplantation.

Note These Variations

- Goal of surgery is complete gross total resection.
- Extended right hepatectomy, extended left hepatectomy, non-anatomic resections.
- Intraoperative ultrasound (IOUS).

Template Operative Dictation

Preoperative Diagnosis Hepatoblastoma/hepatocellular carcinoma/liver mass

D. J. Papandria et al. (eds.), *Operative Dictations in Pediatric Surgery*,
https://doi.org/10.1007/978-3-030-24212-1_64

Postoperative Diagnosis Same as preoperative diagnosis

Findings

1. Hepatic tumor involving the __
2. *Intraoperative ultrasound notable for* ___
3. Frozen section pathologic examination with resection margin *negative/positive at* ___

Procedure(s) Performed *Right/extended right/left/non-anatomic (wedge)* hepatic resection

Anesthesia General endotracheal anesthesia

Specimen *Right/extended right/left/non-anatomic (wedge)* hepatic resection involving segments ___

Estimated Blood Loss ___ mL

Indications This is a/an ___ *-day/week/month/year*-old *male/female* with a hepatic mass. *He/she* was deemed to be a suitable candidate for *right/extended right/left/non-anatomic (wedge)* hepatic resection.

Description of Procedure:

After verifying informed consent, the patient was taken to the operating room and placed in a supine position on the operating table. General endotracheal anesthesia was induced. A time-out was then held verifying the correct patient, operation, operative site, and consent. The patient was then positioned supine with his right side bumped up taking care to pad all pressure points. The abdomen was then prepped and draped in a usual sterile fashion. A right subcostal incision was made and extended over to the left side from midline. Dissection was carried down through the skin and subcutaneous tissues using electrocautery. The muscles were divided and the abdomen was entered safely with no sequela of injury. Once the abdomen was entered, the entire peritoneal cavity was grossly explored and no other areas of disease were found. Specifically, the contralateral liver was smooth without any nodularity or areas of concern. There was no ascites or peritoneal implants.

[Choose One:]

Right hepatectomy: Once this exploration was completed, the liver was then mobilized. The falciform ligament was taken between clamps and ligated and tied. It was then divided over the liver to the level of the hepatic veins using electrocautery. The right side of the liver was then mobilized from its peritoneal attachments using electrocautery. Once this was complete, attention was turned to the hilum of the liver. The gallbladder was then taken off the gallbladder fossa using a top-down technique using a combination of blunt and sharp dissection with electrocautery. Once the infundibulum was reached, the dissection was carried down to the cystic duct. The cystic artery was then divided using electrocautery/tied with 3–0 Vicryl ties and divided, and the cystic duct was ligated using 3–0 Vicryl ties and divided.

Dissection then began at the porta hepatis. The pars flaccida was opened using electrocautery and the portal structures were encircled with a vessel loop for a later Pringle maneuver if necessary. The bile duct was then dissected free from the portal structures and encircled. This was traced out to its bifurcation and the right-sided duct was encircled using a silk tie. Attention was then turned to the hepatic artery which was dissected in a similar fashion identifying it within the portal triad and tracking it proximally to the liver. The portal vein was then dissected free and encircled individually and was then dissected to the level of the bifurcation. Attention was then turned to mobilizing the liver off the inferior vena cava. Care was taken to clip/tie/ligate individual perforating vessels from the inferior vena cava to the liver.

***If IVC is intrahepatic**:* The inferior vena cava was also noted to be intrahepatic with the liver parenchyma meeting posterior to the vena cava. The liver parenchyma was divided using electrocautery to expose the entire inferior vena cava.

***If IOUS performed**:* Intraoperative ultrasound was then performed delineating the margin of resection and clarifying the vascular branches. Ultrasound was used multiple times throughout the case to reorient the anatomy.

At this point, the right arterial branches were divided using 3–0 silk ties and titanium clips. The right bile duct was then ligated in a similar manner. The left portal vein and right portal vein were clearly identified and the right portal vein branch was ligated and divided. A suture ligature was placed on the proximal end using a 3–0 silk. Once this was complete, the liver did appear to demarcate fairly well noting an ischemic right liver. Next, the line of transection was planned and marked using electrocautery. The liver capsule was taken along this line using electrocautery. The hepatic vein/inferior vena cava was then occluded. The liver parenchyma was then taken using a crush clamp technique with cautery and a sealing device, taking care to clip all significantly sized vessels and ductules. Ultrasonography was used to identify the right hepatic vein emptying into the vena cava and the crush clamp technique was used to divide liver parenchyma to this level and the right hepatic vein was isolated and divided using a vascular load of an Endo GIA stapler. Other large veins encountered were divided similarly.

Once this was completed, the cut edge of the liver was noted to be relatively hemostatic. It was made further hemostatic by use of argon beam coagulation. No bile was noted leaking from the liver and it was completely hemostatic. The wound was then irrigated and all vessel loops were released. Once this was completed, fibrillar and thrombin were sprayed in the dissection bed. The abdomen was then closed in layers using a running __-0 PDS suture followed by 3–0/4–0 Vicryl in the Scarpa's and deep dermis and then 5–0 running Vicryl subcuticular suture in the skin. Mastisol, Steri-Strips, and a dry sterile dressing were applied.

***Left hepatectomy*:** Once this exploration was completed, the liver was then mobilized. The falciform ligament was taken between clamps and ligated and tied. It was then divided over the liver to the level of the hepatic veins using electrocautery. The right side of the liver was then mobilized from its peritoneal attachments using electrocautery. Once this was complete, attention was turned to the hilum of the liver. The gallbladder was then taken off the gallbladder fossa using a top-down technique using a combination of blunt and sharp dissection with electrocautery. Once the infundibulum was reached, the dissection was carried down to the cystic duct. The cystic artery was then divided using electrocautery/tied with 3–0 Vicryl ties and divided, and the cystic duct was ligated using 3–0 Vicryl ties and divided.

Dissection then began at the porta hepatis. The pars flaccida was opened using electrocautery and the portal structures were encircled with a vessel loop for a later Pringle maneuver if necessary. The bile duct was then dissected free from the portal structures and encircled. This was traced out to its bifurcation and the left-sided duct was encircled using a silk tie. Attention was then turned to dissecting out the hepatic artery which was dissected in a similar fashion identifying it within the portal triad and tracking it up to the liver. The portal vein was then dissected free and encircled and then it was then dissected out to its bifurcation. Attention was then turned to mobilizing the liver off the vena cava as needed.

***If IOUS performed*:** Intraoperative ultrasound was then performed delineating the margin of resection and clarifying the vascular branches. Ultrasound was used multiple times throughout the case to reorient the anatomy.

At this point, the left arterial branches were divided using 3–0 silk ties and titanium clips. The left bile duct was then ligated in a similar manner. The left portal vein and right portal vein were clearly identified and the left portal branch was ligated and divided. A suture ligature was placed on the proximal end using a 3–0 silk. Once this was complete, the liver did appear to demarcate fairly well noting an ischemic left liver. Next, the line of transection was planned and marked using electrocautery. The liver capsule was taken along this line using electrocautery. The hepatic vein/inferior vena cava was then occluded. The liver parenchyma was then taken using a crush clamp technique with cautery and a sealing device taking care to clip all significantly sized vessels and ductules. Ultrasonography was used to identify the left hepatic vein emptying into a common channel with the middle hepatic vein and the crush clamp technique was used to divide liver parenchyma to this level and this common vein was isolated and divided using a vascular load of an Endo GIA stapler. Other large veins encountered were divided similarly.

Once this was completed, the cut edge of the liver was noted to be relatively hemostatic. *It was made further hemostatic by use of argon beam coagulation*. No bile was noted leaking from the liver and it was completely hemostatic. The wound was then irrigated and all vessel loops were released. Once this was completed, *fibrillar and thrombin* were sprayed in the dissection bed. The abdomen was then closed in layers using a running _-0 PDS suture followed by 3–0/4–0 Vicryl in the Scarpa's and deep dermis and then 5–0 Vicryl running subcuticular suture in the skin. Mastisol, Steri-Strips, and a dry sterile dressing were applied.

Upon completion of the procedure, a debriefing checklist was completed to share information critical to the postoperative care of the patient. The patient tolerated the procedure well, *was extubated in the operating room*, and was transported to the postanesthesia care unit in stable condition thereafter.

Inguinal Hernia Repair

65

Melissa Vanover and Payam Saadai

Indications and Benefits

- Inguinal hernia
- Hydrocele
- Benefits: Reduce risk of incarceration at the level of internal ring, improvement of pain if present

Risks and Alternatives

- Standard risks (bleeding, infection, need for additional procedures, risks of anesthesia)
- Injury to adjacent structures (vas deferens, bowel, bladder, vascular)
- Hematoma, including scrotal swelling
- Recurrence
- Testicular atrophy
- Alternatives: None

M. Vanover
University of California, Davis, Department of Pediatric General, Thoracic and Fetal Surgery, Sacramento, CA, USA
e-mail: mvanover@ucdavis.edu

P. Saadai (✉)
UC Davis Medical Center/Shriners Hospital for Children, Division of Pediatric Surgery, Sacramento, CA, USA
e-mail: psaadai@ucdavis.edu

Essential Steps

Open Inguinal Hernia Repair

1. *Consider regional anesthesia (spinal, epidural, caudal) may be used instead of general anesthesia.*
2. Oblique incision in the skin crease between the anterior superior iliac spine and the pubic tubercle.
3. Expose the external oblique and external inguinal ring.
4. Incise the external oblique lateral to the external ring parallel to its fibers and extend medially through the external inguinal ring.
5. Bluntly clear the undersurface of the external oblique superiorly and inferiorly.
6. Identify the hernia sac on the anteromedial aspect of the *spermatic cord/round ligament*, grasp gently, and elevate.
7. Carefully separate the hernia sac from the *spermatic cord/round ligament*. Dissect the hernia sac free from surrounding structures to the level of the internal inguinal ring.
8. *Open the hernia sac at the most distal aspect/ divide the hernia sac between clamps* and inspect hernia sac for contents.
9. *If hernia contents are present, viability determines if manual reduction should be attempted.*
   - *If viable contents are reduced, continue high ligation repair.*

D. J. Papandria et al. (eds.), *Operative Dictations in Pediatric Surgery*,
https://doi.org/10.1007/978-3-030-24212-1_65

- *If sliding components are identified, ensure they are reduced back into the peritoneal cavity and not included in hernia sac ligation.*
- *If contents cannot be reduced or are of questionable viability, ligate the inferior epigastric vessels and enlarge the internal inguinal ring, ensuring the contents do not slip back into the peritoneal cavity. Resect non-viable contents.*
- *If the internal inguinal ring is enlarged, perform formal repair of the inguinal floor.*

10. *To assess the contralateral side: Place a feeding tube/port through the internal inguinal ring and insufflate the abdomen. Perform diagnostic laparoscopy by passing an endoscope through the ipsilateral internal inguinal ring. Desufflate the abdomen after removing the endoscope.*
11. Twist the proximal hernia sac on itself and doubly ligate to perform high ligation.
12. *In females, close the internal inguinal ring.*
13. *In males, gently pull the testicle(s) back into the scrotum.*
14. Close wound in three layers: external oblique, Scarpa's fascia, skin.

Laparoscopic Inguinal Hernia Repair

1. Monitor at the patient's feet.
2. Decompress the bladder.
3. Induce pneumoperitoneum using a *Veress needle/5-mm port superior to/inferior to/through the base of* the umbilicus.
4. Introduce the laparoscope and inspect the abdomen for pathology or injury.
5. *A 3-mm instrument can be placed in the lower midline or contralateral lower quadrant to assist with exclusion of spermatic cord structures and guiding the spinal needle.*
6. *Hydro-dissection using saline/local anesthetic can be used to develop the preperitoneal plane, as well as assist exclusion of the spermatic cord structures in males.*
7. Small nick incision in the suprapubic midline/at the site on the abdominal wall that corresponds to the location of the internal inguinal ring.
8. Direct purse-string suture around the internal inguinal ring, tied extra-corporeally.
9. *Cauterize the superiolateral margin of the peritoneum just inside of the internal ring to create inflammation and reduce the risk of recurrence.*
10. Remove *port(s)/instrument(s)* and desufflate abdomen.
11. Close incision(s).

Note These Variations

- *In infants, opening of the external ring to gain access to the internal ring is not necessary.*
- Opening hernia sac.
- Management of hernia contents.
- Diagnostic laparoscopy to assess contralateral side.
- Periumbilical incision.
- Number, placement of ports/instruments.
- Intracorporeal or extracorporeal technique.
- Differences by gender.
- *Various laparoscopic techniques have been described including intracorporeal repair and inversion ligation of the hernia sac (in females). This dictation describes just one commonly used technique.*

Template Operative Dictation (Open)

Preoperative Diagnosis *Right/left/bilateral* inguinal hernia(s)

Postoperative Diagnosis *Same as preoperative diagnosis/bilateral inguinal hernias/hydrocele*

Findings Same as postoperative diagnosis

Procedure(s) Performed Inguinal hernia repair

Anesthesia *General/regional/procedural sedation*

Specimen None

Drains None

Implants None

Estimated Blood Loss ___mL

Indications This is a/an ___ *-day/week/month/year*-old *male/female* with *right/left/bilateral groin/scrotal/labial* bulge(s) consistent with inguinal hernia(s).

Procedure in Detail Following satisfactory induction of anesthesia, the patient was placed in the supine position and appropriately padded. Timeout was performed using both pre-induction and pre-incision safety checklists with participation of all present in the operative suite. These confirmed the correct patient, procedure, operative site, and additional critical information prior to the start of the procedure. The lower abdomen and genitals was then prepped and draped in the usual sterile fashion.

The midline, pubic tubercles, and anterior iliac spines were marked. An oblique incision was made in a skin line just superior and lateral to the pubic tubercle on the *right/left* side. Subcutaneous tissues were divided until the external oblique was encountered. The inguinal ligament was bluntly cleared to expose the external inguinal ring. An incision was made in the external oblique in the direction of its fibers and extended medially through the external inguinal ring. Hemostats were placed on the cut edges, and the undersurface of the external oblique bluntly cleared. *The ilioinguinal nerve was identified and preserved.*

The hernia sac was identified, gently grasped, and elevated into the wound. The *spermatic cord/round ligament* was identified and encircled with a *vessel loop/penrose drain.* The hernia sac was carefully dissected free of surrounding structures to the level of the internal inguinal ring. The hernia sac was inspected and found to *be empty/contain bowel/omentum/___*. The hernia sac was *opened at the most distal aspect/divided between two clamps and opened.*

If assessing the contralateral groin: A *small feeding tube/3-mm port* was fed through the internal inguinal ring *and secured in place with 3–0 silk tie* and the abdomen was insufflated. A 70-degree laparoscope was inserted, and the contralateral internal inguinal ring found to be *closed/open.* The laparoscope and *feeding tube/port* were removed and the abdomen desufflated.

A high ligation was performed by twisting the proximal hernia sac on itself and doubly ligating with absorbable suture. [*If internal inguinal ring was enlarged:* The inguinal floor was repaired by reapproximating the conjoint tendon to the shelving edge of the inguinal ligament.]

For male patient: *Inferior traction on the testicle returned the spermatic cord structures to their normal anatomic position.* The external oblique was closed with long-term absorbable suture.

If contralateral hernia was known/identified: The contralateral hernia was then repaired in identical fashion with *no notable findings/findings notable for ___*.

The *wound/wounds* was closed in layers with absorbable suture and covered with a sterile dressing. Upon completion of the procedure, a debriefing checklist was completed to share information critical to the postoperative care of the patient. The patient tolerated the procedure well, *was extubated in the operating room,* and was transported to the postanesthesia care unit in stable condition thereafter.

Template Operative Dictation (Laparoscopic)

Preoperative Diagnosis *Right/left/bilateral* inguinal hernia(s)

Postoperative Diagnosis *Right/left/bilateral* inguinal hernia(s)

Findings Same as postoperative diagnosis

Procedures Performed Laparoscopic inguinal hernia repair

Anesthesia General

Specimen None

Drains None

Implants None

Estimated Blood Loss ___

Indications This is a/an ___ *-day/week/month/year*-old *male/female* with *right/left/bilateral groin/scrotal/labial* bulge(s) consistent with inguinal hernia(s).

Procedure in Detail Following satisfactory induction of anesthesia, the patient was placed in the supine position and appropriately padded. Timeout was performed using both pre-induction and pre-incision safety checklists with participation of all present in the operative suite. These confirmed the correct patient, procedure, operative site, and additional critical information prior to the start of the procedure. The abdomen was then prepped and draped in the usual sterile fashion.

[Choose One:]
If Veress needle: An incision was made *supra-umbilical/infraumbilical/through the base of the umbilicus*. The fascia was elevated and the Veress needle inserted. Proper position was confirmed by aspiration and saline drop test. The abdomen was insufflated and a 5-mm port was inserted.

If trans-umbilical: The base of the umbilicus was inverted, elevated, and incised. Entry into the abdomen was confirmed visually and noted to be clear of adjacent bowel loops. A 5-mm port was inserted under direct vision and the abdomen insufflated.

The laparoscope was introduced, and the peritoneal cavity inspected. There *was/was no* evidence of injury from initial port placement. *Right/left/bilateral* inguinal hernia(s) *was/were* identified *with/without* incarcerated contents.

A stab incision was made in the lower abdomen and a 3 mm Maryland grasper was placed. Hydro-dissection using saline/local anesthetic was performed to develop the preperitoneal space around the internal ring. The location of the internal inguinal ring on the abdominal wall was identified with a finder needle and a small nick was made in the overlying skin. *Using a spinal needle double loop technique,* the hernia sac was encircled with monofilament suture, ensuring the spermatic cord structures were excluded. *The suture was exchanged for long-term absorbable/non-absorbable suture* and doubly tied extracorporeally, completing a high ligation. *The superolateral aspect of the peritoneum just outside of the internal ring was carefully cauterized to decrease the risk of recurrence.*

If contralateral hernia was known/identified: The contralateral hernia was then repaired in identical fashion with *no notable findings/findings notable for* ___.

The *port(s)/instrument(s) was/were* removed and the abdomen desufflated. The umbilical fascia was closed with interrupted absorbable suture. The skin incision(s) *was/were* closed and sterile dressing(s) applied.

Upon completion of the procedure, a debriefing checklist was completed to share information critical to the postoperative care of the patient. The patient tolerated the procedure well, *was extubated in the operating room*, and was transported to the postanesthesia care unit in stable condition thereafter.

Ventral/Incisional Hernia Repair (Open and MIS Approaches)

66

Michaela Kollisch-Singule and Jennifer Stanger

Indications and Benefits

- Large epigastric/ventral/incisional hernia
- Large omphalocele with staged closure
- Benefits: Reduced risk of strangulation/incarceration, cosmesis, reduced pain

Risks and Alternatives

- Standard risks (bleeding, infection, need for additional procedures, risks of anesthesia)
- Injury to adjacent structures (bowel, epigastric arteries)
- Mesh infection/migration
- Recurrent hernia
- Enterocutaneous fistula
- Chronic pain
- Granulomas
- Adhesions
- Alternatives: For non-strangulated/incarcerated hernias, non-operative symptom management, abdominal binder

Essential Steps – MIS

1. Induction of general anesthesia
2. Establish pneumoperitoneum
3. Port placement
4. Reduce hernia sac and contents
5. Freshen fascial edges
6. Assessment of size of fascia defect and need for mesh
7. Hernia Repair
   a. Primary (interrupted transfascial sutures)
   b. Underlay Mesh (fixed in place with tacks and transfascial sutures)
8. Port removal and desufflation
9. Closure
10. Abdominal binder

Essential Steps – Open

1. Induction of general anesthesia
2. Skin incision over hernia
3. Mobilization of hernia sac off fascial edges
4. Enter peritoneum and lyse adhesions
5. Identify and freshen fascial edges
6. Assessment of size of fascia defect and need for mesh
7. ***If {primary closure}*** then closure of fascial edges
8. ***If {mesh closure}***
   a. Underlay (mesh anchored to fascia from peritoneal cavity)

M. Kollisch-Singule (✉) · J. Stanger
SUNY Upstate Medical University, Department of General Surgery, Syracuse, NY, USA
e-mail: KolliscM@upstate.edu; StangerJ@upstate.edu

D. J. Papandria et al. (eds.), *Operative Dictations in Pediatric Surgery*,
https://doi.org/10.1007/978-3-030-24212-1_66

b. Sublay (posterior rectus sheath isolated and closed with mesh superficial to posterior fascia and secured to anterior fascia)

9. Placement of drain
10. Closure
11. Abdominal binder

Note These Variations

- Orogastric/nasogastric tube placement
- Open versus laparoscopic
- Open
  - Scar excision
  - Primary closure versus mesh with underlay, sublay (retrorectus), inlay, onlay approach
- Laparoscopic
  - Primary closure ± mesh
  - Hasson/Veress needle entry
  - Placement of laparoscopic port sites
  - Transfascial suture ± tacking
- Choice of mesh
- Choice of suture
- Drain placement
- Placement of abdominal binder

Template Operative Dictation (Open)

Preoperative Diagnosis Ventral/incisional {recurrent} hernia

Postoperative Diagnosis Same as preoperative diagnosis

Findings Same as postoperative diagnosis

Procedure(s) Performed Open *ventral/incisional* hernia repair {with mesh}

Anesthesia *General and local*

Specimen None

Drains __ *Fr Blake / Jackson Pratt/none*

Implants ___ mesh (__ × __ cm)

Estimated Blood Loss ___ mL

Indications This is a/an ___ *-day/week/month/year*-old *male/female* with a *ventral/incisional hernia* that is *recurrent/painful/incarcerated/strangulated. He/she* was deemed to be a suitable candidate for an open *ventral/incisional* hernia repair.

Procedure in Detail Following satisfactory induction of anesthesia, the patient was placed in the supine position and appropriately padded. {An orogastric tube was placed.} Timeouts were performed using both pre-induction and pre-incision safety checklists with participation of all present in the operative suite. These confirmed the correct patient, procedure, operative site and additional critical information prior to the start of the procedure. The abdomen was then prepped and draped in the usual sterile fashion. Prophylactic antibiotics *were/were not* given.

[Choose One:]
If recurrent hernia with scar: An elliptical incision was created around the scar of the previous hernia and the scar excised.

If primary hernia: A vertical incision was made overlying the hernia.

The dissection was carried deeper through the subcutaneous tissues until the hernia sac was encountered and mobilized. The sac was entered providing access to the peritoneal cavity. {There were adhesions between the *omentum/bowel* and the *hernia sac/anterior abdominal wall* that were taken down *sharply/with electrocautery.*} The hernia contents were fully reduced and the fascial edges were identified and cleared of tissue and hernia sac. Additional fascial defects *were/were not* identified. {The edges were debrided, establishing healthy fascia.} The hernia defect was noted to be __ × __cm.

[Choose One:]
If primary repair: The fascial edges could be brought together under minimal tension. The fascia

was closed with interrupted __ sutures, placed in a full thickness manner.

If underlay repair: A piece of __ mesh measuring __ × -__ cm was selected and trimmed to size. In an underlay fashion, the mesh was anchored at the 6 and 12 o'clock positions with __ suture followed by the 3 and 9 o'clock positions, verifying that it lay flat. Interrupted mattress __ suture was used to secure the mesh circumferentially to the fascia. {The anterior fascia was closed over the mesh with running __ suture.}

If sublay repair: The posterior rectus sheath was identified on either side of the fascia and incised at the edge of the defect. It was dissected laterally, superiorly and inferiorly to establish the lateral rectus space. The same procedure was accomplished on the contralateral side. With the two flaps of the posterior sheath dissected free, it was closed with *interrupted/continuous* __ suture. A __ mesh measuring __ × __ cm was selected, inserted, and trimmed to fit. It was anchored at the 6 and 12 o'clock positions with __ suture followed by the 3 and 9 o'clock positions, verifying that it lay flat. Using interrupted __ mattress sutures, inverting the edges of the mesh, it was circumferentially secured to the anterior rectus sheath. The anterior rectus sheath was trimmed to remove excess sac and scar and closed with an *interrupted/continuous* ___ suture.

Hemostasis was verified. {A __-French __ drain was placed in the *retrorectus/subcutaneous* space and tunneled out laterally through the skin. It was secured to the skin with a __ suture and connected to bulb suction.} The incision was irrigated. It was infiltrated with __mL of __*% lidocaine/Marcaine with/without* epinephrine. The subcutaneous tissues were closed with a __ suture and the skin closed with subcuticular sutures/staples and the incision dressed. *An abdominal binder was placed.*

Upon completion of the procedure, a debriefing checklist was completed to share information critical to the postoperative care of the patient. The patient tolerated the procedure well, *was extubated in the operating room,* and was transported to the postanesthesia care unit in stable condition thereafter.

Template Operative Dictation (Laparoscopic)

Preoperative Diagnosis Incisional/Ventral {recurrent} hernia

Postoperative Diagnosis Same as Preoperative Diagnosis

Findings Same as Postoperative Diagnosis

Procedure(s) Performed Laparoscopic *ventral/incisional* hernia repair {with mesh}

Anesthesia *General and Local*

Specimen None

Drains __ *Fr Blake / Jackson Pratt / None*

Implants ___ mesh (__ × __ cm)

Estimated Blood Loss ___ mL.

Indications This is a/an ___*-day/week/month/year*-old *male/female* with a *ventral/incisional hernia* that is *recurrent/painful/incarcerated/strangulated. He/she* was deemed to be a suitable candidate for a laparoscopic *ventral/incisional* hernia repair.

Procedure in Detail Following satisfactory induction of anesthesia, the patient was placed in the supine position, appropriately padded, and secured to the bed. {An orogastric tube was placed.} Timeouts were performed using both pre-induction and pre-incision safety checklists with participation of all present in the operative suite. These confirmed the correct patient, procedure, operative site, and additional critical information prior to the start of the procedure. The abdomen was then prepped and draped in the usual sterile fashion. Prophylactic antibiotics *were/were not* given.

[Choose One:]

If Hasson technique: An incision was made in the __ quadrant and the incision carried down through the subcutaneous tissues until the anterior fascia was encountered. The fascia was grasped, elevated, and incised, establishing entry into the peritoneal cavity. 0-Vicryl sutures were placed on either side of the fascia and the Hasson cannula inserted. Pneumoperitoneum was established with carbon dioxide and the sutures anchored.

If Veress needle: A small incision was made in the __ quadrant and the Veress needle inserted. After two clicks, appropriate placement into the peritoneal cavity was verified with aspiration followed by a saline drop test. Pneumoperitoneum was established with carbon dioxide with adequate flow. An incision was made in the __ quadrant. The peritoneal cavity was entered with a 5-mm camera mounted in a trocar under direct visualization.

Another 5-mm port was placed under direct visualization in the __ quadrant and a 12-mm port in the __ quadrant equidistant between the two ports. {Additional ports were placed ____.} The patient was rolled to the *right/left*. *Bowel loops/fat/omentum* were visualized herniating through the defect. The herniated contents were mobilized and attachments to the hernia sac were taken down *sharply/with electrocautery*. The fascial defect was cleared of tissue, exposing the edges. The defect measured to be approximately __cm × __cm. Upon clarifying the anatomy of the hernia, the decision was made to proceed with a *primary/mesh* repair.

[Choose One:]

If primary repair: Since an *isolated/small* fascial defect was noted, it was deemed appropriate for a primary repair. The defect was closed using interrupted __ suture with a __ suture passer. The sutures were placed 1 cm apart and approximately 1–2 cm from the fascial edge.

If mesh repair: Since *multiple/large/recurrent* fascial defects were noted, it was deemed appropriate for a mesh repair, which was performed with an intraperitoneal underlay mesh. {The defect was first approximated with several *interrupted/continuous* __ sutures.} A __ mesh measuring __ × __cm was rolled and inserted into the peritoneal cavity through the 12 mm port. The mesh was oriented such that the non-adherent side was facing the bowels. Using a suture passer, transfascial sutures were used to position the mesh over the hernia defect in four quadrants. The sutures were clamped at the level of the skin, anchoring the mesh in place. The mesh was found to lay over the hernia edges with a minimum of a 2 cm overlap.

[Choose One:]

If tacking device: A tacking device was used to secure tacks circumferentially around the mesh, approximately 1 cm from the mesh edge and with 1 cm distance between tacks. {A double-crown technique was used and an additional inner row of tacks were applied to secure the middle aspect of the mesh.} {Additional transfascial __ sutures were placed circumferentially around the mesh at 2–3 cm intervals and pulled out through small skin incisions. The abdomen was partially desufflated and the sutures tied down.}

If transfascial sutures: Transfascial sutures were placed circumferentially around the mesh at 1 cm intervals and pulled out through small skin incisions. The abdomen was partially desufflated and the sutures tied down.

The mesh appeared to lay satisfactorily and was secure. The peritoneal cavity was inspected and hemostasis verified. All trocars were removed under direct visualization. The fascia of the 12-mm port site was closed with __ suture *laparoscopically with a transfascial suture passer/under direct visualization with a figure-of-8 suture*. The port and transfascial suture sites were infiltrated with __mL of __% *lidocaine/marcaine with/without epinephrine* and the skin incisions closed with __ in a subcuticular fashion and dressed with __. *An abdominal binder was applied.*

Upon completion of the procedure, a debriefing checklist was completed to share information critical to the postoperative care of the patient. The patient tolerated the procedure well, *was extubated in the operating room*, and was transported to the post-anesthesia care unit in stable condition thereafter.

Umbilical Hernia Repair

67

Katherine Culbreath and Daniel Rhee

Indications and Benefits

- Incarcerated (non-reducible) umbilical hernia
- Symptomatic umbilical hernia, or large diameters (~2 cm) unlikely to close on own
- Umbilical hernia that fails to close by 4–5 years of age
- Proboscoid or "elephant's trunk" appearance of hernia, suggesting that it will not close on its own
- Benefits: Prevention of incarceration or strangulation. If incarcerated, relief of symptoms due to incarceration or bowel obstruction or ischemia

Risks and Alternatives

- Standard risks (bleeding, infection, need for additional procedures, risks of anesthesia).
- Injury to adjacent structures (bowel).
- Recurrence.
- Alternatives: Continued observation if asymptomatic. Spontaneous closure of the hernia defects are less likely to happen if the child is greater than 5 years of age, the hernia is large, or if the hernia has a proboscoid shape. There is a risk of incarceration; however, this risk is overall small.

K. Culbreath (✉) · D. Rhee
Johns Hopkins Hospital, Department of Surgery, Baltimore, MD, USA
e-mail: kculbre1@jhmi.edu; drhee1@jhmi.edu

Essential Steps

1. Incise the skin in a natural skin crease along the inferior umbilical rim. A supraumbilical incision is also acceptable.
2. Circumferentially dissect around the hernia sac at the level of the anterior abdominal wall fascia, passing the clamp behind the hernia to gain control of the sac.
3. Reduce any contents in the hernia sac into the peritoneal cavity.
4. Divide the hernia sac near its skin attachments, or alternatively the sac can be dissected free.
5. Excise the sac to the rim of the abdominal wall fascia defect.
6. Close the fascial edges of the defect transversely with interrupted sutures.
7. Optional: Suture the middle of the undersurface of the umbilicus to the anterior abdominal wall fascia to invert the umbilicus.
8. Close the skin in the usual fashion.

Note These Variations

- If the contents of the hernia sac are incarcerated, the hernia defect can be enlarged. In patients with acute incarcerated hernias, the hernia sac should be opened and the herniated bowel should be inspected for viability. If the incarcerated hernia contains only

D. J. Papandria et al. (eds.), *Operative Dictations in Pediatric Surgery*,
https://doi.org/10.1007/978-3-030-24212-1_67

omentum, this can be resected instead of enlarging the defect.
- Suture technique for the closure of the hernia defect can be interrupted, running, or "vest over pants" plication. Several suture materials are available to use, but a slowly absorbable suture is recommended in most cases.

Template Operative Dictation (Open)

Preoperative Diagnosis *Umbilical hernia/ incarcerated umbilical hernia/symptomatic umbilical hernia/others*

Postoperative Diagnosis Same

Findings Umbilical hernia

Procedure(s) Performed umbilical hernia repair

Anesthesia *General*

Specimen Hernia sac

Drains None

Implants None

Estimated Blood Loss ___

Indications This is a/an ___-*day/week/month/ year*-old *male/female* with an *asymptomatic/ symptomatic/incarcerated* umbilical hernia. *He/ she* presents for umbilical hernia repair.

Procedure in Detail Following satisfactory induction of anesthesia, the patient was placed in the supine position and appropriately padded. Timeouts were performed using both pre-induction and pre-incision safety checklists with participation of all present in the operative suite. These confirmed the correct patient, procedure, operative site, and additional critical information prior to the start of the procedure. The abdomen was then prepped and draped in the usual sterile fashion.

A skin incision was made along a natural skin crease on the *inferior* umbilical rim. Dissection was carried down along the hernia sac to the anterior abdominal wall fascia. The hernia sac was dissected out circumferentially starting from the lateral sides of the defect working superiorly to get around and control the entire sac using a curved hemostat clamp.

[Choose One:]
If reducible hernia: The contents of the hernia sac were reduced into the peritoneal cavity. The sac was then divided from its skin attachments, being careful to not injure the dermis.

If incarcerated hernia and omentum is found: After unsuccessful attempts to reduce the hernia, the hernia sac was opened and omentum was identified in the hernia sac. After ensuring no bowel was in the hernia, the omentum was divided at its base using 4–0 vicryl ties and electrocautery. The remaining portion of omentum was reduced into the peritoneal cavity.

If incarcerated hernia and bowel is found: After unsuccessful attempts to reduce the hernia, the hernia sac was opened and bowel was identified in the hernia sac. The bowel was inspected for viability. The hernia defect was enlarged adequately to free up the intestine. After ensuring the bowel was viable, it was reduced back into the abdominal cavity.

The hernia sac was excised circumferentially down to the rim of the fascial defect. The fascial edges of the defect were identified and isolated from the subcutaneous tissue and the preperitoneal tissue. The defect was closed transversely with interrupted sutures *using 3–0 (infants) or 2–0 (older children) Vicryl or PDS suture.* All sutures were first laid in place and then tied down sequentially closing the defect, being careful not to incorporate any intra-abdominal contents. *The umbilicus was tacked down to the anterior abdominal wall fascia using a 4–0 vicryl suture to invert the umbilicus*. The skin was closed using *absorbable suture* in a *running subcuticular* technique *and was sealed with skin glue*.

Upon completion of the procedure, a debriefing checklist was completed to share information critical to the postoperative care of the patient. The patient tolerated the procedure well, *was extubated in the operating room*, and was transported to the postanesthesia care unit in stable condition.

68 Silo Placement for Gastroschisis

Jamie E. Anderson and Payam Saadai

Indications and Benefits

- Gastroschisis with inability to reduce abdominal contents.
- Benefits: Using a silo can assist in achieving abdominal closure for gastroschisis over a few days, if unable to achieve primary closure at the time of initial presentation.

Risks and Alternatives

- Standard risks (bleeding, infection, need for additional procedures, risks of anesthesia)
- Bowel ischemia with possible necrosis
- Abdominal compartment syndrome
- Respiratory failure
- Alternatives: Primary sutured or sutureless closure, if able

J. E. Anderson
University of California, Davis, Department of Pediatric General, Thoracic and Fetal Surgery, Sacramento, CA, USA
e-mail: jeanderson@ucdavis.edu

P. Saadai (✉)
UC Davis Medical Center/Shriners Hospital for Children, Division of Pediatric Surgery, Sacramento, CA, USA
e-mail: psaadai@ucdavis.edu

Essential Steps

1. Monitored sedation and analgesia is required, but if the infant is not in respiratory distress and does not have significant intraabdominal pressure, it may not be required to intubate.
2. Preoperative antibiotics are required, as is gastric decompression, typically with a Replogle nasogastric tube.
3. Manually decompress the colon to express meconium from the anus.
4. *To allow for potential sutureless closure in the future, maintain a long umbilical stalk (at least 5 cm) by tying the distal cut end with a permanent suture (0 silk) and removing the plastic clamp. Tuck the umbilical cord either in the silo or in the abdomen, taking care to ensure it is not caught between the silo ring and the fascia.*
5. *Enlarge the abdominal wall defect if necessary to prevent intestinal strangulation, although this is seldom required.*
6. Choose a silicone spring-loaded silo with a ring typically 4–6 cm in diameter, size chosen based on the diameter of the defect.
7. Lubricate the silo with warm normal saline and place the eviscerated intestines into the bag, ensuring the mesentery is not twisted.
8. Compress the ring and place it into the abdomen, ensuring no contents are trapped between the ring and the inside of the abdominal wall.

D. J. Papandria et al. (eds.), *Operative Dictations in Pediatric Surgery*,
https://doi.org/10.1007/978-3-030-24212-1_68

9. Place a dry sterile dressing loosely around the base of the silo and suspend the top of the silo with gentle traction.
10. Reduce the bowel over several days by rolling the top of the silo down, while keeping it suspended. Inspect the bowel regularly through the clear silo to ensure no signs of ischemia.
11. Once the intestines are completely reduced, consider sutureless versus sutured closure.
12. *Complex gastroschisis (including intestinal atresia, perforation, or volvulus) may require additional procedures, including intestinal resection and/or ostomy creation. Those are not discussed in this dictation.*

Note These Variations

- Umbilical stalk is kept long (at least 5 cm) and tucked under the fascia or kept in the silo for possible use as a biologic dressing in a sutureless closure once abdominal contents have been reduced.
- This closure uses a silicone spring-loaded silo. If you do not have access to this, clear silicone plastic sheeting can be used to create a silo. The ends can be sutured directly to the circumference of the abdominal wall defect.

Template Operative Dictation

Preoperative Diagnosis Gastroschisis.

Postoperative Diagnosis Gastroschisis

Findings Evisceration of *stomach/small bowel/colon/ovaries/bladder.* Small bowel *matted/not matted. No atresias noted.*

Procedure(s) Performed Silo placement for gastroschisis

Anesthesia *General endotracheal /procedural sedation*

Specimen None

Drains Replogle nasogastric tube. *Foley catheter*

Implants ___cm silo

Estimated Blood Loss ___mL

Indications This is a/an ___*-hour*-old *male/female* with gastroschisis. Approximately ___% *of small bowel, colon, and stomach* are eviscerated. Eviscerated contents were unable to be completely reduced thus a silo was placed with planned for staged closure.

Procedure in Detail *Intravenous sedation and analgesia was given /general endotracheal anesthesia was induced.* The patient was placed in the supine position. Timeout was performed using both pre-induction and pre-incision safety checklists with participation of all present in the NICU. Preoperative antibiotics *(ampicillin and gentamicin)* were given. A Replogle nasogastric tube *was/had previously been* placed. The abdomen and exposed viscera and umbilicus were prepped *with betadine* and draped in a sterile fashion.

The bowel was inspected. It was *dilated and edematous but pink and viable. No atresias were noted.* The abdominal wall defect was approximately __ cm in diameter, to the right of the umbilicus as expected. Meconium was expressed from the anus using manual decompression of the colon.

Approximately __% of the small bowel/colon was able to be reduced. Due to inability to completely reduce the eviscerated content, the decision was made to place a silo for a staged closure.

Since the abdominal wall defect was quite small, the defect was enlarged by extending it cephalad and caudad by ___ cm in each directly to allow for reduction and prevent intestinal strangulation through the defect.

A *4/5/6* cm-diameter silo was chosen. After lubricating the silo with warm normal saline, the eviscerated intestines were gently placed into the bag, ensuring the mesentery was not twisted. The ring was compressed and placed into the abdomen, ensuring no contents were trapped between the ring and the inside of the abdominal wall. The bowel remained pink and viable. A sterile dressing was loosely secured around the base of the silo. The top of the silo was suspended with gentle traction.

Upon completion of the procedure, a debriefing checklist was completed to share information critical to the postoperative care of the patient. The patient tolerated the procedure well, *remained extubated/intubated*, and *was transported to/remained in* the neonatal intensive care unit in stable condition.

Operative Repair of Gastroschisis 69

Jamie E. Anderson and Payam Saadai

Indications and Benefits

- Gastroschisis repair after abdominal contents have been reduced
- Insufficient length or non-viability of the umbilical cord preventing sutureless closure with the umbilical cord
- Benefits: If able, reduction of intestinal contents into the abdomen soon after birth without the need for silo reduction may reduce morbidity

Risks and Alternatives

- Standard risks (bleeding, infection, need for additional procedures, risks of anesthesia)
- Bowel ischemia with possible necrosis
- Abdominal compartment syndrome
- Respiratory failure
- Alternatives: Silo reduction or sutureless closure, if able

Essential Steps

1. *If abdominal contents cannot be primarily reduced, proceed with silo reduction first.*
2. Monitored sedation and analgesia is required, but if the infant is not in respiratory distress and does not have significant intraabdominal pressure, it may not be required to intubate.
3. Preoperative antibiotics are required, as is nasogastric decompression, typically with a Replogle nasogastric tube.
4. Manually decompress the colon to express meconium from the anus and carefully replace the eviscerated content into the abdomen, taking care to ensure the mesentery is not twisted and there is no damage to the intestines.
5. *Enlarge the abdominal wall defect if necessary to prevent intestinal strangulation, although this is seldom required.*
6. If not enough viable umbilical cord is available, or if the defect required enlargement, a primary sutured closure is indicated.
7. Close the abdominal wall defect primarily, using interrupted full-thickness 3–0 long-term absorbable sutures in an interrupted fashion.
8. *Complex gastroschisis (including intestinal atresia, perforation, or volvulus) may require additional procedures, including intestinal resection and/or ostomy creation. Those are not discussed in this dictation.*

J. E. Anderson
University of California, Davis, Department of Pediatric General, Thoracic and Fetal Surgery, Sacramento, CA, USA
e-mail: jeanderson@ucdavis.edu

P. Saadai (✉)
UC Davis Medical Center/Shriners Hospital for Children, Division of Pediatric Surgery, Sacramento, CA, USA
e-mail: psaadai@ucdavis.edu

D. J. Papandria et al. (eds.), *Operative Dictations in Pediatric Surgery*,
https://doi.org/10.1007/978-3-030-24212-1_69

Note These Variations

- This closure incorporates both the skin and fascia en mass in the repair. Alternatively, a skin flap can be created to separate the skin from the fascia, and each layer can be closed separately with absorbable sutures.

Template Operative Dictation

Preoperative Diagnosis Gastroschisis

Postoperative Diagnosis Gastroschisis

Findings Evisceration of *stomach/small bowel/colon/ovaries/bladder.* Small bowel *matted/not matted. No atresias noted.*

Procedure(s) Performed Repair of gastroschisis

Anesthesia *General endotracheal/Procedural sedation*

Specimen None

Drains Replogle nasogastric tube. *Foley catheter*

Implants None

Estimated Blood Loss ___mL

Indications This is a/an ___-*hour/day*-old *male/female* with gastroschisis *status post silo reduction.*

Procedure in Detail *General endotracheal anesthesia was induced.* The patient was placed in the supine position. Timeouts were performed using both pre-induction and pre-incision safety checklists with participation of all present in the *neonatal intensive care unit/operating room.* Preoperative antibiotics *(ampicillin and gentamicin)* were given. A Replogle nasogastric tube *was/had previously been* placed. *A Foley catheter was placed under sterile technique.* The abdomen and exposed viscera and umbilicus were prepped *with betadine* and draped in a sterile fashion.

[Choose One:]

If previous silo reduction: The silo bag was removed. The remaining exposed small bowel/colon appeared healthy and viable and was reduced.

If primary reduction: The bowel was inspected. It was *dilated and edematous but pink and viable. No atresias were noted.* The abdominal wall defect was approximately __ cm in diameter, to the right of the umbilicus as expected. Meconium was expressed from the anus using manual decompression of the colon. The eviscerated contents were replaced into the abdomen.

The abdominal wall defect was extended cephalad and caudad to allow reduction. This was done via *a sharp skin incision and electrocautery.* The abdominal defect was then closed *vertically/horizontally/in a purse-string fashion.* The defect was closed with *interrupted full-thickness 3–0 long-term absorbable sutures, incorporating both the fascia and skin.* There were no adverse changes in *peak ventilator pressures/tidal volumes* noted after closure. A dry non-adherent sterile dressing and a clear, occlusive bandage were placed. The patient tolerated the procedure well.

Upon completion of the procedure, a debriefing checklist was completed to share information critical to the postoperative care of the patient. The patient tolerated the procedure well, *was extubated/remained intubated,* and *was transported to/remained in* the neonatal intensive care unit in stable condition.

Sutureless Repair of Gastroschisis

70

Jamie E. Anderson and Payam Saadai

Indications and Benefits

- Gastroschisis repair after abdominal contents have been reduced
- Requires sufficient length (>3–5 cm) and viability of the umbilical cord
- Benefits: Reduction of intestinal contents into the abdomen soon after birth without the need for silo reduction may reduce morbidity

Risks and Alternatives

- Standard risks (bleeding, infection, need for additional procedures, risks of anesthesia)
- Bowel ischemia with possible necrosis
- Abdominal compartment syndrome
- Respiratory failure.
- Alternatives: Silo reduction or primary sutured closure

J. E. Anderson
University of California, Davis, Department of Pediatric General, Thoracic and Fetal Surgery, Sacramento, CA, USA
e-mail: jeanderson@ucdavis.edu

P. Saadai (✉)
UC Davis Medical Center/Shriners Hospital for Children, Division of Pediatric Surgery, Sacramento, CA, USA
e-mail: psaadai@ucdavis.edu

Essential Steps

1. *If abdominal contents cannot be primarily reduced, proceed with silo reduction first.*
2. Monitored sedation and analgesia is required, but if the infant is not in respiratory distress and does not have significant intraabdominal pressure, it may not be required to intubate.
3. Preoperative antibiotics are required, as is nasogastric decompression, typically with a Replogle nasogastric tube.
4. Manually decompress the colon to express meconium from the anus and carefully replace the eviscerated content into the abdomen, taking care to ensure the mesentery is not twisted and there is no damage to the intestines.
5. Eviscerate the umbilical cord. This should be long enough to adequately cover the remaining abdominal defect, at least 3–5 cm in length. The cut end should be ligated with a permanent suture (0 silk), rather than a plastic clamp.
6. Use the umbilical cord to cover the abdominal wall defect.
7. Apply liquid adhesive to the skin surrounding the abdominal defect.
8. *If the cord completely covers the defect, covering the cord with Mepilex foam is recommended but not required.*

D. J. Papandria et al. (eds.), *Operative Dictations in Pediatric Surgery*,
https://doi.org/10.1007/978-3-030-24212-1_70

9. Cover the entire defect *and Mepilex* with a large Tegaderm or other occlusive clear bandage.
10. Change the dressing every 3 days or sooner if concern for saturation or evisceration. The umbilical cord will eventually desiccate after the defect is epithelialized.
11. *Complex gastroschisis (including intestinal atresia, perforation, or volvulus) may require additional procedures, including intestinal resection and/or ostomy creation. Those are not discussed in this dictation.*

Note These Variations

- A silo can be used to assist in the reduction of eviscerated viscera, especially if the patient is not intubated. Once the viscera have been completely reduced with the aid of the silo, primary sutureless closure can be performed at the same procedure.
- A Mepilex foam dressing is placed over the cord and defect, but is not required if the cord completely covers the defect.

Template Operative Dictation

Preoperative Diagnosis Gastroschisis

Postoperative Diagnosis Gastroschisis

Findings Evisceration of *stomach/small bowel/colon/ovaries/bladder.* Small bowel *matted/not matted. No atresias noted.*

Procedure(s) Performed Sutureless repair of gastroschisis

Anesthesia *General endotracheal/procedural sedation*

Specimen None

Drains Replogle nasogastric tube. *Foley catheter*

Implants None

Estimated Blood Loss ___mL

Indications This is a/an ___*-hour/day*-old *male/female* with gastroschisis *status post silo reduction.*

Procedure in Detail *General endotracheal anesthesia was induced.* The patient was placed in the supine position. Timeouts were performed using both pre-induction and pre-incision safety checklists with participation of all present in the *neonatal intensive care unit/operating room.* Preoperative antibiotics *(ampicillin and gentamicin)* were given. A Replogle nasogastric tube *was/had previously* been placed. *A Foley catheter was placed under sterile technique.* The abdomen and exposed viscera and umbilicus were prepped *with betadine* and draped in a sterile fashion.

[Choose One:]
If previous silo reduction: *The silo bag was removed. The umbilical cord was eviscerated from under the fascia. The remaining exposed small bowel/colon appeared pink and viable and was reduced.*

If primary reduction: *The eviscerated small intestine/colon/stomach appeared dilated and edematous but pink and viable. No atresias were noted. The meconium was expressed from the anus using manual decompression of the colon. The eviscerated contents were replaced into the abdomen. The end of the umbilical cord was tied with a 0 silk tie and the distal cord and clamp were removed. The remaining length of the umbilical cord was approximately __ cm in length which was adequate to cover the defect.*

The fascial defect was fully covered with the umbilical cord as a biological dressing. Liquid adhesive was applied to the skin. An appropriately sized piece of Mepilex foam dressing was placed over the cord and the defect. Additional liquid adhesive was applied to the surrounding skin and a large Tegaderm was placed over the wound. There were no adverse changes in *peak ventilator pressures/tidal volumes* noted as closure. The patient tolerated the procedure well.

Upon completion of the procedure, a debriefing checklist was completed to share information critical to the postoperative care of the patient. The patient tolerated the procedure well, *remained extubated/intubated*, and *remained in/was transported to* the neonatal intensive care unit in stable condition.

71 Repair of Omphalocele

A. Francois Trappey III and Payam Saadai

Indications and Benefits

- Omphalocele with small to moderate size abdominal wall defect (generally <5 cm)
- Stable patient without major cardiopulmonary comorbidities
- Benefits: Early, single-stage closure of the abdominal wall may reduce morbidity in carefully selected patients

Risks and Alternatives

- Standard risks, such as bleeding, infection, need for additional procedures, and risks of anesthesia.
- Injury to Glisson's capsule or hepatic veins during excision of the omphalocele sac.
- Obstruction of cardiac return during reduction of the liver into the abdomen.
- Abdominal compartment syndrome.
- Respiratory failure.
- *Alternatives*: Various methods of staged closure including scarification with the use of antiseptic ("paint and wait"), skin-only closure with later ventral hernia repair, mesh closure, and other complex abdominal wall closures (Schuster technique, component separation). A silastic silo may be needed in cases of a ruptured omphalocele not amenable to primary closure.

Essential Steps

1. General endotracheal anesthesia.
2. Preoperative antibiotics are required and are usually continued for 48 h postoperatively.
3. A Replogle nasogastric tube, if not already in place, is used for bowel decompression.
4. Excise the omphalocele sac. Separation of the sac from the liver should not be attempted as this can cause major bleeding from Glisson's capsule or underlying hepatic veins. Ligation of the umbilical vessels and urachus will be required during excision of the sac.
5. Reduce the abdominal contents into the abdominal cavity. Some gentle stretching of the abdominal wall may be required.
6. Raise circumferential subcutaneous flaps prior to closure of the abdominal wall in layers using absorbable suture.

A. Francois Trappey III
University of California, Davis, Department of Pediatric General, Thoracic and Fetal Surgery, Sacramento, CA, USA
e-mail: aftrappey@ucdavis.edu

P. Saadai (✉)
UC Davis Medical Center/Shriners Hospital for Children, Division of Pediatric Surgery, Sacramento, CA, USA
e-mail: psaadai@ucdavis.edu

D. J. Papandria et al. (eds.), *Operative Dictations in Pediatric Surgery*,
https://doi.org/10.1007/978-3-030-24212-1_71

Note These Variations

- Attempt can be made to reduce the abdominal contents with the sac intact.
- The fascia can be closed either vertically or transversely.
- The overlying skin can be closed linearly with a purse-string style closure or with a more formal umbilicoplasty.
- Giant omphalocele requires a more complex management not discussed here in detail.

Template Operative Dictation (Open)

Preoperative Diagnosis Omphalocele

Postoperative Diagnosis Omphalocele

Findings Omphalocele with Intact sac

Procedure(s) Performed Repair of omphalocele

Anesthesia General endotracheal

Specimen None

Drains None

Implants None

Estimated Blood Loss ___mL

Indications This is a/an ___-*hour/day*-old *male/female* with a *small/moderate* size omphalocele. He/she was deemed to be a suitable candidate for primary repair of the omphalocele.

Procedure in Detail Following satisfactory induction of general endotracheal anesthesia, the patient was placed in supine position and appropriately padded. Time-outs were performed using both preinduction and preincision safety checklists with participation of all present in the operative suite. These confirmed the correct patient, procedure, operative site, and additional critical information prior to the start of the procedure. Preoperative antibiotics were administered. A nasogastric tube *was/had previously been* placed. The abdomen was then prepped and draped in the usual sterile way.

The omphalocele was measured to be __ cm in size. The sac was resected sharply back to the edge of the defect and off the underlying bowel. The umbilical *vein/arteries/urachus* were ligated during this process with a 3–0 *absorbable/nonabsorbable* suture. Sac adherent to the liver was left in place. The abdominal contents were inspected and no gross abnormalities were noted. The abdominal wall was gently stretched to increase its compliance. The abdominal contents were carefully reduced into the abdominal cavity.

Subcutaneous flaps were mobilized sharply off of the anterior fascia circumferentially. The fascial defect was closed using interrupted 3–0 absorbable sutures in a *transverse/vertical fashion* under minimal tension. These were sequentially tied making sure there were no changes in peak pressure or tidal volume noted on the ventilator with fascial closure. The skin was closed in a *linear/purse-string* fashion. A sterile dressing was applied.

Upon completion of the procedure, a debriefing checklist was completed to share information critical to the postoperative care of the patient. The patient tolerated the procedure well, *was/was not extubated in the operating room,* and was transported to the neonatal intensive care unit in stable condition thereafter.

Interval Laparotomy with Placement of Temporary Closure

72

Carolyn Gosztyla and Howard I. Pryor II

Indications and Benefits

- Abdominal compartment syndrome
- Damage control laparotomy in trauma – penetrating injury, blunt abdominal injury with hemodynamic instability
- Uncontrolled intra-abdominal sepsis
- Benefits: Relief of intra-abdominal compartment hypertension, hemostasis, or source control with rapid progression to the resuscitative phase of care

Risks and Alternatives

- Standard risks, such as bleeding, infection, need for additional procedures, and risks of anesthesia
- Injury to adjacent structures within the abdomen
- Need for additional operative exploration to achieve definitive hemostasis or source control
- *Alternatives*: Abdominal drain

C. Gosztyla
Walter Reed National Military Medical Center, Department of General Surgery, Bethesda, MD, USA

H. I. Pryor II (✉)
Division of Pediatric Surgery, Walter Reed National Military Medical Center, Department of Surgery, Bethesda, MD, USA

Essential Steps

Access to the Abdomen

1. Transverse laparotomy in children whose abdomen is wider than it is long (typically <6 years old)
2. Midline laparotomy incision for all other patients

Abdominal Exploration

1. Four quadrant packing if there is hemoperitoneum with hemodynamic instability
2. Systematic exploration of all quadrants of the abdomen

Temporary Closure

1. Temporary closure performed per surgeon preference: *wound VAC, silo, Bogota bag*
2. Return to ICU for continued resuscitation

Note These Variations

- Damage control operations may be performed in an ICU environment in patients who are too unstable to facilitate transfer to the operating room.

D. J. Papandria et al. (eds.), *Operative Dictations in Pediatric Surgery*,
https://doi.org/10.1007/978-3-030-24212-1_72

- An abdominal drain may be utilized in some scenarios as a temporizing measure in patients who are too unstable to tolerate laparotomy.

Template Operative Dictation (Open)

Preoperative Diagnosis *Abdominal compartment syndrome, abdominal trauma, uncontrolled abdominal sepsis*

Postoperative Diagnosis Same as preoperative diagnosis

Findings Same as postoperative diagnosis

Procedure(s) Performed Interval laparotomy with placement of temporary closure

Anesthesia General

Specimen None

Drains None

Implants None

Estimated Blood Loss XXX ml

Indications This is a/an *XX-day/week/month/year*-old *male/female* presented with *abdominal compartment syndrome/abdominal trauma/intra-abdominal sepsis.* He/she was deemed to be a suitable candidate for interval laparotomy with placement of temporary closure.

Procedure in Detail Following satisfactory induction of anesthesia, the patient was placed in supine position with arms abducted and appropriately padded. Time-outs were performed using both preinduction and preincision safety checklists with participation of all present in the operative suite. These confirmed the correct patient, procedure, operative site, and additional critical information prior to the start of the procedure. The abdomen was then prepped and draped in the usual sterile fashion.

A *midline/transverse* laparotomy incision was made in the skin and was deepened through the subcutaneous tissue and the fascia was incised to expose the peritoneum. The peritoneum was entered sharply.

[Choose One:]

If operation is performed for abdominal compartment syndrome: The abdomen was systematically explored for evidence of ischemia.

If operation is performed for abdominal trauma: Upon entering the abdomen, hemoperitoneum was encountered. Four quadrant packing was placed to provide hemostasis. The abdomen was explored starting in the *RUQ/LUQ/RLQ/LLQ* and moving *clockwise/counterclockwise*. The following injuries were identified: *(Describe the specific operative findings here)* The following interventions were performed: *(Describe the specific operative interventions here).*

If operation is performed for abdominal sepsis: Upon entering the abdomen, *purulent/feculent* peritonitis was encountered. The abdomen was systematically explored for the source. The following findings were encountered: *(Describe the specific operative findings here).* The following interventions were performed to obtain source control: *(Describe the specific operative interventions here).*

After adequate exploration and intervention, the abdomen was left open and a temporary abdominal closure was placed to facilitate transfer to the resuscitative phase of care. A *silo/wound VAC/vacuum pack* was placed.

[Choose One:]

If a silo is placed: A silastic silo was placed in the abdominal wall defect. *The wound edges were dressed with Kerlix/gauze. (Describe the specific operative interventions here)*

If a negative pressure wound therapy dressing is placed: The omentum was draped over the abdominal contents. A plastic sheet was placed over the abdominal contents. Wound VAC sponge was then placed over the plastic sheeting *and was stapled/sutured in place. Adhesive dressing/iodine-impregnated adhesive dressing* was placed over the top and a defect was created to place the

VAC device. The VAC tubing was connected to a negative pressure device and negative pressure was initiated.

If an abdominal vacuum pack is created and placed: Small slits were placed in a variety of locations along a *plastic sheet/sterilized IV bag. The omentum was draped over the abdominal contents.* The *plastic sheet/IV bag* was placed in the subfascial space taking care to cover all abdominal contents and ensure covering is packed along the paracolic gutters. The plastic drape was covered with sterile gauze. Two XX Fr *flat/round Jackson-Pratt/silicone channel drains/Salem sump tubes* were laid on top of the gauze. This assembly was then covered with additional sterile gauze. The wound was covered with sterile towels and an *adhesive/iodine-impregnated adhesive* dressing was used to cover the wound. The abdominal pack was placed on suction and inspected for leaks prior to conclusion of the case.

Upon completion of the procedure, a debriefing checklist was completed to share information critical to the postoperative care of the patient including dressing and packing equipment intentionally left with the peritoneal cavity. The patient remained in critical condition and was transferred to the ICU to facilitate resuscitation with the plan to return to the operating room for reexploration and closure.

73 Flexible Bronchoscopy

Carlos Andrés de la Torre Ramos

Indications and Benefits

- Diagnosis: Phonation anomalies, stridor, persistent wheezing, recurrent or persistent pneumonia, atelectasis, bronchiectasis, localized hyperinflation, hemoptysis, unexplained persistent cough, suspicion of foreign body, and airway burn or trauma
- To obtain samples: Bronchial aspirate, bronchoalveolar lavage, bronchial or transbronchial biopsy (diffuse pulmonary infiltrate, interstitial pneumonia, pulmonary pathology in immunocompromised patients, monitoring rejection post lung transplant, intraluminal tumor, extraluminal mass)
- Therapeutic: Resolution of atelectasis, difficult intubation, instillation of drugs, washes for alveolar proteinosis, foreign body extraction in selected cases, and airway dilations

Risks and Alternatives

- Standard risks, such as bleeding, infection, need for additional procedures, and risks of anesthesia
- Injury to adjacent structures
- Major complications: Pneumothorax, severe desaturation, and apnea
- Minor complications: Epistaxis, laryngospasm, bronchospasm, and transient desaturation
- Fever within the first 24 h
- After biopsy: Pneumothorax and bleeding
- Alternatives: Rigid bronchoscopy, thoracoscopy or thoracotomy for lung biopsy

Essential Steps

1. Supine position. Patient under sedation and spontaneous ventilation
2. *Nasal access*: Topic application of *1%/2%* lidocaine in the right/left naris

Maximum recommended dose of 2% lidocaine: 0.2 ml/kg; and 1% lidocaine: 0.4 ml/kg for the entire procedure

3. Exploration of the oropharynx and larynx (supraglottic space)
4. Inspection of the vocal cords motion
5. Additional instillation of *1%/2%* lidocaine in the vocal cords and subglottic space.
6. Flexible bronchoscope advancement through the larynx into the trachea
7. Examination for mucosal abnormalities, secretions, masses, stenosis, cartilage rings, extrinsic compressions, and/or malacia

C. A. de la Torre Ramos (✉)
University Hospital La Paz, Pediatric Surgery, Madrid, Spain

D. J. Papandria et al. (eds.), *Operative Dictations in Pediatric Surgery*,
https://doi.org/10.1007/978-3-030-24212-1_73

8. Bronchoscope advancement until the carina
9. Additional topic anesthesia with *1%/2%* lidocaine was applied in the carina
10. Systematic exploration of the bronchial tree starting at the right upper lobe and finishing at the left lower lobe bronchi
11. *If indicated: Bronchial aspiration/bronchoalveolar lavage or bronchial/transbronchial biopsy*
12. Bronchoscope withdrawal

Note These Variations

If nasal access: *For stable patients – Topic application of ___cc of 1%/2% lidocaine in the right/left naris prior to start of the procedure. Oxygen administration through nasal cannula. The entire airway is examined. The procedure is performed under sedation and spontaneous ventilation.*

If laryngeal mask access: *When nasal access is not possible or unstable patients – Laryngeal mask provides adequate ventilation, but the supraglottic space cannot be examined. The procedure is performed under sedation and spontaneous ventilation.*

If endotracheal tube access: *Critical patients – Only anatomical aspects of distal trachea and bronchial tree can be explored. Flexible bronchoscope size must be selected to allow correct ventilation through the endotracheal tube.*

If tracheostomy cannula access: *Patients with tracheostomy – The upper airway cannot be explored. The procedure can be performed under sedation with spontaneous ventilation or mechanical ventilation.*

Template Operative Dictation

Preoperative Diagnosis *Stridor and suspicion of tracheomalacia/pneumonia/inhalation injury/___*

Postoperative Diagnosis __

Findings __

Procedures Performed Flexible bronchoscopy

Anesthesia Procedural sedation

Specimen *None/tracheal and bronchial secretions*

Estimated Blood Loss ___

Indications This is a/an __ *-day/week/month/year*-old *male/female* presented with stridor and apneic spells. *He/she* was deemed to be a suitable candidate for flexible bronchoscopy.

Procedure in Detail Following satisfactory induction of anesthesia, the patient was placed in supine position and appropriately padded. Time-outs were performed using both preinduction and preincision safety checklists with participation of all present in the operative suite. These confirmed the correct patient, procedure, operative site, and additional critical information prior to the start of the procedure.

The patient was under sedation with spontaneous ventilation. Topic application of ___ml of *1%/2%* lidocaine was instilled through the right/left naris. We inserted *a 2.2-mm/2.8-mm/3.5-mm/4.9-mm* flexible bronchoscope through the previously instilled naris. The nasopharynx and oropharynx looked normal. The supraglottic (including epiglottis and arytenoids) space was then carefully inspected and was normal. Vocal cords movement and position were normal. Additional topic instillation of ____ml of *1%/2%* lidocaine was instilled to the larynx and subsequently throughout the tracheobronchial tree. The bronchoscope was advanced through the vocal cords easily. The subglottic space did not show any narrowing or abnormalities. The proximal third of the trachea also looked normal and the tracheal rings had normal consistency and diameter at this level. The bronchoscope was then advanced. From the middle third to the carina, a 60% of collapsibility of the tracheal lumen was observed during expiration due to tracheomalacia. No extrinsic compressions were noted during the examination and the tracheal mucosa looked normal. Clear secretions were suctioned. Once in the carina, additional ___ ml of *1%/2%* lidocaine was applied. The bronchoscope was then advanced. A systematic exploration of the entire bronchial tree was done. First, the right upper, middle, and lower lobes and their segments were inspected. Subsequently, the exploration was performed in the left lobes and segments.

[Choose One:]

- ***If bronchial aspirate is indicated:*** Bronchial secretions were obtained through the suction channel and collected in a specimen container. Saline was instilled during the procedure to facilitate aspiration of dense secretions. Samples were sent to microbiology.
- ***If bronchoalveolar lavage is indicated***: (Whether we select the compromised segment, if the anomaly is localized, or the middle or lower right bronchi, if the anomaly is generalized). Instillation of 3 ml/kg of saline divided in three syringes through the working channel was performed. After every instillation samples were suctioned and sent to microbiology, pathology, and biochemistry.
- ***If bronchial or transbronchial biopsy is indicated:*** Under fluoroscopy guidance. Biopsy forceps was advanced to the periphery of the selected segmental bronchi until resistance is encountered. Placement of the biopsy forceps near but not at the lung surface to minimize the risk of pneumothorax. The forceps was withdrawn approximately 1 cm. The forceps was then advanced close to the area where resistance is encountered, and the jaws are closed. The biopsy forceps was firmly retracted to obtain the sample. Four to six samples were obtained from the same lobe. Hemostasis was checked. Fluoroscopy excluded pneumothorax.
- ***If a foreign body is found:*** Refer to Chap. 86 section: *Note These Variations*.

No masses, anatomic distortions, external compressions, bronchomalacia, foreign bodies, or hemorrhage were identified. Bronchial mucosa was normal. The bronchoscope was then withdrawn to the carina and then to the larynx noting the same findings as described above.

Upon completion of the procedure, a debriefing checklist was completed to share information critical to the postoperative care of the patient. The patient tolerated the procedure well and was transported to the postanesthesia care unit in stable condition thereafter.

Rigid Bronchoscopy and Foreign Body Removal

74

Carlos Andrés de la Torre Ramos

Indications and Benefits

- Foreign body aspiration.
- Benefits: Achieve a correct oxygenation and ventilation. Avoid risk of fatal asphyxia or further infections and/or airway stenosis.

Risks and Alternatives

- Standard risks, such as bleeding, infection, need for additional procedures, and risks of anesthesia
- Injury to the airway: Tracheal wall injury leading to pneumothorax and/or cervical subcutaneous emphysema
- Foreign body blockage at the level of the subglottic space and need of an emergency tracheostomy
- Alternatives: Open thoracotomy or cervicotomy for an open-airway surgery

Essential Steps

1. Patient under total anesthesia and fully relaxed. Supine position and slight neck hyperextension
2. Teeth protection placement
3. Direct laryngoscopy with adequate size laryngoscope. Inspection of oral cavity, pharynx, and supraglottic space
4. Intubation with a rigid bronchoscope according to the patient's age with a rod-lens telescope attached to the bronchoscope
5. Connection of the ventilation system through the side port of the bronchoscope
6. Airway inspection of the trachea down to the basal bronchi
7. Aspiration of secretions
8. Extraction of foreign body with forceps
9. Exploration of the airway distally looking for further ones

Subsection 2

1. If foreign body is distally to the carina, a rod-lens telescope longer than the rigid bronchoscope will be needed.
2. Extraction forceps could be either optical forceps mounted on a straightforward telescope or single forceps can be inserted inside the bronchoscope in parallel to the rod-lens telescope.

Note These Variations

- Some authors advocate for flexible bronchoscopy for foreign body removal. The patient is

C. A. de la Torre Ramos (✉)
University Hospital La Paz, Pediatric Surgery, Madrid, Spain

D. J. Papandria et al. (eds.), *Operative Dictations in Pediatric Surgery*, https://doi.org/10.1007/978-3-030-24212-1_74

under spontaneous ventilation. The foreign body extraction is done with a forceps or basket grasping forceps inserted through the working channel. With this technique, the airway is not secured. Also, the forceps fitting in the working channel are smaller than the ones that could be used with a rigid bronchoscope. This technique should not be performed in unstable patients.

Template Operative Dictation (Endoscopic)

Preoperative Diagnosis Foreign body in right main bronchus

Postoperative Diagnosis Same as preoperative diagnosis

Findings Foreign body in the *right mainstem bronchus/___*

Procedure(s) Performed Rigid bronchoscopy and foreign body removal

Anesthesia *General*

Specimen Foreign body: *nut/seed/___*

Estimated Blood Loss __ml

Indications This is a/an __-*day/week/month/year*-old *male/female* presented with clinical suspicion of foreign body aspiration. He/she was deemed to be a suitable candidate for rigid bronchoscopy and foreign body removal.

Procedure in Detail Following satisfactory induction of anesthesia, the patient was placed in supine position with slight neck hyperextension and appropriately padded. Time-outs were performed using both preinduction and preincision safety checklists with participation of all present in the operative suite. These confirmed the correct patient, procedure, operative site, and additional critical information prior to the start of the procedure. The teeth protector was placed. Once the patient was fully sedated and relaxed, a direct laryngoscopy was performed. Oral cavity, pharynx, and supraglottic space were inspected. No foreign body was identified. Under direct visualization, a __ size bronchoscope with a 0° rod-lens telescope was then used to intubate the patient. The ventilator was connected to the side port of the bronchoscope. The trachea from the subglottic space to the carina was inspected and appeared normal. A foreign body and some dense secretions were then identified in the *right mainstem bronchus/___*. A rubber suction catheter was introduced through the working channel of the bronchoscope to aspirate secretions. This maneuver was done carefully to avoid distal displacement of the foreign body. The optic was then removed and an optical forceps mounted on a straightforward telescope was inserted through the bronchoscope. The foreign body was grasped with the forceps.

[Choose One:]

If the size of the foreign body is larger than the bronchoscope lumen: We carefully removed with gentle movements the bronchoscope as well as the optic forceps with the foreign body firmly grasped to avoid loosing it during extraction. Special attention was paid at the level of the subglottic space and the vocal cords area. Once the foreign body was removed, the patient was reintubated to reexplore the airway. We used the same rigid bronchoscope following the protocols as described above.

If the size of the foreign body is smaller than the bronchoscope lumen: The optic forceps grasping the foreign body was removed through the bronchoscope.

The optic was then reinserted to explore the airway. Right and left mainstem, lobar, and segmental bronchi were inspected with no evidence of more foreign bodies. The bronchoscope was removed. The anesthesiologist assumed control over the airway. Upon completion of the procedure, a debriefing checklist was completed to share information critical to the postoperative care of the patient. The patient tolerated the procedure well and was transported to the postanesthesia care unit in stable condition thereafter.

75 Tube Thoracostomy

Carlos Andrés de la Torre Ramos

Indications and Benefits

- Pneumothorax: Spontaneous, traumatic, iatrogenic, and following thoracic procedures
- Hemothorax
- Pleural effusion: transudative, empyema, parapneumonic
- Chylothorax: idiopathic, congenital, secondary
- Benefits: Helps to maintain an optimal ventilation and oxygenation. To drain fluids

Risks and Alternatives

- Standard risks, such as bleeding, infection, need for additional procedures, and risks of anesthesia
- Injury to structures: Intercostal vessels, lung, heart, mediastinum, diaphragm, or subdiaphragm structures
- Alternatives: Thoracoscopy or thoracotomy approaches

Essential Steps

1. Supine position, abduction of the arm and flexion of the elbow.
2. Choose between fourth or fifth intercostal space, anterior or midaxillary line (based on imaging).
3. Skin incision one intercostal space below to the initial selected space.
4. Create subcutaneous tunnel toward the initial selected intercostal space.
5. Enter the pleural space with a mosquito or a Kelly clamp.
6. Spread gently the intercostal muscles.
7. Introduce tube with a trocar or holding the tip with a Kelly clamp through the tunnel created.
8. Push the tube in until all the holes are within 2 cm or 1 inch inside the pleural space.
9. Connect to water seal.
10. Fix to skin with stitch.

Note These Variations

- Seldinger technique: Chest tube placed over a guidewire. Same position of the patient and same intercostal space. Good for drain air and nonviscous fluid. Useful to place at bedside outside the operating room.
- Needle thoracostomy: Indicated in emergency situations. Patient unstable with suspected tension pneumothorax. Supine position. Through second or third intercostal space at midclavicular line. Following the improvement of the patient, proper thoracostomy tube must be placed as described above.

C. A. de la Torre Ramos (✉)
University Hospital La Paz, Pediatric Surgery, Madrid, Spain

D. J. Papandria et al. (eds.), *Operative Dictations in Pediatric Surgery*,
https://doi.org/10.1007/978-3-030-24212-1_75

Template Operative Dictation (Open)

Preoperative Diagnosis Hydropneumothorax

Postoperative Diagnosis Same as preoperative diagnosis

Findings Hydropneumothorax

Procedure(s) Performed Tube thoracostomy

Anesthesia *Preferable sedation and local anesthesia in all children. Adolescents can be performed under local anesthesia only.*

Specimen Sample of liquid for biochemistry and culture

Drains ____ Fr. thoracostomy tube

Estimated Blood Loss ____ml

Indications This is a/an ___ -day/week/month/year-old male/female presented with *right/left* hydropneumothorax. He/she was deemed to be a suitable candidate for tube thoracostomy.

Procedure in Detail Following satisfactory induction of anesthesia, the patient was placed in supine position with abduction of the arm and flexion of the elbow over the head and appropriately padded. Time-outs were performed using both preinduction and preincision safety checklists with participation of all present in the operative suite. These confirmed the correct patient, procedure, operative site, and additional critical information prior to the start of the procedure. The *right/left* hemithorax was then prepped and draped in the usual sterile fashion. A ___ needle was used to infiltrate ___ ml of local anesthesia with mepivacaine 2% prior to the skin incision. A 1-cm skin incision using a Nº 11 or 15 blade was performed at the level of the sixth right intercostal space on the midaxillary line. With a Kelly clamp, subcutaneous dissection toward fifth intercostal space was performed. The upper edge of the inferior rib in the fifth intercostal space was identified.

[Choose One:]

If the chest tube has no trocar attached: The parietal pleura was entered carefully holding the handle with the right hand and left hand firmly close to the tip. Open the Kelly clamp to spread gently the intercostal muscles and parietal pleura. A ___Fr. tube was selected based on the patient age and size. The distal part of the tube was clamped with a mosquito. The Kelly was then used to hold the tube tip and introduce it through the tunnel previously done.

If the chest tube has a trocar attached: The pleural space was entered using the tube trocar in a controlled manner through the tunnel we previously performed.

Once inside the pleural space, the tube was pushed until all the tube holes were inside the pleural space at least 2 cm (or 1 inch).

[Choose One:]

If pneumothorax: Direct the tube anteriorly to the upper part of the pleural cavity.

If hemothorax or pleural effusion: Direct the tube posteriorly.

Fluid samples were obtained to be sent to biochemistry and microbiology. The tube was unclamped and connected to the water seal system device. A 3/0 silk was used to perform a purse-string stitch to fix the tube to the skin.

Upon completion of the procedure, a debriefing checklist was completed to share information critical to the postoperative care of the patient. The patient tolerated the procedure well, *was awaken in the operating room,* and was transported to the postanesthesia care unit in stable condition thereafter.

76 Pulmonary Bleb Resection and Pleurodesis (Open and MIS Approaches)

Ekene A. Onwuka and Christopher K. Breuer

Indications and Benefits

- Persistent pneumothorax or air leak for 3–5 days following chest tube or pigtail placement
- Recurrent pneumothorax following initial episode treated with air evacuation
- Recurrent spontaneous pneumothorax in patients with underlying lung diseases with high propensity for developing pneumothoraces (such as cystic fibrosis), or initial pneumothorax in those with underlying disease that is severe or progressive
- Benefits: Low recurrence rate.

Risks and Alternatives

- Standard risks (bleeding, infection, need for additional procedures, risks of anesthesia).
- Injury to adjacent structures (pulmonary artery, pulmonary vein, intercostal bundle, aorta, diaphragm, liver, spleen).
- Respiratory failure secondary to chemical pleurodesis (particularly with talc).
- Arrhythmias, cardiac arrest, chest pain, and hypotension following chemical pleurodesis.
- Systemic inflammatory reaction following chemical pleurodesis.
- Patients with chronic progressive pulmonary diseases, such as cystic fibrosis, may require additional thoracic procedures over their lifetime, including lung transplant, which will be significantly more difficult after pleurodesis.
- Alternatives: Tube thoracostomy with chemical pleurodesis via tube, endobronchial valve placement.

Essential Steps

1. Lung isolation by anesthesia (either via double-lumen endotracheal tube or endoscopically placed bronchial blocker)
2. Safe entry into thoracic cavity (either via thoracotomy incision for open or thoracoscopic port sites for VATS)
3. Careful evaluation of the lung for bullous disease
4. Resection of bullae with Endo GIA staple loads
5. Mechanical or chemical (or both) pleurodesis
6. Chest tube placement
7. Closure

E. A. Onwuka
The Ohio State University Wexner Medical Center, Department of General Surgery, Columbus, OH, USA
e-mail: ekene.onwuka@osumc.edu

C. K. Breuer (✉)
Nationwide Children's Hospital, Department of Pediatric Surgery, Columbus, OH, USA
e-mail: christopher.breuer@nationwidechildrens.org

D. J. Papandria et al. (eds.), *Operative Dictations in Pediatric Surgery*,
https://doi.org/10.1007/978-3-030-24212-1_76

Note These Variations

- Bleb resection plus mechanical pleurodesis
- Bleb resection plus chemical pleurodesis

Template Operative Dictation (Open)

Preoperative Diagnosis *Right/left* spontaneous pneumothorax, bleb disease

Postoperative Diagnosis Same as preoperative diagnosis

Findings ___

Procedure(s) Performed *Right/left* thoracotomy, wedge resection of *right/left upper/middle/lower* lobe bleb, *mechanical/chemical* pleurodesis

Anesthesia General

Specimen *Right/left upper/middle/lower* wedge resection

Drains ___Fr Argyle chest tube

Implants None

Estimated Blood Loss ___

Indications This is a/an ___*-day/week/month/year*-old *male/female* with *left/right persistent/recurrent* spontaneous pneumothorax. *He/she* was deemed to be a suitable candidate for thoracotomy, blebectomy, and *mechanical/chemical* pleurodesis.

Procedure in Detail Following satisfactory induction of anesthesia, the patient was placed in the *right/left* lateral decubitus position and appropriately supported with a bean bag. *His/her* arms and legs were appropriately oriented and pressure points padded. Time-outs were performed using both preinduction and preincision safety checklists with participation of all present in the operative suite. These confirmed the correct patient, procedure, operative site, and additional critical information prior to the start of the procedure. Perioperative antibiotics were administered and the *right/left* chest was then prepped and draped in the usual sterile fashion. The lung on the operative side was then isolated by anesthesia with the use of *a ___Fr dual-lumen endotracheal tube/endoscopically deployed bronchial blocker*.

The skin was incised with a #15 scalpel from the anterior axillary line to the posterior axillary line, just inferior to the scapula. The subcutaneous layer was divided with the Bovie electrocautery. The latissimus dorsi muscle was then divided. The serratus anterior muscle was preserved. We entered the *right/left* thorax at the level of the *fourth/fifth/sixth* intercostal space. We then divided the *fourth/fifth/sixth* rib posteriorly with a linear bone cutter. A rib spreader was placed in the incision for exposure. The thoracic cavity was inspected to ensure there were no entry injuries.

The lung was grasped with ringed forceps to rotate the various lobes for complete visualization. Special care was taken to thoroughly inspect the lung apices. A bleb was identified at the ___ of the *superior/middle/lower* lobe. The bleb was surgically resected using ___ applications of the Endo GIA stapler *purple/black* load. The specimen was removed and sent for permanent histology.

[Choose One:]
If mechanical pleurodesis is performed: Next a mechanical pleurodesis was performed. The parietal pleura was mechanically excoriated using a Bovie scratch pad. The scratch pad was grasped with a ringed forceps and rubbed against the chest wall, from the apex to the base of the thoracic cavity. There was a small amount of bleeding, which was controlled with cautery in several areas.

If chemical pleurodesis is performed: Next a chemical pleurodesis was performed. ___*mg of doxycycline/tetracycline/fibrin glue/a talc powder slurry* was instilled into the thoracic cavity.

A ___ Fr chest tube was placed in the eighth intercostal space and secured with a ___ suture. The right lung was then reexpanded under direct vision. The thoracotomy incision was closed in multiple layers. A total of ___ intercostal #1 vicryl sutures were placed to reapproximate the ___ and ___ ribs. The serratus anterior and latissimus dorsi muscle layers were reapproximated with a running ___ vicryl suture. The adipose tissue layer was reapproximated with a *running/interrupted* ___ vicryl suture. The skin was reapproximated with a running ___ vicryl suture. A sterile dressing was placed on the incision.

Upon completion of the procedure, a debriefing checklist was completed to share information critical to the postoperative care of the patient. The patient tolerated the procedure well, *was extubated in the operating room*, and was transported to the postanesthesia care unit in stable condition thereafter. Surgical counts were correct × ___.

Template Operative Dictation (Thoracoscopic)

Preoperative Diagnosis *Right/left* spontaneous pneumothorax, bleb disease

Postoperative Diagnosis Same as preoperative diagnosis

Findings ___

Procedure(s) Performed Video-assisted thoracoscopic surgery (VATS), wedge resection of *right/left upper/middle/lower* lobe bleb, *mechanical/chemical* pleurodesis

Anesthesia General

Specimen *Right/left upper/middle/lower* wedge resection

Drains ___Fr Argyle chest tube

Implants None

Estimated Blood Loss ___

Indications This is a/an ___*-day/week/month/year*-old *male/female* with a *left/right persistent/recurrent* spontaneous pneumothorax. *He/she* was deemed to be a suitable candidate for thoracoscopic blebectomy and *mechanical/chemical* pleurodesis.

Procedure in Detail Following satisfactory induction of anesthesia, the patient was placed in the *right/left* lateral decubitus position and appropriately supported with a bean bag. *His/her* arms and legs were appropriately oriented and pressure points padded. Time-outs were performed using both preinduction and preincision safety checklists with participation of all present in the operative suite. These confirmed the correct patient, procedure, operative site, and additional critical information prior to the start of the procedure. Perioperative antibiotics were administered and the *right/left* chest was then prepped and draped in the usual sterile fashion. The lung on the operative side was then isolated by anesthesia with the use of *a ___Fr dual-lumen endotracheal tube/endoscopically deployed bronchial blocker*.

A/an ___-mm incision was placed at the level of the *seventh/eight* interspace in the *mid/posterior* axillary line and carried down to the fascia and over the rib using blunt dissection with a hemostat. The pleural space was entered, a/an ___-mm trocar was placed and CO_2 insufflation initiated to a pressure of 8 mmHg. The thoracoscope was introduced into the chest and a cursory survey of the thoracic contents revealed no traumatic sequelae of access and confirmation of collapse of the operative lung. Local anesthetic infiltration and stab incisions were then placed at ___ additional trocar sites, followed by ___-mm trocars located in the ___ interspace in the ___ line. Trocars were introduced under thoracoscopic vision.

The pleural cavity was explored and the lung was grasped with ringed forceps to rotate the various lobes for complete visualization. Special care was taken to thoroughly inspect the lung apices. A bleb was identified at the ___ of the *superior/middle/lower* lobe. The bleb was surgically resected using ___ applications of the Endo GIA stapler, *purple/black* load. The specimen was removed from the anterior thoracoscopic port and sent for permanent histology.

[Choose One:]

If mechanical pleurodesis is performed: Next a mechanical pleurodesis was performed. The parietal pleura was mechanically excoriated using a Bovie scratch pad throughout the chest. The scratch pad was grasped with a ringed forceps and rubbed against the chest wall, from the apex to the base of the thoracic cavity. There was a small amount of bleeding, which was controlled with cautery in several areas.

If chemical pleurodesis is performed: Next a chemical pleurodesis was performed. ___*mg of doxycycline/tetracycline/fibrin glue/a talc powder slurry* was instilled into the thoracic cavity.

A ___Fr chest tube was placed through the ___ port and, under direct visualization, directed toward the apex. At this point, all trocars were removed under vision and sites were noted to be hemostatic. The lung was then slowly reinflated by anesthesia and thoracoscopy was terminated. The chest tube was secured to the skin using ___ and hooked to a Pleur-evac. The port sites were closed at the fascia using *running/interrupted* ___ vicryl and the skin at all port sites closed with ___. All sites were then dressed with Steri-Strips.

Upon completion of the procedure, a debriefing checklist was completed to share information critical to the postoperative care of the patient. The patient tolerated the procedure well, *was extubated in the operating room*, and was transported to the postanesthesia care unit in stable condition thereafter. Surgical counts were correct × ___.

Pectus Excavatum Repair (Open and MIS Approaches)

77

Kate Savoie and Brian D. Kenney

Indications and Benefits

- Pectus excavatum with two or more of the following criteria:
  - Progressive or symptomatic
  - Restrictive lung disease evident on pulmonary function tests
  - Cardiac compression or displacement on CT
  - Haller index >3.25
  - Cardiac abnormalities (i.e., mitral valve prolapse, bundle branch block)
  - Recurrence after previous repair
- Benefits: Potentially improved lung capacity, correction of obvious deformity, correct placement of heart within the mediastinum

Risk and Alternatives

- Risks: Pneumothorax, infection, pneumonia, wound dehiscence, cardiac injury, sternal nonunion (open)
- Alternatives: Vacuum bell (potentially no lasting benefit)

K. Savoie (✉) · B. D. Kenney
Nationwide Children's Hospital, Department of Pediatric Surgery, Columbus, OH, USA
e-mail: Kate.savoie@nationwidechildrens.org; Brian.Kenney@nationwidechildrens.org

Essential Steps

Minimally Invasive Approach

1. Mark the extent of the defect on the chest wall.
2. Two transverse lateral incisions to level of muscle fascia placed at the location of maximum excursion.
3. Develop subcutaneous pockets laterally to medially from incisions to point of maximal excursion.
4. Develop lateral subcutaneous pockets to hold ends of pectus bar.
5. Introduce trocar into chest cavity bilaterally; inspect thoracic cavity and confirm pneumothorax.
6. Introduce lower anterior chest wall trocar bilaterally under direct vision; remove the lateral trocars.
7. Bluntly enter thoracic cavity at point of maximum excursion.
8. Develop substernal space.
9. Place the tunneling device into subcutaneous tunnel; visualize passage of the tunneling device across mediastinum and into left chest.
10. Pass the tunneling device through left chest wall and into subcutaneous pocket.
11. Attach pectus bar to the tunneling and visualize passage across the mediastinum.
12. Once in place, flip pectus bar into position.
13. Confirm hemostasis.
14. Secure to chest wall.
15. Close muscle and subcutaneous tissues over bar struts.
16. Remove pneumothorax.
17. Close trocar port.

D. J. Papandria et al. (eds.), *Operative Dictations in Pediatric Surgery*,
https://doi.org/10.1007/978-3-030-24212-1_77

Open Approach

1. Transverse incision inferior to and in between nipples.
2. Create myocutaneous flaps from Angle of Louis to xiphoid process.
3. Elevate pectoralis muscles off of sternum to expose deformed cartilages from chondrosternal joint to costochondral junction.
4. Incise periosteum over cartilaginous portion of involved ribs.
5. Remove cartilaginous portion of involved ribs.
6. Develop substernal plane.
7. Perform wedge osteostomy/osteomoties where sternum reflects posteriorly.
8. Pull sternum into correct position.
9. Pass sternal bar behind sternum and bend to fit chest wall.
10. Close the osteotomy.
11. Secure bar in place.
12. Reapproximate muscles, securing to sternal periosteum.
13. Close subcutaneous tissues and skin.

Notes These Variations

- For the minimally invasive approach: A single thoracic port can be introduced into the right thoracic cavity, rather than the bilateral approach. The bilateral approach aids in visualization of the bar crossing the mediastinum.
- For the minimally invasive approach: A third incision can be made over the xiphoid process to aid in sternal elevation and/or substernal dissection.
- For the open approach: Instead of a horizontal incision a 7-cm vertical incision and placement of a wound protector/retractor has been described.
- For the open approach: A drain can be left at the surgeons discretion.
- Some patients require multiple bars to correct the deformity. This may require separate incisions for placement of the additional bars.

Template Operative Dictation (Minimally Invasive Approach)

Preoperative Diagnosis Pectus excavatum

Postoperative Diagnosis Same as preoperative diagnosis

Findings Same as postoperative diagnosis

Anesthesia *General/regional/procedural sedation*

Specimen None

Drains {Drains}

Implants ____ cm *performed/ modified* pectus bar

Estimated Blood Loss ____

Indications This is *a/an* ___-year-old *male/ female* with pectus excavatum. He/she was deemed to be a suitable candidate for a Nuss procedure to correct this.

Procedure in Detail Following satisfactory induction of anesthesia, the patient was placed in a supine position with gel rolls on either side of the spine. The arms were left in an untucked position and appropriately padded. Time-outs were performed using both preinduction and preincision safety checklists with participation of all present in the operative suite. These confirmed the correct patient, procedure, operative site, and additional critical information prior to the start of the procedure. The chest was then prepped and draped in the usual sterile fashion.

The extent of the deformity was marked on the chest wall and the point of maximum excursion identified. A __-cm incision was then made on the lateral chest wall bilaterally at the level of maximum excursion. The dissection was carried down through the subcutaneous tissues to the level of the pectoralis fascia. A subcutaneous tunnel was then created along the anterior chest wall, tunneling anterior to the apex of the deformity.

The thoracic cavity was then entered with a __-mm blunt trocar bilaterally and the pleural cavity visualized. The mediastinum was readily visualized. A __-mm trocar was then placed in the most anterior portion of the lower chest wall. The thoracoscope was moved to this trocar and the previous trocars removed. A second thoracoscope was then placed into the left pleural cavity to allow for simultaneous visualization for the remainder of the procedure. A clamp was then introduced through the previous subcutaneous tunnel on the right side and passed bluntly into the thoracic cavity at the apex of the defect under direct visualization. The pericardium was then bluntly dissected away from the sternum.

The clamp was removed and a pectus bar passing device passed through the tunnel under direct visualization. This was then advanced under the sternal defect into the left chest and then out of the left anterior chest wall, entering the previously made subcutaneous tunnel, and then through the left chest wall incision.

An umbilical tape is then secured to the tunneling device and passed through a 34-French chest tube. The chest tube is then pulled through the tunnel. At this time, the pectus bar is bent into correct conformation for the deformity and then secured to the umbilical tape on the left side of the patient. The end of the bar is placed into the chest tube. The chest tube and umbilical tape is then pulled from the right side of the body to move the bar into correct position while protecting the mediastinum.

Once the bar was in place, it was flipped into position. The bar was then anchored bilaterally in three locations with ___ (long-lasting/absorbable) sutures under thoracoscopic visualization by completely encircling the rib. The muscle was then imbricated over the bar at each incision site using __ vicryl suture. The subcutaneous tissue was closed with a *running/interrupted* __-0 vicryl stitch. The skin was closed with a ___-0 *monocryl/vicryl*. The wounds were dressed with *Dermabond/Steri-Strips and gauze*. The pneumothorax was released with a red rubber tube placed through the anterior trocar under water seal. An on-table chest X-ray confirmed no obvious pneumothorax. All trocars were withdrawn and the incisions closed and dressed.

All counts were correct at the end of the case and the attending of record was present and scrubbed for *all/key* portions of the case.

Upon completion of the procedure, a debriefing checklist was completed to share information critical to the postoperative care of the patient. The patient tolerated the procedure well, *was extubated in the operating room*, and was transported to the postanesthesia care unit in stable condition. A postextubation chest X-ray was obtained and *no/a small/a large* pneumothorax identified. *The pneumothorax was observed with serial chest X-rays/ treated with tube thoracostomy.*

Template Operative Dictation (Open Approach)

Preoperative Diagnosis Pectus excavatum

Postoperative Diagnosis Same as **p**reoperative diagnosis

Findings Same as postoperative diagnosis

Anesthesia General

Specimen None

Drains {Drains}

Implants ___ cm *preformed/modifiable* pectus bar

Estimated Blood Loss ____

Indications This is a/an ___-year-*old male/ female* with pectus excavatum. He/she was evaluated and deemed to be a suitable candidate for an open Nuss procedure.

Procedure in Detail Following satisfactory induction of anesthesia, the patient was placed in a supine position with gel rolls on either side of the spine. The arms were then tucked and appropriately padded. Time-outs were performed using both preinduction and preincision safety checklists with participation of all present in the operative suite. These confirmed the correct patient, procedure, operative site, and additional critical information prior to the start of the procedure. The chest was then prepped and draped in the usual sterile fashion.

A transverse incision was placed ___ *cm below the nipple line/at the fourth intercostal space/within the projected inframammary fold.* Dissection was carried down to the pectoralis muscles and skin flaps mobilized bilaterally with electrocautery from the Angle of Louis to the xiphoid process. The pectoralis muscles in their entirety were then bluntly dissected off of the sternum starting at the free area just anterior to the chondrosternal junction. As the dissection continued, the pectoralis minor and serratus anterior were also reflected in continuity to the muscle flap until costochondral junction of the third to fifth ribs were identified. The periosteum was incised in an H-type incision and periosteal elevators were then used to remove the cartilaginous portions of the ___ to ___ ribs. The xiphoid process was then excised and substernal blunt dissection performed. The posterior angulation of the sternum was identified and osteotomies performed to remove a wedge of sternum at this level. The sternum was then mobilized anteriorly to the correct position. A pectus bar was then placed under the sternum, with the struts located below the myocutaneous flaps. The osteotomy was closed with a ___-0 vicryl. The bar was shaped to the anterior chest wall. Hemostasis was achieved and the muscles reapproximated and secured to the sternum with a ___-0 vicryl suture. The subcutaneous space was closed with *interrupted/running* ___-0 vicryl and the skin reapproximated with ___-0 *monocryl/vicryl.* The incision was cleaned and dried, after which *Dermabond/Steri-Strips and gauze* were applied.

All counts were correct at the end of the case and the attending of record was present and scrubbed for *all/key* portions of the case.

Upon completion of the procedure, a debriefing checklist was completed to share information critical to the postoperative care of the patient. The patient tolerated the procedure well, *was extubated in the operating room*, and was transported to the postanesthesia care unit in stable condition.

Ravitch Procedure (Open Approach for Chest Wall Deformities)

78

Carlos Andrés de la Torre Ramos

Indications and Benefits

- Pectus excavatum
- Pectus carinatum
- Pectus arquatum (Currarino–Silverman syndrome)
- Mixed chest wall deformities

Risks and Alternatives

- Standard risks (bleeding, infection, need for additional procedures, risks of anesthesia)
- Injury to adjacent structures (heart, lung, diaphragm). Pneumothorax, pericardial effusion
- Unaesthetic results: Hypertrophic scar, recidive
- Overcorrection
- Chest wall constriction
- Alternatives: Nuss procedure or conservative treatment for pectus excavatum. Abramson technique or bracing therapy for pectus carinatum

Essential Steps

1. *Vertical midsternum or bilateral submammary* skin incision. Subcutaneous dissection until the pectoralis fascia is identified.
2. Detachment of the pectoralis major muscle and rectus abdominis off from anterior chest wall.
3. Exposure of costal cartilages, sternum, and xiphoid.
4. Longitudinal incision on the anterior aspect of the perichondrium from third to seventh costal cartilage bilaterally.
5. Bilateral subperichondrial resection of malformed costal cartilages using a periostotome.
6. *Transverse or oblique* outer table sternotomy with oscillating saw at the sternal–manubrial junction *(sternotomy location sometimes depends on the subtype deformity).*
7. Inner sternal table fracture and manual correction of the malformation.
8. Fixation of the corrected sternum at the level of the fracture with an absorbable *osteosynthesis mesh, wires, or nonabsorbable plates.*
9. The xiphoid is then resected *if needed* to achieve a better esthetic result.
10. Check for pleural injury using saline on the surgical field and Valsalva maneuver.
11. Closure of the perichondrial sheath with running absorbable suture.
12. Redon-type drain on the surgical bed.
13. Reinsertion of pectoralis and rectus muscles to the sternum.
14. Closure of subcutaneous layer and skin.

C. A. de la Torre Ramos (✉)
University Hospital La Paz, Pediatric Surgery, Madrid, Spain

D. J. Papandria et al. (eds.), *Operative Dictations in Pediatric Surgery*,
https://doi.org/10.1007/978-3-030-24212-1_78

Template Operative Dictation

Preoperative Diagnosis Pectus carinatum not suitable for bracing or minimal invasive technique.

Postoperative Diagnosis Pectus carinatum

Findings Same as postoperative diagnosis

Procedure Performed Ravitch procedure

Anesthesia *General*

Specimen Abnormal costal cartilages and xiphoid process

Drains Redon-type drain on the surgical bed

Implants Absorbable osteosynthesis mesh

Estimated Blood Loss ____ ml

Indications This is a/an ___-day/week/month/year-old male/female with pectus carinatum. He/she was deemed to be a suitable candidate for Ravitch procedure.

Procedure in Detail Following satisfactory induction of anesthesia, the patient was placed in supine position with arms adducted and appropriately padded. Time-outs were performed using both preinduction and preincision safety checklists with participation of all present in the operative suite. These confirmed the correct patient, procedure, operative site, and additional critical information prior to the start of the procedure. The thorax was then prepped and draped in the usual sterile fashion. A *vertical midsternal skin incision/bilateral submammary* skin incision was performed. A subcutaneous dissection was begun until the pectoralis major fascia is reached. The pectoralis major muscles are dissected free and elevated from their sternal and inferior rib insertions with electrocautery bilaterally. The rectus abdominis muscles are also dissected off from their attachment to the sternum upon the malformation was exposed. Costal cartilages from third to seventh were abnormal and the sternal bone presented a severe protrusion from the manubriosternal junction. Longitudinal incisions over the perichondrium with electrocautery were performed bilaterally from the third to the seventh rib. Once the perichondrium was opened and the cartilages exposed, a subperichondrial dissection with a periostotome was performed.

[Choose One:]
If the patient presents a mild costal cartilage deformity: The malformed costal cartilages are only partially resected to achieve mobilization of the sternum.

***If the patient presents a severe costal cartilage deformity*:** All the malformed costal cartilages are fully resected to achieve mobilization of the sternum and good cosmetic result.

Once the cartilages were resected and the sternum was released, a sternotomy was performed using an oscillating saw.

[Choose One:]
If the sternal deformity is symmetric: A transverse sternotomy of the outer sternal table was performed at the level of the manubriosternal junction.

If the sternal malformation is asymmetric and the sternum is rotated: An oblique sternotomy following the angulation of the malformation was performed. This way allows correction of the sternal elevation and derotation at the same time.

The inner table of the sternum remained untouched. With manual manipulation, the inner table was fractured in a controlled manner and the malformation was then corrected. The sternum was fixed in the corrected position at the level of the fracture with *absorbable osteosynthesis mesh, absorbable plates, or wires.*

[Choose One:]
If the xiphoid is malformed: The xiphoid was also malformed. It was resected with electrocautery to achieve a better cosmetic result.

If the xiphoid is normal: The xiphoid appeared normal and was left in place.

Pleural integrity was checked instilling saline in the surgical field and asking the anesthesiologist for Valsalva maneuvers. No air leaks were noted. Hemostasis was checked. The previously incised perichondrium sheaths were closed with 4/0 running absorbable sutures. A ___Fr Redon drain was left on the surgical field. The drain was fixed to the skin with a purse-string 3/0 silk suture.

Pectoralis muscles and rectus abdominis were refixed to the sternum and ribs. Subcutaneous tissue was closed with running 4/0 absorbable suture. Skin was closed with running subcuticular suture. A compressive dressing was applied.

Upon completion of the procedure, a debriefing checklist was completed to share information critical to the postoperative care of the patient. The patient tolerated the procedure well, *was extubated in the operating room*, and was transported to the postanesthesia care unit in stable condition thereafter.

Repair of Pectus Carinatum

79

Kate Savoie and Brian D. Kenney

Indications and Benefits

- Pectus carinatum failing bracing therapy
- Pectus carinatum with severe asymmetry

Risk and Alternatives

- Risks: Pneumothorax, infection, pneumonia, wound dehiscence, cardiac injury, sternal non-union (open), sternal necrosis
- Alternatives: Bracing (standard therapy)

Essential Steps

1. Transverse incision inferior to and in between nipples.
2. Create myocutaneous flaps from angle of Louis to xiphoid process.
3. Elevate pectoralis muscles off of sternum to expose deformed cartilages from chondro-sternal joint to costochondral junction.
4. Incise periosteum over cartilaginous portion of involved ribs.
5. Remove cartilaginous portion of involved ribs.
6. Perform osteotomy.
7. Fashion and place piece of removed cartilage into osteotomy to maintain correct positioning of sternum.
8. Perform sternal plating.
9. Plicate perichondrial sheets.
10. Reapproximate muscles.
11. Close subcutaneous tissues and skin.

K. Savoie (✉) · B. D. Kenney
Nationwide Children's Hospital, Department of Pediatric Surgery, Columbus, OH, USA
e-mail: Kate.savoie@nationwidechildrens.org; Brian.Kenney@nationwidechildrens.org

Notes These Variations

- A minimally invasive technique similar to the minimally invasive pectus excavatum repair exists; however, with this method the bar stays anterior to the sternum and compresses the defect down. A modification of this technique called the "sandwich technique" includes a substernal stabilization bar in addition to the external compression bar.
- A drain can be left at the surgeons discretion.

Template Operative Dictation (Open Approach)

Preoperative Diagnosis Pectus carinatum

Postoperative Diagnosis Same as preoperative diagnosis

Findings Same as postoperative diagnosis

D. J. Papandria et al. (eds.), *Operative Dictations in Pediatric Surgery*,
https://doi.org/10.1007/978-3-030-24212-1_79

Anesthesia General

Specimen None

Drains {Drains}

Implants None

Estimated Blood Loss ____

Indications This is a/an ___-year-old *male/female* with pectus carinatum. He/she was evaluated and deemed to be a suitable candidate for an open repair of *his/her* pectus carinatum.

Procedure in Detail Following satisfactory induction of anesthesia, the patient was placed in a supine position. The arms were then tucked and appropriately padded. Time-outs were performed using both preinduction and preincision safety checklists with participation of all present in the operative suite. These confirmed the correct patient, procedure, operative site, and additional critical information prior to the start of the procedure. The chest was then prepped and draped in the usual sterile fashion.

A transverse incision was placed ___ *cm below the nipple line/within the projected inframammary fold.* Dissection was carried down to the pectoralis muscles and myocutaneous flaps mobilized bilaterally with electrocautery from the Angle of Louis to the xiphoid process. The pectoralis muscles in their entirety were then bluntly dissected off the sternum starting at the free area just anterior to the chondrosternal junction. As the dissection continued, the pectoralis minor and serratus anterior were also reflected in continuity to the muscle flap until costochondral junction of the third to fifth rib were identified. The periosteum is incised in an H-type incision and periosteal elevators were then used to remove the cartilaginous portions of the ___ to ___ ribs.

A substernal blunt dissection performed *after excision of the xiphoid process.* The posterior angulation of the sternum was identified and osteotomies performed to remove a wedge of sternum at this level. A sternal plate was then placed at the level of the ostomy for stabilization and fixated to the periosteum with ___-0 vicryl sutures. The perichondrial sheets were then plicated with ___-0 vicryl sutures in an interrupted fashion. The muscles were then reapproximated with ____-0 *interrupted/running* vicryl sutures.

The subcutaneous space was closed with *interrupted/running* ___-0 vicryl and the skin reapproximated with ___-0 *monocryl/vicryl.* The incision was cleaned and dried, after which *Dermabond/Steri-Strips and gauze* were applied.

All counts were correct at the end of the case and the attending of record was present and scrubbed for *all/key* portions of the case.

Upon completion of the procedure, a debriefing checklist was completed to share information critical to the postoperative care of the patient. The patient tolerated the procedure well, *was extubated in the operating room,* and was transported to the postanesthesia care unit in stable condition. A postextubation chest X-ray was obtained and *no/a small/a large* pneumothorax identified. *The pneumothorax was observed with serial chest X-rays/treated with tube thoracostomy.*

Transabdominal Repair of Congenital Diaphragmatic Hernia (Open and MIS Approaches)

80

Dominic J. Papandria and Karen A. Diefenbach

Indications and Benefits

- Congenital diaphragmatic hernia.
- Benefits: Restoration of normal respiratory mechanics, partial correction of pulmonary hypoplasia.

Risks and Alternatives

- Standard risks (bleeding, infection, need for additional procedures, and risks of anesthesia).
- Injury to adjacent structures (lung parenchyma, phrenic nerve, abdominal viscera).
- Recurrence of hernia.
- Chest wall deformity and scoliosis.
- Alternatives: Thoracic approach for repair, delayed repair until further medically optimized.

Essential Steps

1. Patient positioning in modified supine position (bump at costovertebral location on side of hernia).
2. Safe access to the abdomen.
3. Reduction of the abdominal viscera into the abdominal cavity.
4. Assessment of the size of the defect and the need for patch repair.
5. Mobilization of the posterior leaflet of the diaphragm.
6. Closure of the defect.
7. Closure of incision(s).

Note These Variations

- Thoracic approach is most common for minimally invasive technique, while abdominal approach most common for open technique.
- The use of a patch for large defects is common, but patch reinforcement has also been used in primary repairs.
- Not all surgeons leave a drain or chest tube. Considerations include need for drainage of the cavity, the presence of a patch. Care should be taken not to shift the mediastinum with suction applied to the drain.

D. J. Papandria
Department of Surgery, Emory University, Atlanta, GA, USA
e-mail: dominic.papandria@emory.edu

K. A. Diefenbach (✉)
Nationwide Children's Hospital, Columbus, OH, USA
e-mail: Karen.Diefenbach@nationwidechildrens.org

D. J. Papandria et al. (eds.), *Operative Dictations in Pediatric Surgery*,
https://doi.org/10.1007/978-3-030-24212-1_80

Template Operative Dictation (Open)

Preoperative Diagnosis Congenital diaphragmatic hernia.

Postoperative Diagnosis Same as preoperative diagnosis.

Findings Same as postoperative diagnosis.

Procedure(s) Performed *Laparoscopic/open* repair of congenital diaphragmatic hernia, *right/left.*

Anesthesia General.

Specimen None.

Drains *None/__ Fr chesttube/__ Fr Blake.*

Implants *None/polytetrafluoroethylene prosthetic patch.*

Estimated Blood Loss ___.

Indications This is a/an ___*-day/week/month/year*-old *male/female* with a *right/left* congenital diaphragmatic hernia. *He/she* was deemed to be a suitable candidate for *laparoscopic/open* repair of congenital diaphragmatic hernia.

Procedure in Detail Following satisfactory induction of anesthesia, the patient was placed in a modified supine position with a bump under the *right/left* costovertebral angle and appropriately padded. Time-outs were performed using both preinduction and preincision safety checklists with participation of all present in the operative suite. These confirmed the correct patient, procedure, operative site, and additional critical information prior to the start of the procedure. The entire abdomen and inferior aspect of the chest was then prepped and draped in the usual sterile fashion.

[Choose One:]

If laparoscopic (MIS) approach: A/an ___-mm incision was made at the level of the umbilicus being careful to avoid injury to the umbilical vessels. A/an ___-mm port was placed through this incision. Once intra-abdominal placement was verified, the abdomen was insufflated to a pressure of ___ mmHg. Two additional ports were placed under direct vision, a/an ___-mm port in the left lower quadrant lateral to the rectus muscle just below the level of the umbilicus and a/an ___-mm port in the right upper quadrant just to the right of midline.

If open approach: A/an ___-mm subcostal incision was made a fingerbreadth below the *right/left* costal margin. The incision was extended down through the subcutaneous tissue using electrocautery for hemostasis. The fascia and underlying muscle was divided and the peritoneum entered and opened the full length of the incision.

{Continue dictation}.

Inspection of the abdominal cavity was performed and the abdominal viscera including the *small bowel, colon, stomach, liver, and spleen* {choose all that apply} were reduced into the abdominal cavity being careful to avoid injury to these structures. The posterior leaflet of the diaphragm was mobilized using electrocautery for hemostasis. In addition, the pleuroperitoneal attachments were separated using electrocautery along the circumference of the defect. Once this was accomplished, the size of the defect was assessed as well as the laxity of the diaphragm to determine if a primary repair was feasible or if a prosthetic patch was indicated.

[Choose One:]

If primary repair: Based on the size of the defect and the presence of sufficient laxity of the diaphragm to achieve a tension-free repair, a primary repair of the defect was performed. Interrupted ___-0 *Ethibond* sutures were placed from *medial to lateral/lateral to medial* to close the defect. A total of ___ sutures were placed. Care was taken at the posterior–lateral margin of the defect to ensure adequate tissue closure. *This required ___ suture(s) to be placed around the adjacent rib.*

If repair with prosthetic patch: Based on the size of the defect and the absence of adequate diaphragmatic tissue to achieve a primary repair, the defect was closed using a/an ___ cm × ___ cm prosthetic patch of ___ *mm Gortex*. The defect was measured and the patch trimmed to allow for adequate coverage with some residual laxity of the patch. Interrupted ___*-0 Ethibond/*___ *Gortex* suture was used to secure the patch circumferentially. Care was taken at the posterior–lateral margin of the defect to ensure adequate tissue closure. *This required ___ suture(s) to be placed around the adjacent rib.*

{Continue dictation}.

Once the defect was closed, the area was inspected for hemostasis.

[Choose One:]

If laparoscopic approach: The ports were then removed and the fascia closed at all port sites using a ___-0 Vicryl suture. The skin was closed using a ___*-0 Vicryl/monocryl/*___ *suture.*

If open approach: The fascia was closed using interrupted ___-0 Vicryl sutures. The subcutaneous tissue was closed using a running ___-0 Vicryl, and the skin was closed using a running ___*-0 Vicryl/monocryl* subcuticular stitch.

{Continue dictation}.

Dressings were applied to the incision(s). All counts were correct at the end of the procedure. Upon completion of the procedure, a debriefing checklist was completed to share information critical to the postoperative care of the patient. The patient tolerated the procedure well, *was extubated in the operating room*, and was transported to the postanesthesia care unit in stable condition thereafter.

81 Thoracic Repair of Congenital Diaphragmatic Hernia (Open and MIS Approaches)

Dominic J. Papandria and Karen A. Diefenbach

Indications and Benefits

- Congenital diaphragmatic hernia
- Benefits: Restoration of normal respiratory mechanics, partial correction of pulmonary hypoplasia

Risks and Alternatives

- Standard risks (bleeding, infection, need for additional procedures, and risks of anesthesia)
- Injury to adjacent structures (lung parenchyma, phrenic nerve, abdominal viscera)
- Recurrence of hernia
- Chest wall deformity and scoliosis
- Alternatives: Abdominal approach for repair, delayed repair until further medically optimized

Essential Steps

1. Patient positioning: lateral decubitus position (side of hernia up)
2. Safe access to the chest
3. Reduction of the abdominal viscera into the abdominal cavity
4. Assessment of the size of the defect and the need for patch repair
5. Mobilization of the posterior leaflet of the diaphragm
6. Closure of the defect
7. Closure of incision(s)

Note These Variations

- Thoracic approach is most common for minimally invasive technique, while abdominal approach is most common for open technique.
- The use of a patch for large defects is common, but patch reinforcement has also been used in primary repairs.
- Not all surgeons leave a drain or chest tube. Considerations include need for drainage of the cavity, the presence of a patch. Care should be taken not to shift the mediastinum with suction applied to the drain.

D. J. Papandria
Department of Surgery, Emory University, Atlanta, GA, USA
e-mail: dominic.papandria@emory.edu

K. A. Diefenbach (✉)
Nationwide Children's Hospital, Columbus, OH, USA
e-mail: Karen.Diefenbach@nationwidechildrens.org

D. J. Papandria et al. (eds.), *Operative Dictations in Pediatric Surgery*,
https://doi.org/10.1007/978-3-030-24212-1_81

Template Operative Dictation (Open)

Preoperative Diagnosis Congenital diaphragmatic hernia

Postoperative Diagnosis Same as preoperative diagnosis

Findings Same as postoperative diagnosis

Procedure(s) Performed *Thoracoscopic/open* repair of congenital diaphragmatic hernia, *right/left*

Anesthesia General

Specimen None

Drains *None/__ Fr chest tube/__ Fr Blake*

Implants *None/polytetrafluoroethylene prosthetic patch*

Estimated Blood Loss ___

Indications This is a/an ___*-day/week/month/year*-old *male/female* with a *right/left* congenital diaphragmatic hernia. *He/she* was deemed to be a suitable candidate for *thoracoscopic/open* repair of congenital diaphragmatic hernia.

Procedure in Detail Following satisfactory induction of anesthesia, the patient was placed in *right/left* lateral decubitus and appropriately padded. Time-outs were performed using both preinduction and preincision safety checklists with participation of all present in the operative suite. These confirmed the correct patient, procedure, operative site, and additional critical information prior to the start of the procedure. The *right/left* chest and axilla were then prepped and draped in the usual sterile fashion and the lung isolated on the operative side by anesthesia.

[Choose One:]
If thoracoscopic (MIS) approach: A/an ___-mm incision was made in the anterior axillary line at the level of the tip of the scapula. Blunt dissection was used to enter the chest cavity in a controlled fashion. A/an ___ port was placed through this incision into the chest cavity. Once intrathoracic placement was verified, the chest was insufflated to a pressure of ___ mmHg to facilitate visualization and reduction of the abdominal viscera into the abdominal cavity. Two additional ports were placed under direct vision, one in the anterior axillary line two rib spaces below the initial port and the other just posterior and inferior to the tip of the scapula.

If thoracotomy: A/an ___-mm anterolateral thoracotomy incision was made in the sixth intercostal space and extended down through the subcutaneous tissue using electrocautery for hemostasis. The latissimus dorsi muscle was mobilized from the fascia and retracted posteriorly. The serratus anterior muscle was separated from its posterior insertion and retracted anteriorly. The incision was extended down to the level of the ribs and the chest entered just above the seventh rib in the sixth intercostal space. The intercostal muscles and pleura were opened to the full length of the incision and the Finochietto retractor used to spread the ribs for exposure.

Inspection of the pleural cavity revealed a hypoplastic *left/right* lung and the *small bowel, colon, stomach, liver, and spleen* (choose all that apply). The abdominal viscera were reduced into the abdominal cavity being careful to avoid injury to these structures. The posterior leaflet of the diaphragm was mobilized using electrocautery for hemostasis. In addition, the pleuroperitoneal attachments were separated using electrocautery along the circumference of the defect. Once this was accomplished, the size of the defect was assessed as well as the laxity of the diaphragm to determine if a primary repair was feasible or if a prosthetic patch was indicated.

[Choose One:]

If primary repair: Based on the size of the defect and the presence of sufficient laxity of the diaphragm to achieve a tension-free repair, a primary repair of the defect was performed. Interrupted ___-0 *Ethibond* sutures were placed from *medial to lateral/lateral to medial* to close the defect. A total of ___ sutures were placed. Care was taken at the posterior–lateral margin of the defect to ensure adequate tissue closure. *This required ___ suture(s) to be placed around the adjacent rib.*

If repair with prosthetic patch: Based on the size of the defect and the absence of adequate diaphragmatic tissue to achieve a primary repair, the defect was closed using a ___-cm × ___-cm prosthetic patch of ___ *mm Gortex*. The defect was measured and the patch trimmed to allow for adequate coverage with some residual laxity of the patch. Interrupted ___*-0 Ethibond/___ Gortex* suture was used to secure the patch circumferentially. Care was taken at the posterior–lateral margin of the defect to ensure adequate tissue closure. *This required ___ suture(s) to be placed around the adjacent rib.*

Once the defect was closed, the area was inspected for hemostasis. *A ___-Fr chest tube/drain was placed and secured at its exit with a ___-0 silk/nylon/___ and a dressing applied.*

[Choose One:]

If thoracoscopic approach: The ports were then removed and the fascia closed at all port sites using a ___-0 Vicryl suture. The skin was closed using a ___*-0 Vicryl/monocryl/___ suture.*

If thoracotomy: The retractor was removed and the ribs reapproximated using interrupted ___-0 Vicryl/Ethibond/___ sutures being careful to avoid obliteration of the intercostal space. The posterior insertion of the serratus anterior muscle was reapproximated using interrupted ___-0 Vicryl sutures. The subcutaneous tissue was closed using a running ___-0 Vicryl, and the skin was closed using a running ___*-0 Vicryl/monocryl* subcuticular stitch.

Dressings were applied to the incision(s). All counts were correct at the end of the procedure. Upon completion of the procedure, a debriefing checklist was completed to share information critical to the postoperative care of the patient. The patient tolerated the procedure well, *was extubated in the operating room*, and was transported to the postanesthesia care unit in stable condition thereafter.

82 Lobar Resection of Congenital Pulmonary Malformations (Open and MIS Approaches)

Rita D. Shelby, Dominic J. Papandria, and Karen A. Diefenbach

Indications and Benefits

- Symptomatic, persistent, or enlarging congenital pulmonary airway malformation (CPAM)
- Intralobar pulmonary sequestration
- Congenital lobar emphysema
- Benefits: Resolution of respiratory insufficiency, resolution of recurrent pulmonary infections, prevention of malignant transformation

Risks and Alternatives

- Standard risks (bleeding, infection, need for additional procedures, risks of anesthesia)
- Injury to adjacent structures (airways, lung parenchyma, pulmonary arteries or veins)
- Chest wall deformity and scoliosis for open approach
- Persistent air leak, bronchopleural fistula
- Bronchial injury
- Conversion to open thoracotomy for MIS procedure
- Alternatives: Observation (for small stable lesions without respirator compromise)

Essential Steps

1. Positioning for right or left lobar resection
2. Port placement
3. Dissection in adjacent fissure(s)
4. Isolation, ligation, and division of arterial supply to lobe
5. Isolation, ligation, and division of venous supply to lobe
6. Isolation, ligation, and division of bronchial branches to lobe
7. Removal from chest cavity
8. Chest tube placement
9. Closure of incision
10. Postoperative CXR

Note These Variations

- Congenital lobar emphysema is often managed with observation if asymptomatic.
- Method of ligation and division of systemic vessels is surgeon dependent.

R. D. Shelby
Nationwide Children's Hospital, Ohio State University Wexner Medical Center, Department of Pediatric Surgery, Columbus, OH, USA

D. J. Papandria
Department of Surgery, Emory University, Atlanta, GA, USA
e-mail: dominic.papandria@emory.edu

K. A. Diefenbach (✉)
Nationwide Children's Hospital, Columbus, OH, USA
e-mail: Karen.Diefenbach@nationwidechildrens.org

D. J. Papandria et al. (eds.), *Operative Dictations in Pediatric Surgery*,
https://doi.org/10.1007/978-3-030-24212-1_82

- Positioning depends on procedure type, open versus MIS, and location of lobe to be removed.
- Variation to the MIS procedure include a hybrid procedure utilizing a mini thoracotomy for direct manipulation and removal of the specimen.

Template Operative Dictation

Preoperative Diagnosis *Congenital pulmonary airway malformation/congenital lobar emphysema/pulmonary sequestration*

Postoperative Diagnosis Same as preoperative diagnosis

Findings Same as postoperative diagnosis

Procedure(s) Performed *Thoracoscopic/open right/left upper/middle/lower* lobectomy

Anesthesia General

Specimen *Right/left upper/middle/lower* lobe

Drains *None/__ Fr Argyle chest tube/__ Fr Blake*

Implants None

Estimated Blood Loss ___ ml

Indications This is a/an ___*-day/week/month/year*-old *male/female* with a *congenital pulmonary airway malformation/congenital lobar emphysema/pulmonary sequestration* involving the *right/left upper/middle/lower* lobe. *He/she* was deemed to be a suitable candidate for lobectomy.

Procedure in Detail Following satisfactory induction of anesthesia, intubation proceeded to allow for single lung ventilation. The patient was then placed in *right/left* lateral decubitus. Care was taken to position the head, neck, arms, hips, and legs in neutral positions with all pressure points appropriately padded. Time-outs were performed using both preinduction and preincision safety checklists with participation of all present in the operative suite. These confirmed the correct patient, procedure, operative site, and additional critical information prior to the start of the procedure. The *right/left* chest and axilla were then prepped and draped in the usual sterile fashion and the lung isolated on the operative side by anesthesia.

[Choose One]:
If thoracoscopic approach: A/an ___-mm incision was made in the anterior axillary line of the fifth intercostal space and blunt dissection used to enter the chest cavity. A/an ___-mm port was inserted through this incision and once intrathoracic placement was confirmed, the chest was insufflated to a pressure of ___ mmHg, until pneumothorax and complete collapse of the lung is achieved. Two additional ports were placed under direct vision, a/an __-mm port in the anterior axillary line two rib spaces below the first incision and a/an ___-mm port ___ cm *posterior and inferior/anterior and inferior* to the tip of the scapula.

If open approach: A posterolateral, muscle-sparing incision was then made at the anticipated location of the fifth intercostal space and extended posteriorly approximately ___ cm. The incision carried down through the subcutaneous tissue with electrocautery. The latissimus dorsi muscle was mobilized at its anterior margin retracted posteriorly. The serratus anterior muscle was mobilized from its posterior insertion and retracted to expose the ribs and intercostal muscles. The rib spaces were counted and the fifth intercostal space identified. This was divided along the attachments to the inferior ribs. Then a Finochietto retractor was placed into chest cavity to fully expose the operative field.

{Continue dictation}

After inspection of the lung, the *right/left* lung is then mobilized. Then the inferior pulmonary ligament and any pleuropulmonary adhesions are released. Once the lung is free, attention is turned to the hilum. Attention is turned to the fissure adjacent to the lobe to be resected. If the fissure is incomplete, the pulmonary parenchyma is dissected, sealed with a bipolar sealing device, and divided to expose the branches of the pulmonary artery supplying the abnormal lobe. These vessels are isolated and double ligated with ___-*0 Silk ties/bipolar sealing device/endoclips/endoscopic stapler* until the fissure is completely separated from the normal parenchyma. Branches of the *superior/inferior* pulmonary vein are identified and preserved. The branch supplying the affected lobe is then dissected from proximal to distal until the main branches within the parenchyma of this lobe are isolated and dissected circumferentially. These branches are then double ligated with ___-*0 Silk ties/bipolar sealing device/endoclips/endoscopic stapler* and divided preserving the bronchus in situ and in continuity before the lobe is completely mobilized. The bronchus is dissected distally into the parenchyma of the lobe before ligating to assure there is no compression or injury to the bronchi to the remaining lung. The bronchus is then *ligated and divided using the endoscopic stapler/sharply and the bronchial stump oversewn using interrupted sutures of* ___-*0 PDS/vicryl/prolene.*

[Choose One]:

If thoracoscopic approach: The anterior–inferior port site is enlarged to ___ mm and the specimen removed from the chest cavity, morcelating the tissue if necessary. This is done under direct vision to verify that the entire specimen is removed, which is then sent to pathology for further evaluation. The pleural cavity was inspected and noted to be hemostatic. *Intercostal rib blocks are performed for regional anesthetic affect using ___ % ___ with epinephrine to the intercostal spaces involved with the incisions.* A ___ *Fr chest/Blake drain* was then placed through the anterior–inferior incision and directed posteriorly and superiorly toward the apex. The fascia and skin are approximated around the tube and the chest tube/drain secured using a ___-*0 Silk/Nylon/___ suture*. The lung is then re-expanded under direct visualization. The remaining ports were removed and the fascia closed with ___-0 vicryl suture. The skin was closed with ___-*0 vicryl/monocryl* suture.

If open approach: The specimen is then removed and sent to pathology for further evaluation. The pleural cavity was inspected and noted to be hemostatic. *Intercostal rib blocks are performed for regional anesthetic affect using ___ % ___ with epinephrine to the intercostal spaces involved with the incision.* A ___ *Fr chest/Blake drain* was then placed through a separate anterior chest incision and directed posteriorly and superiorly toward the apex. It was secured with a ___-*0 Silk/Nylon/___ suture.* The lung is then re-expanded under direct visualization.

The Finochietto retractor was then removed and the ribs reapproximated with interrupted ___-0 *vicryl/___* sutures being careful not to obliterate the intercostal space. The serratus anterior muscle was reapproximated to its posterior insertion using interrupted ___-0 __sutures. The latissimus dorsi muscle was returned to its normal position and the subcutaneous tissue was approximated using a running ___-0 __ suture. The skin was closed using a running ___-0 ___suture.

{Continue dictation}

The skin was cleaned and dried and *Dermabond/Steri-Strips and an occlusive dressing* applied. The chest tube was dressed and connected to suction. Upon completion of the procedure, a debriefing checklist was completed to share information critical to the postoperative care of the patient. The patient tolerated the procedure well, *was extubated in the operating room/transported intubated*, and was transported to the *postanesthesia care/critical care* unit in stable condition thereafter. A postoperative chest X-ray was obtained confirming adequate expansion on the lung and correct placement of the chest tube.

Extralobar Resection of Congenital Pulmonary Malformations (Open and MIS Approaches)

83

Kate Savoie, Dominic J. Papandria, and Karen A. Diefenbach

Indications and Benefits

- Extralobar pulmonary sequestration
- Congenital bronchopulmonary cyst
- Benefits: Resolution of respiratory insufficiency, resolution of recurrent pulmonary infections, prevention of malignant transformation

Risks and Alternatives

- Standard risks (bleeding, infection, need for additional procedures, risks of anesthesia)
- Injury to adjacent structures (airways, lung parenchyma, pulmonary arteries or veins, or other systemic vessels)
- Scoliosis when an open procedure is performed
- Alternatives: Observation (for small stable lesions without respiratory compromise)

K. Savoie
Nationwide Children's Hospital, Department of Pediatric Surgery, Columbus, OH, USA

D. J. Papandria
Department of Surgery, Emory University, Atlanta, GA, USA

K. A. Diefenbach (✉)
Nationwide Children's Hospital, Columbus, OH, USA
e-mail: Karen.Diefenbach@nationwidechildrens.org

Essential Steps

1. Safe access to the chest
2. Port placement
3. Safe ligation and division of systemic vessels
4. Resection of abnormal bronchopulmonary cyst or extralobar sequestration
5. Removal from chest cavity
6. Closure of incisions

Note These Variations

- Method of ligation and division of systemic vessels is surgeon dependent.
- Some centers observe these lesions.

Template Operative Dictation

Preoperative Diagnosis *Right/left congenital bronchopulmonary cyst/extralobar pulmonary sequestration.*

Postoperative Diagnosis Same as preoperative diagnosis

Findings Same as postoperative diagnosis

Procedure(s) Performed *Thoracoscopic/open* resection of *right/left* congenital pulmonary mal-

D. J. Papandria et al. (eds.), *Operative Dictations in Pediatric Surgery*,
https://doi.org/10.1007/978-3-030-24212-1_83

formation, *bronchopulmonary cyst/extralobar sequestration*

Anesthesia General

Specimen Bronchopulmonary *cyst/sequestration*, to pathology

Drains *None/__ Fr Argyle chest tube/__ Fr Blake*

Implants None

Estimated Blood Loss ___ ml

Indications This is a/an ___*-day/week/month/year*-old *male/female* with a *right/left*-sided congenital pulmonary malformation. Based on preoperative imaging, this is a suspected *bronchopulmonary cyst/pulmonary sequestration. He/she* was deemed to be a suitable candidate for lobectomy via thoracotomy.

Procedure in Detail Following satisfactory induction of anesthesia, the patient was placed in *right/left* lateral decubitus and appropriately padded. Time-outs were performed using both preinduction and preincision safety checklists with participation of all present in the operative suite. These confirmed the correct patient, procedure, operative site, and additional critical information prior to the start of the procedure. The *right/left* chest and axilla were then prepped and draped in the usual sterile fashion and the lung isolated on the operative side by anesthesia.

[Choose One]:

If an open approach was performed: A posterolateral, muscle-sparing incision was then made at the anticipated location of the fifth intercostal space and extended posteriorly approximately ___ cm. The incision carried down through the subcutaneous tissue with electrocautery. The latissimus dorsi muscle was mobilized at its anterior margin retracted posteriorly. The serratus anterior muscle was mobilized from its posterior insertion and retracted to expose the ribs and intercostal muscles. The rib spaces were counted and the fifth intercostal space identified. This was incised using and a Finochietto retractor placed into chest cavity.

If a thoracoscopic approach was performed: A/an ___-mm incision was made in the anterior axillary line of the fifth intercostal space and blunt dissection used to enter the chest cavity. A/an ___-mm port was inserted through this incision and once intrathoracic placement was confirmed, the chest was insufflated to a pressure of ___ mmHg. Two additional ports were placed under direct vision, a/an __-mm port in the anterior axillary line two rib spaces below the first incision and a/an ___-mm port ___ cm *posterior and inferior* to the tip of the scapula.

{Continue dictation}

Inspection of the chest cavity revealed the anomalous tissue in the *paraspinal/posterior costophrenic sulcus*.

[Choose One]:

For bronchopulmonary cysts: The cystic structure was dissected circumferentially from its adventitial attachments being careful to preserve hemostasis. There was no systemic vessel identified. Once completely mobilized, the cyst was brought out of the chest cavity and sent to pathology for further evaluation.

For extralobar sequestrations: The inferior pulmonary ligament was divided and the extralobar sequestration was identified in the posterior costophrenic sulcus. The systemic vessels were identified and the arterial supply isolated. The artery was dissected to have adequate length to maintain control of the vessel after division. The artery was ligated with a *hemoclip/endoclip/suture ligature/vascular staple load* and was divided with good hemostasis. Additional arterial branches were *not identified/identified and were ligated and divided in the same manner*. The remaining attachments including the venous drainage were ligated and divided using *electrocautery/a bipolar sealing device/___-0 ___ sutures* with good hemostasis. It was then removed from the pleural cavity and sent to pathology.

{Continue dictation}

The pleural cavity was inspected and noted to be hemostatic. *A ___-Fr chest tube was then placed through a separate anterior chest incision/ the anterior and inferior port site and directed posteriorly and superiorly toward the apex. It was secured at the exit site using ___-0 Silk/Nurolon/ Nylon sutures and then connected to water seal.*

If an open approach was performed: The Finochietto retractor was then removed and the ribs reapproximated with interrupted ___-0 vicryl sutures being careful not to obliterate the intercostal space. The serratus anterior muscle was reapproximated to its posterior insertion using interrupted ___-0 vicryl sutures. The latissimus dorsi muscle was returned to its normal position and the subcutaneous tissue was approximated using a running ___-0 vicryl suture. The skin was closed using a running ___-0 *vicryl/ monocryl* subcuticular stitch.

If a thoracoscopic approach was performed: The remaining ports were removed and the fascia closed using a ___-0 vicryl suture. The skin at these incisions was closed using a ___-0 *vicryl/ monocryl* suture.

{Continue dictation}

The skin was cleaned and dried and *Dermabond/Steri-Strips and an occlusive dressing* applied. The chest tube was dressed and connected to suction.

Upon completion of the procedure, a debriefing checklist was completed to share information critical to the postoperative care of the patient. The patient tolerated the procedure well, *was extubated in the operating room/transported intubated*, and was transported to the *postanesthesia care/critical care* unit in stable condition thereafter. A postoperative chest X-ray was obtained confirming adequate expansion on the lung and correct placement of the chest tube.

Thymectomy and Aortopexy

84

Joseph Adam Sujka and Shawn D. St. Peter

Indications and Benefits

- Indication: Life-threatening tracheal obstruction secondary to severe tracheomalacia
- Benefit: Improvement in tracheal obstruction and tracheomalacia

Risks and Alternatives

- Standard risks (bleeding, infection, need for additional procedures, risks of anesthesia)
- Injury to adjacent structures (phrenic nerve, pericardium, aorta, innominate artery, thymus)
- Alternatives: Continuous positive airway pressure (CPAP), tracheopexy

Essential Steps

Open

1. Upper sternal edge, angle of Louis, xiphisternum, and sternal midline were marked.
2. Skin incision made from the upper sternum to the angle of Louis.
3. Blunt blind dissection of the retrosternal space.
4. Sternotomy performed.
5. Thymectomy performed, with identification of the phrenic nerve.
6. Pretracheal space dissected.
7. Pericardium opened extending to the origin of the brachiocephalic artery. Stay sutures were placed along the four corners of the two flaps.
8. Pledgeted stitches passed into the aortic wall at the origin of the innominate artery and through the pericardial edge at the level of the pericardial reflection.
9. Pericardium closed.
10. Stitches passed inside out through each half of the sternum. Sternum reapproximated.
11. Stitches tied down.
12. Completion of sternotomy and wound closure.

Thoracoscopic

1. Induce pneumothorax, place ports, and insert scope.
2. Visualize the triangle formed by the internal mammary vessels, phrenic nerve, and pericardium inferiorly.
3. Open the mediastinal pleura and mobilize the thymus.
4. Create a stab incision over the midsternum at the level of the ascending aorta.
5. Pass three sutures through the sternum and secure one to each structure:

J. A. Sujka (✉) · S. D. St. Peter
Children's Mercy Hospital, Department of Pediatric Surgery, Kansas City, MO, USA
e-mail: sspeter@cmh.edu

D. J. Papandria et al. (eds.), *Operative Dictations in Pediatric Surgery*,
https://doi.org/10.1007/978-3-030-24212-1_84

   (a) Pericardial reflection on the aorta.
   (b) Innominate artery adventitia.
   (c) Ascending aorta adventitia.
6. Tie down stitches confirming elevation of aorta with scope.
7. Close midsternum stab incisions.
8. Ports were removed and sites closed.

Template Operative Dictation (Open) [1]

Preoperative Diagnosis *Tracheomalacia*

Postoperative Diagnosis Same as preoperative diagnosis

Findings Same as postoperative diagnosis

Procedure(s) Performed Thymectomy and aortopexy

Anesthesia General

Specimen None

Drains None

Estimated Blood Loss ___

Indications This is a/an ___-*day/week/month/year*-old *male/female* with tracheomalacia. He/she was deemed to be a suitable candidate for thymectomy and aortopexy.

Procedure in Detail Following satisfactory induction of anesthesia, the patient was placed in supine position. Time-outs were performed using both preinduction and preincision safety checklists with participation of all present in the operative suite. These confirmed the correct patient, procedure, operative site, and additional critical information prior to the start of the procedure. The chest was then prepped and draped in the usual sterile fashion.

The upper sternal edge, angle of Louis, xiphisternum, and sternal midline were marked. A skin incision was made from the upper sternum to the angle of Louis. This incision was deepened to the anterior sternal plate staying in the midline. The sternum was elevated and a blunt blind dissection of the retrosternal space was performed via insertion of a dissector below the sternal posterior plate. Once this was complete, an oscillating saw was used to perform an upper sternotomy. Hemostasis was obtained and a small spreader was inserted between the two sternal halves.

The thymus was carefully removed via dissection of the thymic capsule. The phrenic nerve was identified along the lateral aspect of the thymic capsule and care was taken to avoid its course during thymectomy. We also identified the pleura and brachiocephalic vein deep to the thymus and were careful to avoid injuring these structures. Dissection was carried down the midline to the pretracheal space. The trachea was identified via digital palpation. Lateral to the trachea, the innominate artery and vein were carefully exposed.

Inferior to the left innominate vein and over the origin of the ascending aorta, the pericardium was opened with a vertical incision extending to the origin of the brachiocephalic artery. Stay sutures were placed along the four corners of the two flaps and fixed bilaterally by Kelly clamps. *Two 3–0 or 4–0 double-needle Prolene "U" stitches reinforced with Teflon pledgets* were passed into the aortic wall at the origin of the innominate artery and through the pericardial edge at the level of the pericardial reflection. Care was taken to have each stitch deep enough inside the aortic wall to not tear it without entering the lumen.

The pericardium was closed with interrupted stitches. Both needles of each U stitch were passed inside out through each half of the sternum with the effect of lifting the aortic arch. The stitches were kept in place with a rubber clamp and not tied down. Next, the sternum was reapproximated with multiple *0 vicryl stitches*. At this time, the Teflon pledgets were positioned and the U stitch sutures gently tied on the anterior surface of the sternum.

The muscle in the midline was reapproximated and the subcutaneous layer and skin were closed with running *5–0 monocryl suture*. Upon completion of the procedure, a debriefing checklist was completed to share information critical to the postoperative care of the patient. The patient tolerated the procedure well, *was extubated in the operating room*, and was transported to the post-anesthesia care unit in stable condition thereafter.

Template Operative Dictation (Thoracoscopic – Infant) [2]

Preoperative Diagnosis *Tracheomalacia*

Postoperative Diagnosis Same as preoperative diagnosis

Findings Same as postoperative diagnosis

Procedure(s) Performed Thoracoscopic thymectomy and aortopexy.

Anesthesia General

Specimen None

Drains None

Estimated Blood Loss ___

Indications This is a/an ___*-day/week/month/year*-old *male/female* with *tracheomalacia*. He/she was deemed to be a suitable candidate for thoracoscopic thymectomy and aortopexy.

Procedure in Detail Following satisfactory induction of anesthesia, the patient was placed in supine position with the left chest elevated by 15°. Time-outs were performed using both preinduction and preincision safety checklists with participation of all present in the operative suite. These confirmed the correct patient, procedure, operative site, and additional critical information prior to the start of the procedure. The chest was then prepped and draped in the usual sterile fashion. A 5-mm port was placed in the midaxillary line at the level of the nipple. The thorax was insufflated with carbon dioxide to a pressure of 8 mmHg. Two additional ports were placed, one superior and the other inferior and anterior.

A triangle formed by the internal mammary vessels anteriorly, phrenic nerve posteriorly, and pericardium inferiorly was visualized. Care was taken to avoid damage to the phrenic nerve. The mediastinal pleura in the center of this triangle was opened with electrocautery. The thymus was mobilized posteriorly until the ascending aorta with its pericardial reflection and the innominate artery was clearly seen.

Once exposure was adequate, a small stab incision was made in the skin and soft tissue overlying the midsternum at the level of the ascending aorta. Three 3–0 Ethibond sutures on a V-5 needle were driven through the stab incision and through the sternum sequentially. The first needle was driven through the sternum and secured to the pericardial reflection on the aorta with care being taken to only include the adventitia and not the vessel wall. The needle was then pushed through the sternum a few millimeters from the other part of the suture. The second and third sutures were placed in a similar fashion. One was secured to the adventitia of the innominate artery and the second the adventitia of the ascending aorta. The sutures were tied extracorporeally and the aorta was visualized to be elevated against the sternum.

The stab incisions were closed with *Steri-Strips*. The ports were removed under direct visualization and the port sites were closed everting vicryl sutures and covered with Steri-Strips. Upon completion of the procedure, a debriefing checklist was completed to share information critical to the postoperative care of the patient. The patient tolerated the procedure well.

Template Operative Dictation (Thoracoscopic – Adolescent) [3]

Preoperative Diagnosis *Tracheal stenosis/tracheomalacia*

Postoperative Diagnosis Same as preoperative diagnosis

Findings Same as postoperative diagnosis

Procedure(s) Performed Thoracoscopic thymectomy and aortopexy

Anesthesia General

Specimen None

Drains None

Estimated Blood Loss ___

Indications This is a/an ___-*day/week/month/year*-old *male/female* with *tracheal stenosis/tracheomalacia*. He/she was deemed to be a suitable candidate for thoracoscopic thymectomy and aortopexy.

Procedure in Detail Following satisfactory induction of anesthesia, the patient was placed in supine position with the left chest elevated by 15°. Time-outs were performed using both preinduction and preincision safety checklists with participation of all present in the operative suite. These confirmed the correct patient, procedure, operative site, and additional critical information prior to the start of the procedure. The chest was then prepped and draped in the usual sterile fashion. A 5-mm port was placed in the midaxillary line at the level of the nipple. The thorax was insufflated with carbon dioxide to a pressure of 8 mmHg. Two additional ports were placed, one superior and the other inferior and anterior.

A triangle formed by the internal mammary vessels anteriorly, phrenic nerve posteriorly, and pericardium inferiorly was visualized. Care was taken to avoid damage to the phrenic nerve. The mediastinal pleura in the center of this triangle was opened with electrocautery. The thymus was mobilized posteriorly until the ascending aorta with its pericardial reflection and the innominate artery was clearly seen.

Once exposure was adequate, a 0 silk suture was introduced and passed through the pericardial reflection on the aorta with care being taken to only include the adventitia and not the vessel wall. The needle was then passed through the back of the sternum and both ends were brought out through the inferior port, the port was removed and replaced to maintain function while holding the suture. The second and third sutures were placed in a similar fashion. One was secured to the adventitia of the innominate artery and the second the adventitia of the ascending aorta. The sutures were tied extracorporeal knot and the knot pusher to secure them down. The aorta was visualized to be elevated against the sternum.

The ports were removed under direct visualization and the port sites were closed with everting vicryl sutures and covered with Steri-Strips. Upon completion of the procedure, a debriefing checklist was completed to share information critical to the postoperative care of the patient. The patient tolerated the procedure well.

References

1. Elliott MJ, Speggiorin S, Torre M. Anterior aortopexy for tracheomalacia. Oper Tech Thorac Cardiovasc Surg. 2011;16:309–21. https://doi.org/10.1053/j.optechstcvs.2011.06.003.
2. Holcomb GW, Georgeson K, Rothenberg S. Atlas of pediatric laparoscopy and thoracoscopy. Philadelphia, PA: Saunders/Elsevier; 2008.
3. van der Zee DC, Straver M. Thoracoscopic aortopexy for tracheomalacia. World J Surg. 2015;39:158–64. https://doi.org/10.1007/s00268-014-2798-2.

Ligation of Patent Ductus Arteriosus

85

Mitchell R. Ladd and Alejandro V. Garcia

Indications and Benefits

- Clinically significant patent ductus arteriosus refractory to medical management
- Asymptomatic patent ductus arteriosus that has not spontaneously closed by age 2 years
- Benefits: Improved hemodynamics, reduced risk of bacterial endocarditis, reduced risk of pulmonary hypertension

Risks and Alternatives

- Standard risks (bleeding, infection, need for additional procedures, risks of anesthesia)
- Injury to adjacent structures (lung, heart, aorta, pulmonary arteries, trachea, recurrent laryngeal nerve)
- Alternatives: Observation, medical management, endovascular occlusion

M. R. Ladd
Johns Hopkins Hospital, Department of General Surgery, Baltimore, MD, USA

A. V. Garcia (✉)
Johns Hopkins University, Department of Pediatric Surgery, Baltimore, MD, USA
e-mail: agarci41@jhmi.edu

Essential Steps

1. Place the patient in right lateral decubitus (i.e left side up).
2. Gain access to the thoracic cavity (either thoracoscopically or via thoracotomy).
3. Retract the left lung.
4. Identify the recurrent laryngeal nerve and preserve it.
5. Circumferentially dissect out the ductus arteriosus.
6. Test clamp the ductus arteriosus.
7. Clip or ligate the ductus arteriosus.
8. Close the thoracic cavity.

Note These Variations

- Thoracoscopic or open depending on experience
- Chest tube placement in select cases
- Conversion from thoracoscopic to open procedure in the case of bleeding

Template Operative Dictation (Thoracoscopic)

Preoperative Diagnosis *Clinically significant patent ductus arteriosus refractory to medical management/patent ductus arteriosus in a 2-year-old child*

D. J. Papandria et al. (eds.), *Operative Dictations in Pediatric Surgery*,
https://doi.org/10.1007/978-3-030-24212-1_85

Postoperative Diagnosis Same as preoperative diagnosis

Findings Same as postoperative diagnosis

Procedure(s) Performed Ligation of patent ductus arteriosus

Anesthesia General

Drains *Chest tube*

Estimated Blood Loss ___

Indications This is a/an ___-*day/week/month/year*-old *male/female* with a *clinically significant patent ductus arteriosus/persistently patent ductus arteriosus*. *He/she* was deemed to be a suitable candidate for ligation of patent ductus arteriosus.

Procedure in Detail Following satisfactory induction of anesthesia, the patient was placed in the right lateral decubitus position and appropriately padded. Time-outs were performed using both preinduction and preincision safety checklists with participation of all present in the operative suite. These confirmed the correct patient, procedure, operative site, and additional critical information prior to the start of the procedure. The left thorax was then prepped and draped in the usual sterile fashion.

A/an ___-cm incision was made in the left fifth intercostal space in the posterior axillary line. A thoracoscope was placed through this incision. Insufflation was turned on to 4 mmHg with a flow rate of 1 L/min. Then, a second ___ cm incision was made in the fifth intercostal space in the midaxillary line. Through this incision, a fan retractor inserted and used to retract the left lung. With retraction, the aorta, left subclavian artery, patent ductus arteriosus, and recurrent laryngeal nerve were visualized. After retraction of the lung, insufflation was discontinued. Next, a third ___ cm incision was made in the fifth intercostal space posteriorly inferior to the tip of the scapula. A curved dissector was used through this final incision to carefully circumferentially dissect out the patent ductus arteriosus near its junction with the aorta taking care not to put excessive traction on the recurrent laryngeal nerve. Once the patent ductus arteriosus was isolated, it was test clamped while monitoring preductal and postductal oxygen saturations. After test clamping confirmed that the structure was the patent ductus arteriosus, two clips were applied with a clip applier through the posterior incision. The thoracic cavity was then inspected for hemostasis or evidence of lung injury from retraction.

[Choose One:]

If lung injury present: Due to the lung *injury/laceration* observed, a ___-French chest tube was placed through the *anterior/middle/posterior* incision under direct visualization. The incisions were then closed in the typical fashion. The chest tube was then placed on ___ cm of water suction. The needle and sponge counts were correct after closure.

If lung injury absent: The incisions were closed in the typical fashion. Just prior to closure of the final muscle layer of the final incision, positive inspiratory pressure was applied to fully inflate the lung and evacuate any residual pneumothorax. The needle and sponge counts were correct after closure.

Upon completion of the procedure, a debriefing checklist was completed to share information critical to the postoperative care of the patient. The patient tolerated the procedure well, *was extubated in the operating room*, and was transported to the postanesthesia care unit in stable condition thereafter.

Template Operative Dictation (Open)

Preoperative Diagnosis *Clinically significant patent ductus arteriosus refractory to medical management/patent ductus arteriosus in a 2-year-old child*

Postoperative Diagnosis Same as preoperative diagnosis

Findings Same as postoperative diagnosis

Procedure(s) Performed Open ligation of patent ductus arteriosus

Anesthesia General

Drains *Chest tube*

Estimated Blood Loss ___

Indications This is a/an __*-day/week/month/year*-old *male/female* with *clinically significant patent ductus arteriosus/persistently patent ductus arteriosus. He/she* was deemed to be a suitable candidate for open ligation of patent ductus arteriosus.

Procedure in Detail Following satisfactory induction of anesthesia, the patient was placed in the right lateral decubitus position and appropriately padded. Time-outs were performed using both preinduction and preincision safety checklists with participation of all present in the operative suite. These confirmed the correct patient, procedure, operative site, and additional critical information prior to the start of the procedure. The left thorax was then prepped and draped in the usual sterile fashion.

A left posterolateral thoracotomy was made in the left fifth intercostal space. After entry into the thoracic cavity, the ribs were gently spread with an appropriately sized Finochietto retractor. The left lung was then gently retracted using a malleable retractor and the aorta, left subclavian artery, patent ductus arteriosus, and recurrent laryngeal nerve were visualized. The patent ductus arteriosus was carefully circumferentially dissected near its junction with the aorta using a Rienhoff/tonsil/right angle clamp being careful not to apply too much traction to the recurrent laryngeal nerve. Once the ductus arteriosus was dissected out, it was test clamped with a Debakey/bulldog clamp while monitoring preductal and postductal saturations. After test clamp confirmed that the structure was the ductus arteriosus, it was *clipped/ligated* with *clip applier/___ stitches*. The thoracic cavity was then inspected for any lung injury or bleeding.

[Choose One:]
If lung injury present: Due to the lung *injury/laceration* observed, a ___-French chest tube was placed through a separate incision below the thoracotomy and placed under direct visualization. The thoracotomy was then closed in layers in the usual fashion. The chest tube was the placed on ___ cm water suction. The needle and sponge counts were correct after closure.

If lung injury absent: The thoracotomy was closed in the typical fashion. Just prior to closure of the muscle layer, positive inspiratory pressure was applied to fully inflate the lung and evacuate any residual pneumothorax. The needle and sponge counts were correct after closure.

Upon completion of the procedure, a debriefing checklist was completed to share information critical to the postoperative care of the patient. The patient tolerated the procedure well, *was extubated in the operating room*, and was transported to the postanesthesia care unit in stable condition thereafter.

Thymectomy (Open and MIS Approaches)

86

Stefan Scholz and Alejandro V. Garcia

Indications and Benefits

- Nonthymomatous (juvenile/ocular) myasthenia gravis.
- Thymoma.
- Partial thymectomy reserved for diagnostic biopsy of lymphoma.
- Robot-assisted thymectomy offers a three-dimensional view and articulating wrists that may provide greater access to the superior portion of the thymus and the contralateral side offering a refinement of the mediastinal dissection and possibly a more complete removal of thymic tissue.
- Benefits: Remission of symptoms of myasthenia gravis, resection of thymoma

Risks and Alternatives

- Standard risks (bleeding, infection, need for additional procedures, risks of anesthesia).
- Injury to the pericardium, the heart, or the phrenic nerve.
- Injury to the great vein of Keynes, the largest thymic vein originating from the left brachiocephalic vein, causing massive bleeding.
- Incomplete thymectomy for myasthenia gravis.
- Alternatives: Traditional techniques such as cervical collar incision or median sternotomy. Median sternotomy is largely reserved today for resection of large thymic tumors. A right-sided thoracoscopic or robotic approach may be chosen for more right-sided tumors.

Essential Steps

Open Thymectomy (Transsternal or Transcervical)

1. Place the patient in supine position with a transverse shoulder roll behind the scapulae and the head in extension.
2. *Transsternal:* A midline incision is made starting one fingerbreadth below the suprasternal notch. The incision is taken down to the fourth intercostal space (this can be taken down to below xiphoid process if needed).
3. The space posterior to the manubrium and xiphoid is dissected bluntly using finger dissection.
4. The sternum is divided using a reciprocating or oscillating saw.

S. Scholz (✉)
University of Pittsburgh School of Medicine, Children's Hospital of Pittsburgh, Department of Pediatric Surgery, Pittsburgh, PA, USA
e-mail: stefan.scholz@chp.edu

A. V. Garcia
Johns Hopkins University, Department of Pediatric Surgery, Baltimore, MD, USA

D. J. Papandria et al. (eds.), *Operative Dictations in Pediatric Surgery*,
https://doi.org/10.1007/978-3-030-24212-1_86

5. Both pleural spaces are opened and the phrenic nerves identified, and the mediastinal pleural is pushed to the sides until the thymus and left innominate vein are in view.
6. Mobilization of the thymus begins at the level of the diaphragm and is carried cranially carefully dissecting the gland off the pericardium.
7. The arterial branches to the thymus arising from the internal thoracic arteries should be ligated appropriately. The thymic veins drain into the innominate vein and are easily identified and ligated as the inferior lobes are elevated.
8. Once separated off the anterior surface of the innominate vein, the superior horns should be carefully dissected avoiding injury to the inferior parathyroid glands. Small venous branches between the thymic horns and the inferior thyroid plexus should be divided.
9. The sternum is approximated with stainless steel wires, and the soft tissue is closed with absorbable sutures in layers.
10. *Transcervical:* A transverse curvilinear incision approximately 2 cm above the sternal notch is made. The platysma is cut, and both superior and inferior skin flaps are raised using electrocautery.
11. The strap muscles are separated and retracted laterally, and the upper poles of the thymus should be visualized.
12. The thymus is elevated and separated off the trachea, thyroid gland, and inferiorly to the sternal notch.
13. The prethymic plane is separated from the sternum bluntly, and the sternum is elevated with a retractor. The dissection is carried down posterior to the thymus until the innominate vein is exposed, and the branches are ligated, the remaining parts of the operating are similar to the transternal approach.

Thoracoscopic Thymectomy (Standard Left or Right)

1. Place the patient in a right lateral 30-degree decubitus position supported with a bean bag.
2. Selective right lung ventilation is established with either right mainstem intubation, bronchial blocker, or double-lumen endotracheal intubation.
3. Alternatively, after endotracheal intubation, the left lung is collapsed using valved trocars and low pressure CO_2 insufflation into the left hemithorax.
4. The mediastinum is accessed through the left chest, and a 30° telescope is used.
5. All three trocars are placed along the submammary fold. The telescope port (5 mm) is placed in the anterior axillary line in the fourth intercostal space.
6. The two working ports (3 or 5 mm) are placed slightly anterior and posterior on either side of the telescope port.
7. Using scissors or monopoly hook cautery, the pleura is incised well anterior to the phrenic nerve, which is used as a reference point, at the lateral border of the left lobe of the thymus. The pink-yellow and lobular appearance of the thymus can be easily distinguished from the surrounding mediastinal fat (which is minimal in very young children).
8. Dissection of the thymus is performed en block and can be performed bluntly, with hook cautery or a fine energy device.
9. The inferior horn of the left lobe of the thymus is freed from the sternum anteriorly and the pericardium posteriorly.
10. The aortocaval groove is dissected free.
11. The right inferior horn is then gently pulled into the field and freed in a similar manner.
12. The arterial supply, originating mostly from left and right internal thoracic arteries to the superior pole of each lobe, is identified and divided (hook, energy device, clips).
13. The dissection is carried superiorly toward the thoracic inlet where smaller and larger veins (the great vein of Keynes), draining directly into the left brachiocephalic (innominate) vein, are identified (usually, there are between two and four thymic veins, which may be short). Those must be divided (clips, energy device) without injury to the innominate vein. This allows the superior extent of

the gland to be carefully mobilized from the thoracic inlet.

14. The intact gland is then removed through one of the port sites in a specimen bag.
15. The entire mediastinum is inspected carefully for hemostasis as well as to assure complete removal of the gland.
16. A rib block is performed under direct vision using dilute local anesthetic.
17. All ports are removed, the pneumothorax evacuated, and the port sites close.
18. Placing a chest tube is usually not necessary.

Robotic Thymectomy

1. The robotic procedure follows the same operative steps as above.
2. Two robotic 5-mm working trocars and an 8.5-mm robotic camera trocar are utilized. Due to the size of the ports, the robot is not used for infants or very small children.

Note These Variations

- Trocar placement may be adjusted depending on the anatomy and the size of the patient.
- If selective lung ventilation is employed, (valved) trocars may not need to be used.
- A right-sided approach may offer a better access to the thoracic inlet and the thymic veins, which drain into the innominate vein and need to be securely divided.
- Dissection with an energy device should only be performed in a safe distance from the phrenic nerve.
- Complete resection on the thymus in one piece should be commented on by the pathologist.

Template Operative Dictation

Preoperative Diagnosis *Myasthenia gravis/thymic mass*

Postoperative Diagnosis Same

Findings None

Procedure Performed *Left thoracoscopic/robotic thymectomy*

Anesthesia General anesthesia

Specimen Complete thymus en block

Drains None

Implants None

Estimated Blood Loss Minimal

Indications This is a/an ___ *-day/week/month/year*-old *male/female* with *myasthenia gravis/thymic mass* required thymectomy. *He/she* was deemed to be a suitable candidate for thymectomy.

Procedure in Detail Following satisfactory induction of anesthesia, the patient was placed on the right side in a right lateral 30-degree decubitus position supported with a bean bag and appropriately padded. *If* open *the patient is kept supine.* Timeouts were performed using both pre-induction and pre-incision safety checklists with participation of all present in the operative suite. These confirmed the correct patient, procedure, operative site, instrumentation, and additional critical information prior to the start of the procedure.

The chest was then prepped and draped in the usual sterile fashion, and a broad-spectrum antibiotic was given intravenously.

If open: *A sternotomy or transcervical incision is performed in standard fashion.*

If thoracoscopic: *All three trocars are placed along the submammary fold. The 5-mm camera port is placed in the anterior axillary line in the fourth intercostal space, and the two 5-mm working ports are placed slightly anterior and posterior to the telescope port.*

If robotic: *All three trocars are placed along the submammary fold. The 8.5-mm robotic camera port is placed in the anterior axillary line in the fourth intercostal space and the two 5-mm robotic working ports are placed slightly anterior and posterior to the telescope port.*

The mediastinum is then accessed through the left chest and a 30° telescope is used. The left phrenic nerve is identified as well as the thymus. Using monopoly hook cautery, the pleura is incised well anterior to the phrenic nerve in a safe distance at the lateral border of the left lobe of the thymus. The pink-yellow and lobular appearance of the thymus was easily distinguished from the small amount of surrounding mediastinal fat. Dissection of the thymus was performed en block bluntly and with hook cautery. The inferior horn of the left lobe of the thymus was freed from the sternum anteriorly and the pericardium posteriorly, and the aortocaval groove was dissected free. The right inferior horn was then gently pulled into the field and freed in a similar manner. The arterial supply of the thymus is identified and divided with hook cautery. The dissection was carried superiorly toward the thoracic inlet where several veins draining directly into the left innominate vein were identified. The larger veins were clipped toward the innominate vein, and then, all veins were divided with hook cautery. This allows the superior extent of the gland to be carefully mobilized from the thoracic inlet. After the thymus was dissected free completely, the intact gland was then removed through one of the port sites in a specimen bag. The specimen was sent to pathology labeled "complete thyroid gland en bloc" and the pathologist asked to comment in his report on complete resection. The entire mediastinum was inspected carefully for hemostasis and complete removal of the gland was, again, confirmed. *A rib block is then performed under direct vision using dilute local anesthetic.* All ports were removed, the pneumothorax evacuated, and the port sites close with absorbable sutures. Sterile dressings were placed.

A debriefing checklist was completed to share information critical to the postoperative care of the patient. The patient tolerated the procedure well, *was extubated in the operating room,* and was transported to the post-anesthesia care unit in stable condition.

Pulmonary Decortication (Open and MIS Approaches)

87

Ekene A. Onwuka and Christopher K. Breuer

Indications and Benefits

- Large multiloculated parapneumonic effusion or those with thick pleural peel.
- Uniloculated or multiloculated empyema failing to resolve with tube thoracostomy and antibiotics.
- Parapneumonic effusion or empyema with continued signs of infection with failure of adequate pulmonary drainage.
- Consolidated hemothorax.
- Lung entrapment secondary to empyema with pleural rind or hemothorax.
- Benefits: Allows full expansion of lung after adhesiolysis and decortication, assists with infection control, and chest tubes can be optimally placed under direct vision.

Risks and Alternatives

- Standard risks (bleeding, infection, need for additional procedures, risks of anesthesia)
- Injury to adjacent structures (pulmonary artery, pulmonary vein, intercostal bundle, aorta, diaphragm, liver, spleen)
- Persistent air leak following decortication
- Alternatives: Interventional radiology-guided placement of drains, tube thoracostomy with instillation of fibrinolytic agents

Essential Steps

1. Lung isolation by anesthesia (either via dual lumen endotracheal tube or endoscopically placed bronchial blocker)
2. Safe entry into thoracic cavity (either via thoracotomy incision for open technique, or thoracoscopic port sites for VATS)
3. Release of adhesions between lung and chest wall. Ensure all lobes mobilized
4. Aspiration of pleural fluid for culture
5. Drainage of any loculated collections
6. Chest tube placement under direct visualization
7. Closure

Note These Variations

- Procedure can be done with intercostal nerve block at end of case for pain control

E. A. Onwuka
The Ohio State University Wexner Medical Center, Department of General Surgery, Columbus, OH, USA

C. K. Breuer (✉)
Nationwide Children's Hospital, Department of Pediatric Surgery, Columbus, OH, USA
e-mail: christopher.breuer@nationwidechildrens.org

D. J. Papandria et al. (eds.), *Operative Dictations in Pediatric Surgery*,
https://doi.org/10.1007/978-3-030-24212-1_87

Template Operative Dictation (Open)

Preoperative Diagnosis *Right/left empyema/ loculated effusion/hemothorax*

Postoperative Diagnosis Same as preoperative diagnosis

Findings ___

Procedure(s) Performed *Right/left* thoracotomy, total pulmonary decortication, intercostal nerve blocks

Anesthesia General

Specimen None

Drains ___Fr Argyle chest tube × 2

Implants None

Estimated Blood Loss ___ml

Indications This is a/an ___ *-day/week/month/ year*-old *male/female* with *left/right* empyema/ *loculated effusion/hemothorax. He/she* was deemed to be a suitable candidate for thoracotomy and decortication.

Procedure in Detail Following satisfactory induction of anesthesia, the patient was placed in the *right/left* lateral decubitus position and appropriately supported with a bean bag. *His/her* arms and legs were appropriately oriented and pressure points padded. Timeouts were performed using both pre-induction and pre-incision safety checklists with participation of all present in the operative suite. These confirmed the correct patient, procedure, operative site, and additional critical information prior to the start of the procedure. Perioperative antibiotics were administered, and the *right/left* chest was then prepped and draped in the usual sterile fashion. The lung on the operative side was then isolated by anesthesia with the use of *a ___Fr dual-lumen endotracheal tube/ endoscopically deployed bronchial blocker*.

The skin was incised with a scalpel from the anterior to the posterior axillary line, just inferior to the scapula. The subcutaneous layer was divided with the Bovie electrocautery. The latissimus dorsi muscle was then also divided. The serratus anterior muscle was preserved. We entered the *right/left* thorax at the level of the *4th/5th/6th* intercostal space. We then divided the *4th/5th/6th* rib posteriorly with a linear bone cutter. A rib spreader was placed in the incision for exposure. The thoracic cavity was inspected to ensure that there were no entry injuries.

We started by dissecting the *right/left* lung off of the chest wall using the Bovie electrocautery. Once our lung was freed from adhesions, we then drained any loculated pockets of *pleural fluid/old blood*. Some fluid was aspirated and sent for culture. The fibrinous exudate on the pleural surface of the lung was debrided with an empty ring clamp and the Bovie electrocautery. Some of the fibrinous exudate was also sent for culture. The *right/left* thoracic cavity was then irrigated with ___ mL of saline solution. All lobes were completely mobilized at the conclusion of the decortication, and all pockets of fluid were completely drained. Posterior intercostal nerve blocks were performed from T-10 to T-3 using an injection of ___.

An anterior and a posterior ___ Fr chest tube was placed in the 8th intercostal space and secured with a ___ suture. The *right/left* lung was then re-expanded under direct vision. The thoracotomy incision was closed in multiple layers. A total of ___ intercostal #1 Vicryl sutures were placed to re-approximate the ___ and ___ ribs. The serratus anterior and latissimus dorsi muscle layers were re-approximated with a running ___ Vicryl suture. The adipose tissue layer was re-approximated with a *running/interrupted* ___ Vicryl suture. The skin was re-approximated using a running ___ Vicryl suture. A sterile dressing was placed on the incision, and the chest tube was connected to the Pleur-evac system.

Upon completion of the procedure, a debriefing checklist was completed to share information critical to the postoperative care of the patient. The patient tolerated the procedure well, was extubated in the operating room, and was transported to the post-anesthesia care unit in stable condition thereafter. Surgical counts were correct × ___.

Template Operative Dictation (Thoracoscopic)

Preoperative Diagnosis *Right/left empyema/loculated effusion/hemothorax*

Postoperative Diagnosis Same as preoperative diagnosis

Findings ___

Procedure(s) Performed Video-assisted thoracoscopic surgery (VATS), total pulmonary decortication, intercostal nerve blocks

Anesthesia General

Specimen *Right/left upper/middle/lower* wedge resection

Drains ___Fr Argyle chest tube × 2

Implants None

Estimated Blood Loss ___ml

Indications This is a/an ___ *-day/week/month/year*-old *male/female* with a *left/right* empyema/*loculated effusion/hemothorax. He/she* was deemed to be a suitable candidate for thoracoscopic total pulmonary decortication.

Procedure in Detail Following satisfactory induction of anesthesia, the patient was placed in the *right/left* lateral decubitus position and appropriately supported with a bean bag. *His/her* arms and legs were appropriately oriented and pressure points padded. Timeouts were performed using both pre-induction and pre-incision safety checklists with participation of all present in the operative suite. These confirmed the correct patient, procedure, operative site, and additional critical information prior to the start of the procedure. Perioperative antibiotics were administered, and the *right/left* chest was then prepped and draped in the usual sterile fashion. The lung on the operative side was then isolated by anesthesia with the use of *a ___Fr dual-lumen endotracheal tube/endoscopically deployed bronchial blocker.*

A/an ___ mm incision was placed at the level of the *seventh/eight* interspace in the *mid-/posterior* axillary line and carried down to the fascia and over the rib using blunt dissection with a hemostat. The pleural space was entered, a/an ___ mm trocar was placed, and CO_2 insufflation initiated to a pressure of 8 mmHg. The thoracoscope was introduced into the chest, and a cursory survey of the thoracic contents revealed no traumatic sequelae of access and confirmation of collapse of the operative lung. Local anesthetic infiltration and stab incisions were then placed at ___ additional trocar sites, followed by ___ mm trocars located in the ___ interspace in the ___ line. Trocars were introduced under thoracoscopic vision.

The fibrinous exudate on the pleural surface of the lung was debrided with an empty ring clamp. Some of the fibrinous exudate was sent for culture. Adhesions to the chest wall were taken down using a combination of blunt dissection and Bovie electrocautery. Any loculated collections of fluid were drained after aspirating a sample for culture. The thoracic cavity was irrigated with ___ mL of saline solution. All lobes were completely mobilized at the conclusion of the decortication, and all pockets of fluid were completely drained. Intercostal nerve blocks were performed from T-10 to T-3 with ___.

Anterior and posterior ___ Fr chest tubes were placed through the port sites and, under direct visualization, directed toward the apex. The lung was then slowly re-inflated by anesthesia, and thoracoscopy was terminated. The chest tubes were secured to the skin using ___ and hooked to a Pleur-evac. The port sites were closed at the fascia using *running/interrupted ___ vicryl, and the skin at all port sites* closed with ___. All sites were then dressed with Steri-strips.

Upon completion of the procedure, a debriefing checklist was completed to share information critical to the postoperative care of the patient. The patient tolerated the procedure well, *was extubated in the operating room*, and was transported to the post-anesthesia care unit in stable condition thereafter. Surgical counts were correct × ___.

88 Exploratory Laparotomy, Right/Left Nephrectomy, Paraaortic/Paracaval Lymph Node Dissection

Sara A. Mansfield and Jennifer H. Aldrink

Indications

- Wilms tumor or other renal mass

Risks

- Standard risks (bleeding, infection, need for additional procedures, risks of anesthesia)
- Injury to adjacent structures (IVC, bowel, liver, spleen)
- Bowel obstruction
- Recurrence

Note These Variations

- Children with bilateral renal masses may receive neoadjuvant chemotherapy prior to local control with nephron-sparing surgery.
- Since many children with Wilms tumor will receive adjuvant chemotherapy, placement of a central venous access device should be considered at the time of nephrectomy. Reference to current treatment protocols are encouraged.
- Thrombus that extends into the vena cava can often be withdrawn from the IVC by opening the IVC after gaining proximal and distal control.
- If tumor invades the colon or other organs except adrenal gland, initial biopsy only is indicated.
- Occasionally a small portion of the diaphragm is removed en bloc with the tumor, or the diaphragm may be inadvertently entered. This can usually be repaired primarily. The resultant pneumothorax can be evacuated prior to closure of the diaphragm defect with a tube under saline irrigation and a Valsalva maneuver, thereby eliminating the need for a chest tube in most cases.

Template Operative Dictation

Preoperative Diagnosis *Right/left* renal mass

Postoperative Diagnosis Same as preoperative diagnosis

Findings Describe intraoperative findings, specifically presence of peritoneal metastases,

S. A. Mansfield
The Ohio State University Wexner Medical Center, Department of General Surgery, Columbus, OH, USA

J. H. Aldrink (✉)
Nationwide Children's Hospital, The Ohio State University College of Medicine, Division of Pediatric Surgery, Department of Surgery, Columbus, OH, USA
e-mail: Jennifer.Aldrink@nationwidechildrens.org

D. J. Papandria et al. (eds.), *Operative Dictations in Pediatric Surgery*,
https://doi.org/10.1007/978-3-030-24212-1_88

presence or absence of renal vein and/or IVC thrombus, presence or absence of liver nodules

Procedure(s) Performed Exploratory laparotomy, right/left nephrectomy, paraaortic/paracaval lymph node dissection

Anesthesia General endotracheal

Specimen *Left/right* kidney, paraaortic/paracaval lymph nodes

Estimated Blood Loss ___

Indications This is a/an ___ *-day/week/month/year*-old *male/female* with an abdominal mass. Imaging revealed a *left/right* kidney mass concerning for a Wilms tumor. *He/she* was deemed to be a suitable candidate for exploratory laparotomy, right/left nephrectomy, paraaortic/paracaval lymph node dissection.

Procedure in Detail After informed consent was obtained, the patient was taken to the operating room and placed supine on the operating table. After the induction of general endotracheal anesthesia, a Foley catheter was placed, epidural catheter was placed, and appropriate IVs and monitoring lines were placed. All pressure points were carefully padded. A bump or roll was placed under the *right/left* flank to elevate the retroperitoneum. The abdomen was prepped and draped in the usual sterile fashion. A surgical timeout was performed. The patient was given preoperative antibiotics.

A *left/right supraumbilical transverse abdominal incision/midline laparotomy/subcostal incision* was created with a 15 blade scalpel. Cautery was used to dissect through subcutaneous tissues and down through the fascial layers. The abdomen was entered without incident. There *was/was no* ascites (describe nature of ascites). The mass was immediately apparent with the *left/right* colon draped over it. A thorough examination of the abdomen revealed *no evidence of peritoneal nodules and no evidence of liver metastases*. We began by mobilizing the *left/right* colon medially with care taken to preserve the thinned out mesentery. Once appropriate exposure of the mass was performed, the lateral attachments to the kidney were divided using both *cautery/LigaSure*™ and blunt dissection as applicable. The posterior attachments were likewise dissected from the retroperitoneum and psoas muscle. The dissection continued superiorly, separating the kidney/mass from the *liver/spleen* using cautery or ligasure as applicable. The adrenal gland was identified and was *carefully separated from the mass and preserved /was intimately adherent to the mass and removed en bloc*. The ureter was identified at the inferomedial aspect of the kidney, and a vessel loop was placed around this for identification. The medial dissection was carefully performed, and the *right/left* renal artery and vein were identified. These were encircled with vessel loops. The *right/left* renal vein was carefully palpated. *There was no evidence of tumor thrombus within the renal vein or IVC*. The artery was ligated with ___ *suture ligature/___ ties* on the proximal and distal ends, and divided. *Titanium hemoclips were placed for additional hemostasis*. The renal vein was similarly ligated with ___ *suture ligature/___ ties* and divided. The ureter was then dissected down to the pelvic brim and ligated this with ___. *No tumor was palpated within the ureter*. The ureter was divided sharply. The specimen was sent *fresh/frozen* to Pathology for analysis. *Preliminary report was Wilms tumor*.

We then turned our attention to *paraaortic/paracaval* lymph node dissection. Lymph nodes were sequentially dissected from the renal hilar region to the bifurcation using cautery and hemoclips as appropriate. Additional lymph nodes within the IVC and *paraaortic/paracaval* region were sampled and sent to pathology. Hemostasis was excellent. The bowel was placed in its normal anatomic position. The colon mesentery was re-inspected and found to be intact. The fascia was closed in two layers with running ___ PDS. Scarpa's layer was closed with ___-0 Vicryl. Deep dermal layer was closed with ___-0 Vicryl. The skin was closed with ___-0 Vicryl in a running, subcuticular fashion. *Steri-Strips/Dermabond* and sterile dressings were applied. All sponge, instrument, and needle counts were correct at the end of the case.

Upon completion of the procedure, a debriefing checklist was completed to share information critical to the postoperative care of the patient. The patient tolerated the procedure well, *was extubated in the operating room*, and was transported to the post-anesthesia care unit in stable condition thereafter.

89 Abdominal Resection of Neuroblastoma

Sara A. Mansfield and Jennifer H. Aldrink

Indications and Benefits

- Low-risk neuroblastomas
- Intermediate- and high-risk neuroblastomas in combination with multimodal therapy and based on resectability on imaging (image-defined risk factors)
- Benefits: Local control of tumor

Risks and Alternatives

- Standard risks (bleeding, infection, injury to adjacent structures, need for additional procedures, risks of anesthesia).
- Chylous ascites from extensive retroperitoneal dissection resulting in lymphatic leakage.
- Tumor manipulation may rarely result in intraoperative catecholamine extravasation resulting in significant alterations in hemodynamics.
- Postoperative intussusception, postoperative small bowel obstruction.
- Recurrence.
- Alternatives: Multiagent chemotherapy is the basis of all treatment regimens for advanced stage and high-risk neuroblastomas.

Note These Variations

- Because of the heterogeneity of disease presentation and tumor stage, no single treatment regimen can be used to effectively treat all neuroblastomas. Patient management should be individualized and protocol based using risk-group stratifications and the biologic characteristics of the tumor as predictors of outcome.
- For tumors involving major midline vessels, particularly on or near the celiac axis and diaphragm, a thoracoabdominal approach may allow for maximal safe exposure.
- Smaller localized adrenal or pelvic neuroblastomas may be safely approached laparoscopically, at the discretion of the surgeon.
- Preservation of vital structures (i.e., kidney, spleen) should be achieved whenever possible during resection of these tumors.
- Resection of neuroblastoma achieves R1; margins are invariably positive given the

S. A. Mansfield
The Ohio State University Wexner Medical Center, Department of General Surgery, Columbus, OH, USA

J. H. Aldrink (✉)
Nationwide Children's Hospital, The Ohio State University College of Medicine, Division of Pediatric Surgery, Department of Surgery,
Columbus, OH, USA
e-mail: Jennifer.Aldrink@nationwidechildrens.org

D. J. Papandria et al. (eds.), *Operative Dictations in Pediatric Surgery*,
https://doi.org/10.1007/978-3-030-24212-1_89

infiltrative nature. On occasion, it may be necessary to split the tumor to achieve improved visualization. This does not alter the patient's stage in any way.
- Goal of surgery is complete gross total resection.

Template Operative Dictation (Open)

Preoperative Diagnosis Neuroblastoma

Postoperative Diagnosis Same as preoperative diagnosis

Findings Same as postoperative diagnosis

Procedure(s) Performed Abdominal resection of neuroblastoma

Anesthesia *General/regional/procedural sedation*

Specimen {Specimen}

Estimated Blood Loss ___

Indications This is a/an ___ *-day/week/month/year*-old *male/female* with *Known neuroblastoma who now presents for surgial resection following neoadjuvant chemotherapy. An adrenal mass who presents for resection. A pelvic mass who presents for* resection. A pelvic mass who presents for resection. He/she was deemed to be a suitable candidate for abdominal resection of neuroblastoma.

Procedure in Detail Following satisfactory induction of anesthesia, the patient was placed in supine and appropriately padded. Appropriate antibiotics were administered. A Foley catheter was placed. Appropriate hemodynamic monitoring devices were ensured. Timeouts were performed using both pre-induction and pre-incision safety checklists with participation of all present in the operative suite. These confirmed the correct patient, procedure, operative site, and additional critical information prior to the start of the procedure. The abdomen was then prepped and draped in the usual sterile fashion.

A *midline/transverse abdominal/subcostal/chevron/thoracoabdominal* incision was made with a 15-blade scalpel. The subcutaneous tissue was divided with electrocautery, followed by the fascia and peritoneum. The abdomen was then explored. *There was no evidence of metastatic disease.* The primary tumor was found to be ___. Regional lymph nodes were noted to be ___.

Tedious dissection of the tumor was then performed, with great care taken to preserve the vascular structures. Hemostasis was achieved with *hemoclips/electrocautery*. Planes between {adjacent structures} were developed. *Describe actual location, structures involved, isolation of vascular structures, operative findings. Gross total resection of all visible and palpable tumor was performed. Comment on any intraoperative frozen pathology analysis as required.*

Upon completion of the procedure, a debriefing checklist was completed to share information critical to the postoperative care of the patient. The patient tolerated the procedure well, *was extubated in the operating room*, and was transported to the post-anesthesia care unit in stable condition thereafter.

90 Right/Left Thoracotomy/ Thoracoscopy, Resection of Paraspinal Thoracic Neuroblastoma

Sara A. Mansfield and Jennifer H. Aldrink

Indications and Benefits

- Thoracic mass, suspected neuroblastic in origin

Risks and Alternatives

- Standard risks (bleeding, infection, need for additional procedures, risks of anesthesia)
- Injury to adjacent structures (upper cervical nerve roots resulting in Horner syndrome, vascular structures, thoracic duct, phrenic nerve)
- Recurrence

Template Operative Dictation (Open)

Preoperative Diagnosis *Right/left* paraspinal/thoracic mass

S. A. Mansfield
The Ohio State University Wexner Medical Center, Department of General Surgery, Columbus, OH, USA

J. H. Aldrink (✉)
Nationwide Children's Hospital, The Ohio State University College of Medicine, Division of Pediatric Surgery, Department of Surgery, Columbus, OH, USA
e-mail: Jennifer.Aldrink@nationwidechildrens.org

Postoperative Diagnosis Same as preoperative diagnosis

Findings Describe intraoperative findings

Procedure(s) Performed Right/left thoracotomy/thoracoscopy, resection of paraspinal thoracic neuroblastoma

Anesthesia *General/regional/procedural sedation*

Specimen *Right/left* paraspinal/thoracic mass

Drains ___ chest tube

Estimated Blood Loss ___

Indications This is a/an ___ *-day/week/month/year*-old *male/female* with a paraspinal mass suspicious for a neuroblastic tumor. He/she was deemed to be a suitable candidate for right/left thoracotomy/thoracoscopy, resection of paraspinal thoracic mass.

Procedure in Detail After verifying informed consent, the patient was taken to the operating room and placed supine upon the operating table. Following satisfactory induction of anesthesia, lung isolation was achieved with the use of a double lumen endotracheal tube/right/left mainstem positioning. The patient was placed in *right/left*

D. J. Papandria et al. (eds.), *Operative Dictations in Pediatric Surgery*, https://doi.org/10.1007/978-3-030-24212-1_90

lateral position and appropriately padded. Timeouts were performed using both pre-induction and pre-incision safety checklists with participation of all present in the operative suite. These confirmed the correct patient, procedure, operative site, and additional critical information prior to the start of the procedure. The *right/left* chest was then prepped and draped in the usual sterile fashion.

For thoracotomy: A transverse incision using a 15-blade scalpel was made along the rib just inferior to the tip of the scapula. Dissection was carried down through the skin and subcutaneous tissues, and then, flaps were raised above the muscle layer. The muscles were then split along their fibers, separating the latissimus from the serratus anterior. A submuscular plane was then developed. With the scapula gently retracted, the chest wall was palpated for the optimal entry point. The *fourth/fifth* intercostal space was then entered under direct visualization and following the achievement of single lung ventilation. Once the thoracic space was entered uneventfully, an appropriately sized Finochietto retractor was then placed, taking care to protect the skin. *A second retractor was placed to retract the muscle and soft tissues from the wound.*

For thoracoscopy: An incision was made using a 15-blade scalpel just inferior to the tip of the scapula. Following the achievement of single lung ventilation, the thoracic cavity was entered bluntly with a hemostat. A *5/10-mm trocar/port* was placed through this incision, and a 5-mm camera was inserted. The thoracic cavity was perused. No injury from entrance was identified. CO2 was insufflated to acheive a pressure of 3 mmHg. The mass was visible in the expected location. *Two/three* additional ports were placed under direct visualization and following the infiltration of local anesthetic (*describe locations*).

For both approaches: The paraspinal mass was noted ___. Dissection began by taking the pleura from around the edges of the mass circumferentially using electrocautery. A top-down and lateral mobilization approach was then performed, taking care to cauterize and LigaSure vascular structures as the mass was taken from the posterior chest wall. With the mass somewhat mobilized, the medial vascular structures were carefully dissected free from the tumor. *Describe the association with vital structures and the dissection.* Once the mass was completely resected, it was placed within an endoscopic retreival bag and removed. The specimen was sent as a *fresh/frozen* specimen to pathology for analysis. *For thoracoscopy, the tumor as placed within an endocatch bag and removed through one of the incisions. This required enlargement of the incision for tumor extraction.* The tumor bed was made hemostatic by use of electrocautery as needed. *No lymphadenopathy was noted/lymph nodes were identified and removed sequentially using cautery and clips as appropriate.* No lymphatic leak was identified. *Thrombin spray was applied to the wound bed.* A ___Fr straight Argyle chest tube was then placed through the sixth intercostal space and laid posterolaterally. It was secured to the skin using __*–0 Prolene/nylon/Ethibond* suture. The chest wall was then closed as follows: **For thoracotomy:** __*-0* Vicryl pericostal sutures, __*-0* Vicryl interrupted sutures to close the muscle layers back together, and interrupted __*-0 Vicryl* sutures in the Scarpa fascia. The deep dermis was closed with interrupted __*-0 Vicryl* sutures, and a __*-0* running *Vicryl* was used subcuticularly to close the skin. **For thoracoscopy:** __*-0 Vicryl* was used to close the fascia of 10-mm port site. All skin incisions were closed using __*-0 Vicryl suture.* Mastisol and Steri-Strips and dry sterile dressing applied as well as a chest tube dressing. Chest tube was placed to −20 cm of suction on the Pleur-evac. The patient tolerated the procedure well, was rolled supine, and was extubated in the operating room. CXR is pending at the time of this dictation.

91 Right/Left Thoracoscopy/Thoracotomy, Resection of Pulmonary Nodule(s)

Sara A. Mansfield and Jennifer H. Aldrink

Indications and Benefits

- Isolated or oligometastatic sarcoma
- Persistent pulmonary nodules in the setting of Wilms tumor, hepatoblastoma, or other malignancy

Risks

- Standard risks (bleeding, infection, need for additional procedures, risks of anesthesia)
- Injury to pulmonary vasculature, injury to lung parenchyma
- Persistent air leak
- Chylous effusion

Note These Variations

- Lobectomy may be required for lesions close to the hilum or for multiple lesions within a single lobe.
- Preoperative wire or other localization techniques by radiology may be beneficial in locating smaller or deeper nodules.

S. A. Mansfield
The Ohio State University Wexner Medical Center, Department of General Surgery, Columbus, OH, USA

J. H. Aldrink (✉)
Nationwide Children's Hospital, The Ohio State University College of Medicine, Division of Pediatric Surgery, Department of Surgery, Columbus, OH, USA
e-mail: Jennifer.Aldrink@nationwidechildrens.org

Template Operative Dictation (Open)

Preoperative Diagnosis Metastatic ___ to the lung

Postoperative Diagnosis Same as preoperative diagnosis

Findings Describe number and location of each nodule removed, if possible

Procedure(s) Performed *Right/left thoracoscopy/thoracotomy*, resection of pulmonary nodule(s)

Anesthesia *General/regional/procedural sedation*

Specimen {Specimen}

Drains ___ Fr chest tube

Estimated Blood Loss ___

Indications This is a/an ___-*day/week/month/year*-old *male/female* with an *intrapleural mass/pulmonary metastases* in the *right/left* chest. *He/*

D. J. Papandria et al. (eds.), *Operative Dictations in Pediatric Surgery*,
https://doi.org/10.1007/978-3-030-24212-1_91

she was deemed to be a suitable candidate for *thoracoscopy/thoracotomy* and resection of pulmonary nodule(s).

Procedure in Detail The patient was brought to the operating room and laid in supine position. Following satisfactory induction of anesthesia, a double-lumen endotracheal tube for single-lung ventilation/the endotracheal tube positioned deep in the *right/left* mainstem bronchus and accurate placement confirmed with bronchoscopy. Appropriate hemodynamic monitors and lines were placed. Preoperative antibiotics were administered. The patient was placed in *right/left* lateral position with flexion, and all pressure points were appropriately padded. Timeouts were performed using both pre-induction and pre-incision safety checklists with participation of all present in the operative suite. These confirmed the correct patient, procedure, operative site, and additional critical information prior to the start of the procedure. The chest was then prepped and draped in the usual sterile fashion.

If open: A posterolateral thoracotomy incision was made using a 15-blade scalpel approximately 1 cm inferior to the scapula tip. Electrocautery was utilized to dissect through the subcutaneous tissues down to the chest wall muscular fascia. Subcutaneous flaps were created above the fascial plans both superiorly and inferiorly with electrocautery. Using a muscle sparing approach, dissection continued to the chest wall. The scapula was bluntly but gently lifted with the aid of a retractor, and the ribs counted to allow for accurate entrance into the chest cavity through the *4th/5th/6th* intercostal space. Single-lung ventilation was established.

If thoracoscopic: After single-lung ventilation was established, an incision was made using a 15-blade scalpel, approximately 1–2 cm inferior to the scapula tip. A hemostat was used to gain entrance bluntly into the thoracic cavity, and a 5-mm trocar was placed through this incision. A 5-mm 30-degree camera was placed through this trocar, and the thoracic cavity was perused. No injury was identified upon entrance. *Additional 5/10-mm ports were placed ___.*

The nodule was *visually identified/palpated*. It was located ___.

If stapled resection: A wedge resection of the tumor was performed with a *30/45/60* mm ___ *load* of the linear stapler cutter. A total of __ loads were used.

If nonstapled resection: A wedge resection of the tumor was performed using cautery dissection followed by repair of the defect with __-0 *PDS* suture in a *running locking/interrupted* fashion.

The specimen was placed in a retrieval bag and removed through the 10-mm port. The staple line was re-examined and found to be hemostatic. Both lungs were then ventilated and filled normally without evidence of an air leak. A ___ Fr chest tube was inserted into the *inferior port site/a separate stab incision* and positioned posterolaterally toward the apex. This was secured to the skin using ___ *Prolene/nylon* suture. Ports were removed under direct visualization. The 10-mm port site was closed with 3-0 vicryl in the fascial layer. *The skin of all port sites was closed using ___suture.* The chest wall was then closed as follows:

__*-0* Vicryl pericostal sutures, __*-0* Vicryl interrupted sutures to reapproximate the muscle layers, interrupted ___-0 Vicryl sutures in the Scarpa fascia, __*-0* vicryl in the deep dermis, and a ___-0 running Vicryl in a subcuticular fashion to close the skin. Mastisol, Steri-Strips, and dry sterile dressing applied as well as a chest tube dressing. Chest tube was placed to −20 cm of suction on the Pleur-evac.

Upon completion of the procedure, a debriefing checklist was completed to share information critical to the postoperative care of the patient. The patient tolerated the procedure well, *was extubated in the operating room*, and was transported to the post-anesthesia care unit in stable condition thereafter.

92 Adrenalectomy (Open and MIS Approaches)

Sara A. Mansfield and Jennifer H. Aldrink

Indications and Benefits

- Neuroblastic tumor (ganglioneuroma, ganglioneuroblastoma, localized neuroblastoma)
- Functional adrenal cortical adenoma
- Adrenal cortical carcinoma
- Pheochromocytoma
- Other adrenal mass
- Benefits:
  - Resolution steroid hypersecretion or catecholamine overproduction
  - Resection of malignancy

Risks

- Standard risks (bleeding, infection, need for additional procedures, risks of anesthesia)
- Injury to adjacent structures (***If left:*** spleen, distal pancreas, stomach; ***if right:*** injury to right hepatic vein or inferior vena cava)
- Diaphragmatic injury leading to pneumothorax
- Injury to renal hilar vessels
- Tumor rupture with spillage and seeding
- Bleeding from large raw surface in the retroperitoneum or from accessory lumbar veins

Essential Steps

1. Preoperative optimization (e.g., hydration, electrolyte correct, blood pressure control, stress dose steroids if cortisol producing).
2. Supine with bump or lateral positioning with appropriate padding.
3. Visualization of the adrenal gland:
   (a) ***If left:*** Mobilize the splenic flexure of the colon, and if required mobilize the spleen and tail of pancreas.
   (b) ***If right:*** Mobilize the triangular ligament and elevate the right lobe of the liver, dissect the right border of the inferior vena cava.
4. Dissect retroperitoneal structures including Gerota's fascia, renal hilum, and paraaortic or paracaval space.
5. Identify, secure, and divide the adrenal vein.
6. If tumor is secretory, minimize instrumentation of the gland until vein ligation.

S. A. Mansfield
The Ohio State University Wexner Medical Center, Department of General Surgery, Columbus, OH, USA

J. H. Aldrink (✉)
Nationwide Children's Hospital, The Ohio State University College of Medicine, Division of Pediatric Surgery, Department of Surgery, Columbus, OH, USA
e-mail: Jennifer.Aldrink@nationwidechildrens.org

D. J. Papandria et al. (eds.), *Operative Dictations in Pediatric Surgery*,
https://doi.org/10.1007/978-3-030-24212-1_92

Note These Variations

- Local extension or invasion, concern for malignancy particularly with lymph node involvement, large neoplasms, major vascular invasion, or extensive adhesions from prior abdominal procedures are relative contraindications to a minimally invasive approach.
- If the spleen and pancreas cannot be mobilized due to malignant involvement from an adrenal tumor, then the spleen and distal pancreas may need to be removed en bloc.
- Large malignant tumors on the right may require en bloc resection of a liver segment (segment VIII) and possibly the kidney.
- If adrenalectomy done for adrenal cortical carcinoma, a paraaortic/paracaval lymph node dissection should also be done.
- For patients who have had extensive abdominal procedures who are not laparoscopic candidates and in whom an anterior approach would be difficult due to adhesions, an open posterior approach is an option. However, a posterior approach should not be utilized for large tumors with local invasion.

Template Operative Dictation

Preoperative Diagnosis *Adrenal mass/pheochromocytoma/functional adrenal tumor/neuroblastic tumor/adrenal carcinoma*

Postoperative Diagnosis Same as preoperative diagnosis

Findings Same as postoperative diagnosis/describe findings

Procedure(s) Performed Adrenalectomy

Anesthesia *General/regional/procedural sedation*

Specimen {Specimen}

Estimated Blood Loss ___

Indications This is a/an ___ *-day/week/month/year*-old *male/female* with *adrenal mass/pheochromocytoma/functional adrenal tumor/neuroblastic tumor/adrenal carcinoma.* He/she was deemed to be a suitable candidate for adrenalectomy.

Procedure in Detail Following satisfactory induction of anesthesia, monitoring lines and a Foley catheter were placed. The patient was placed in ***if laparoscopic:*** *left/right semilateral position or lateral position* and ***if open:*** supine with bump under *right/left* side to allow slight medial rotation. The patient was appropriately padded along all pressure points. Timeouts were performed using both pre-induction and pre-incision safety checklists with participation of all present in the operative suite. These confirmed the correct patient, procedure, operative site, and additional critical information prior to the start of the procedure. *Appropriate antibiotics were administered.* The abdomen was then prepped and draped in the usual sterile fashion.

If laparoscopic: The abdomen was approached under direct vision using *an open cut-down/Veress needle* at the *umbilicus/half way between the anterior iliac spine and the umbilicus.* A 5-mm-port was placed, CO_2 was insufflated to achieve pneumoperitoneum of 15 mmHg, and a 5-mm, 30-degree laparoscope was inserted. The abdomen was perused, and no injuries were identified from entry. Next, a *5-mm* working port was placed lateral to the initial port in the mid-axillary line; an additional 5-mm trocar was placed in the subxiphoid region for liver retraction. Lastly, a 5-mm working port was placed in the posterior axillary line.

If left: Exploration of the abdominal cavity laparoscopically was carried out followed by mobilization of the splenic flexure of the colon by incising the white line of Toldt using the *cautery/scissors/LigaSure™ device/harmonic scalpel.* Attention was then turned to the mobilization of the spleen. The splenorenal and retroperitoneal attachments of the spleen were divided with *electrocautery/scissors/LigaSure device/harmonic scalpel.*

This incision of the peritoneum was carried out to the level of the left diaphragm allowing visualization of the fundus of the stomach. Facilitated by the effect of gravity and the weight of the spleen, the spleen and tail of the pancreas were then rotated medially by gentle dissection of the loose areolar space between the pancreas and the retroperitoneum. Care was taken to avoid injury to the splenic vein during the course of this dissection.

At this point, the suprarenal tissue and its contents (adrenal gland and retroperitoneal fat) were visible. Gerota's fascia, the upper border of the left kidney, and the left renal hilum were then identified and dissected. Dissection of the left renal vein and its upper border led to the identification of the left adrenal vein which was dissected and divided using a *clip or energy device*. The dissection was then carried out along the medial aspect of the adrenal gland down to the level of the quadratus lumborum muscle in the retroperitoneum indicating complete removal of all the fat in the suprarenal space. *An accessory adrenal vein running along the medial aspect of the gland and draining into the phrenic vein was encountered and divided.* Using *electrocautery/energy device*, the retroperitoneal fat of the left suprarenal space was elevated off the superior pole of the left kidney. The dissection of all the suprarenal tissue was then completed in a stepwise fashion. The arterial supply of the left adrenal gland was controlled and divided as it was encountered along this dissection until the gland and its surrounding tissues were completely mobilized.

If right: Exploration of the abdominal cavity was carried out followed by mobilization of the triangular ligament of the liver and *elevation/rotation* of the right hepatic lobe medially using a *5-mm-curved tip retractor/liver retractor/laparoscopic kitner* and electrocautery to allow exposure of the IVC and the adrenal gland in the retroperitoneum. If needed, the hepatic flexure of the colon was mobilized and retracted inferior and medially.

Dissection of the right border of the IVC was then carried out by incising the peritoneal reflection overlying the suprarenal tissues along the right border of the IVC to the diaphragm using *hook electrocautery/energy device*. Care was taken not to injure the IVC or right hepatic vein in this dissection. Gentle dissection along the right border of the IVC led to the identification of the right adrenal vein, which was then *ligated and divided/secured with an endoscopic stapler with a vascular load, energy device, or clip*. The dissection along the right border of the IVC was then carried further posteriorly until reaching the quadratus lumborum muscle and then inferiorly until reaching the right renal hilum with clear identification of the right renal vein. The right suprarenal tissues were then dissected and removed en bloc. Using *electrocautery/energy device*, the retroperitoneal fat of the right suprarenal space was elevated off its superior attachments to the diaphragm, the superior pole of the right kidney, and gently dissected off the lateral abdominal wall. The posterior dissection was carried out to the level of the right quadratus lumborum muscle ensuring complete removal of all the adrenal gland and suprarenal tissue as one block. The arterial supply of the right adrenal gland was controlled and divided using an appropriate energy source, as it was encountered along this dissection. Care was taken not to injure any accessory right renal arteries. Care was also taken to avoid injury to the capsule of the adrenal gland.

Irrigation of the operative bed was then carried out with the confirmation of hemostasis. The adrenal gland and all surrounding fat were then placed in a specimen retrieval bag and extracted *after enlarging the umbilical/other port* via *a muscle-splitting incision*. The extraction site was then sutured closed in layers using an *-0 PDS/Vicryl___* stitch. Re-insufflation of the abdominal cavity was then carried out and hemostasis was confirmed. The trocars were removed under direct vision. The skin of all incisions was closed with ___*-0 Vicryl*. The patient tolerated the procedure well. There were no complications and blood loss was *minimal/__*. Instrument and sponge counts were correct. A debriefing checklist was completed to share information critical to postoperative care of the patient. The patient was extubated and returned to the post-anesthesia care unit in stable condition.

If open: The abdomen was approached via a standard *extended subcostal/transverse laparotomy/midline* incision. The incision was deepened through the skin and subcutaneous tissue. Scarpa's fascia was opened and the incision taken down to the level of the abdominal wall. Using electrocautery, the abdominal wall musculature was divided. The external, internal, and transversalis fascia were divided using electrocautery. Exploration of the abdominal cavity was then carried out with no evidence of metastatic disease noted.

If left: The splenic flexure and descending colon was mobilized along the white line of Toldt. The attachment of the omentum to the distal transverse was also divided using electrocautery, allowing access into the lesser sac to further facilitate the complete takedown of the splenic flexure. Once the splenic flexure of the colon was completely mobilized, the splenorenal and retroperitoneal attachments of the spleen were divided with electrocautery. The splenophrenic attachments were also divided and the spleen along with the tail of the pancreas rotated medially. Care was taken to avoid any injury to the splenic vein in the course of this dissection.

Once the splenic flexure of the colon, the tail of the pancreas, and the spleen were rotated medially, exposure of the adrenal gland in the retroperitoneum was achieved. Gerota's fascia, the upper border of the left kidney, and the left renal hilum were identified and dissected. Dissection of the left renal vein and its upper border lead to the identification of the left adrenal vein, which was doubly ligated and divided. Using *electrocautery/an appropriate energy device*, the retroperitoneal fat of the left suprarenal region was elevated of the superior pole of the left kidney and gently dissected off the lateral abdominal wall and then posteriorly off the left quadratus lumborum muscle. The arterial supply of the left adrenal gland was controlled and divided as it was encountered along this dissection. The cephalad attachments of the adrenal and retroperitoneal tissue to the left diaphragm were then divided. The left adrenal gland was then gently retracted laterally to allow for the completion of the medial dissection. The medial dissection was carried as far medially as possible to ensure complete gross total resection. Care was taken to avoid injury to the capsule of the adrenal gland. The medial dissection was carried out by removing all of the contents of the suprarenal region up to the paravertebral space. *If cancer: An en bloc dissection of the paraaortic/paracaval nodes was also carried out as part of the medial extent of the dissection of the suprarenal region.* The specimen was then removed en bloc.

Irrigation of the suprarenal region was carried out, and confirmation of hemostasis was achieved. The spleen and pancreatic tail were then allowed to return back to their normal anatomical position. Closure of the abdomen in layers was then carried out using a running *__-0 PDS/ Vicryl/___ stitch*, followed by re-approximation of Scarpa's fascia using *__-0 Vicryl*. *__-0 Vicryl* was used to reapproximate the deep dermal layer, and *__-0 Vicryl* was used to close the skin in a subcuticular fashion. The patient tolerated the procedure well. There were no complications, and the blood loss was minimal. The instrument and sponge count was correct. A debriefing checklist was completed to share information critical to postoperative care of the patient. The patient was extubated and returned to the recovery room in stable satisfactory condition.

If right: The triangular ligament of the liver was mobilized, and rotation of the right hepatic lobe medially allowed exposure of the IVC and of the adrenal gland in the retroperitoneum. The right colon was mobilized along the white line of Toldt and reflected medially to expose the duodenum, which was then Kocherized to expose the right adrenal gland and IVC. Dissection of the right border of the IVC was then carried out by incising the peritoneal reflection overlying the suprarenal tissue along the right border of the IVC up to the diaphragm. Care was taken not to injure the right hepatic vein. Gentle dissection along the right border of the IVC led to the identification of the right adrenal vein which was then ligated and divided. The dissection along the right border of the IVC was then carried further posteriorly until reaching the quadratus lumborum muscle and then inferiorly until reaching the right renal hilum.

The right suprarenal tissue was then dissected and removed as one block. Using *electrocautery/energy device*, the retroperitoneal fat of the right suprarenal lodge was elevated off the superior pole of the right kidney and gently dissected off the lateral abdominal wall, posteriorly off the right quadratus lumborum muscle, and superiorly off the diaphragm. The arterial supply of the right adrenal gland was controlled and divided as it was encountered along this dissection. Care was taken not to injure any accessory right renal arteries. Care was also taken to avoid injury to the capsule of the adrenal gland. *If cancer: An en bloc dissection of the paraaortic/ paracaval nodes was also carried out as part of the medial extent of the dissection of the suprarenal tissue. The specimen is then removed en bloc (when indicated for ACC).*

Irrigation of the suprarenal region was carried out, and confirmation of hemostasis was achieved. The spleen and pancreatic tail were then allowed to return back to their normal anatomical position. Closure of the abdomen in layers was then carried out using a running *__-0 PDS/ Vicryl/___ stitch*, followed by re-approximation of Scarpa's fascia using *__-0 Vicryl*. *__-0 Vicryl* was used to reapproximate the deep dermal layer, and *__-0 Vicryl* was used to close the skin in a subcuticular fashion. The patient tolerated the procedure well. There were no complications, and the blood loss was minimal. The instrument and sponge counts were correct. A debriefing checklist was completed to share information critical to postoperative care of the patient. The patient was extubated and was returned to the recovery room in stable satisfactory condition.

Wide Local Excision of Malignant Melanoma With or Without Sentinel Lymph Node Biopsy

93

Jennifer H. Aldrink

Indications and Benefits

- Melanoma
- Benefits: Potential for cure and local control of tumor, as well as accurate staging of the nodal basin for prognostic information

Risks and Alternatives

- Standard risks (bleeding, infection, injury to adjacent structures, need for additional procedures, risks of anesthesia)
- Lymphatic leak/seroma/lymphedema (if sentinel lymph node biopsy performed)
- Recurrence

Note These Variations

- Recommended margins should be followed as per the recommendations by the National Comprehensive Cancer Network guidelines (see https://www.nccn.org/professionals/physician_gls/pdf/melanoma.pdf).
- For appropriate lesions ($\geq$0.75 mm depth and clinically negative nodal basin; <0.75 mm with ulceration or other high-risk features), sentinel lymph node biopsy should be performed.
- Skin grafting or other coverage may be required if primary closure is not achievable.
- The specimen should be carefully oriented so that margins are able to be accurately assessed by the pathologist.
- Some surgeons utilize vital blue dye to identify sentinel lymph nodes, but this is not required.
- In general, the residual background counts following sentinel lymph node removal should be 10% or less than the counts obtained from the hottest removed node.

Template Operative Dictation (Open)

Preoperative Diagnosis Melanoma, *location*

Postoperative Diagnosis Same as preoperative diagnosis

Findings Same as postoperative diagnosis

Procedure(s) Performed Wide local excision of malignant melanoma *with sentinel lymph node biopsy*

J. H. Aldrink (✉)
Nationwide Children's Hospital, The Ohio State University College of Medicine, Division of Pediatric Surgery, Department of Surgery,
Columbus, OH, USA
e-mail: Jennifer.Aldrink@nationwidechildrens.org

D. J. Papandria et al. (eds.), *Operative Dictations in Pediatric Surgery*,
https://doi.org/10.1007/978-3-030-24212-1_93

Anesthesia *General/regional/procedural sedation*

Specimen {Specimen}

Estimated Blood Loss ___

Indications This is a/an ___*-day/week/month/year*-old *male/female* with a concerning skin lesion, biopsy of which demonstrated melanoma. He/she was deemed to be a suitable candidate for wide local excision of malignant melanoma with or without sentinel lymph node biopsy.

Procedure in Detail After verifying informed consent, the patient was taken to the operating room and placed supine on the operating table. *General endotracheal/laryngeal mask* anesthesia was induced. The *location* was then prepped and draped in the usual sterile fashion. A *1-cm/2-cm* margin was measured from the lesion in all directions. A *circular/elliptical* incision was then created using a 15-blade scalpel, and dissection was carried down with electrocautery to the level of the muscular fascia. The specimen was then removed from the deep layer using electrocautery after orienting the specimen appropriately with marking sutures. Once this was complete, the wound was made hemostatic and *a wound vac was applied/the wound was closed in multiple layers using __-0 vicryl/nylon/monocryl* suture. Sterile dressings were applied.

If sentinel lymph node biopsy is performed: Preoperatively radiotracer had been injected into the area of the lesion and *lymphoscintigraphy/SPECT CT* demonstrating uptake by a lymph node in the *location. Lymphazurin or other vital blue dye was injected into the subcutaneous tissues adjacent to the lesion.* A handheld gamma probe was used to identify an appropriate level incision which was made in the *location.* Dissection was taken down through the skin and subcutaneous tissues including scarpa's fascia using electrocautery. The gamma probe was used to localize a lymph node which was sequentially dissected from surrounding tissues, ligated at the hilum, and removed. The count on this after removal was ___ maximum on the gamma probe. *Additional nodes were identified of the following radioactive counts ___/no additional nodes were identified.* The specimens were passed off for pathology after labeling them independently as follows: ___. The wound was irrigated and made hemostatic with electrocautery. This wound was then closed using interrupted *__-0 Vicryl sutures* in the Scarpa's fascia, interrupted *__-0 Vicryl sutures* in the deep dermis, and a running *__-0 Vicryl suture.* Sterile dressings were applied.

Upon completion of the procedure, a debriefing checklist was completed to share information critical to the postoperative care of the patient. The patient tolerated the procedure well, *was extubated in the operating room*, and was transported to the post-anesthesia care unit in stable condition thereafter.

Right/Left Thyroid Lobectomy/Total

94

Sara A. Mansfield and Jennifer H. Aldrink

Indications and Benefits

- Thyroid nodule
- Thyroid cancer
- Grave's disease
- Toxic multinodular goiter
- Multiple endocrine neoplasia type II

Risks and Alternatives

- Standard risks (bleeding, infection, need for additional procedures, risks of anesthesia)
- Injury to adjacent structures (recurrent laryngeal nerve, external branch of the superior laryngeal nerve, vascular structures, trachea, parathyroid glands)
- Hypothyroidism
- Hypocalcemia (temporary or permanent)
- Hoarseness (temporary or permanent)
- Hematoma with airway compromise

Essential Steps

1. Develop subplatysmal flaps.
2. Divide the strap muscles in the midline.
3. Ligate and divide the middle thyroid vein.
4. Preserve the external branch of the superior laryngeal nerve.
5. Ligate and divide the superior pole vessels.
6. Mobilize the inferior pole of the thyroid.
7. Identify and preserve the recurrent laryngeal nerve.
8. Divide the inferior thyroid artery and branches distally.
9. Identify and preserve the superior and inferior parathyroid glands.
10. Dissect the thyroid free of the trachea.
11. Divide the thyroid lobe at the isthmus or continue to contralateral lobe if total thyroidectomy.

Note These Variations

- Intraoperative recurrent laryngeal nerve monitoring
- Drain placement

S. A. Mansfield
The Ohio State University Wexner Medical Center, Department of General Surgery, Columbus, OH, USA

J. H. Aldrink (✉)
Nationwide Children's Hospital, The Ohio State University College of Medicine, Division of Pediatric Surgery, Department of Surgery, Columbus, OH, USA
e-mail: Jennifer.Aldrink@nationwidechildrens.org

D. J. Papandria et al. (eds.), *Operative Dictations in Pediatric Surgery*,
https://doi.org/10.1007/978-3-030-24212-1_94

- Central neck lymph node dissection for appropriate patients
- Lateral cervical lymph node dissection for differentiated thyroid carcinoma and known nodal disease

Template Operative Dictation

Preoperative Diagnosis Thyroid nodule, thyroid malignancy, Graves disease, MEN2A/2B syndrome, goiter

Postoperative Diagnosis Same as preoperative diagnosis

Findings Same as postoperative diagnosis

Procedure(s) Performed Right/left thyroid lobectomy/total

Anesthesia General

Specimen *Thyroid lobe/thyroidectomy*

Drains {Drains}

Estimated Blood Loss ___

Indications This is a/an ___*-day/week/month/year*-old *male/female* with a thyroid nodule/maignancy/Grave's disease/goiter/MEN 2A/B syndrome. *He/she* was deemed to be a suitable candidate for right/left thyroid lobectomy/total.

Procedure in Detail Timeouts were performed using both pre-induction and pre-incision safety checklists to verify correct patient, procedure, site, and additional critical information prior to beginning the procedure. Following induction of general anesthesia *with a recurrent laryngeal nerve monitoring endotracheal tube*, both arms were tucked at the sides and all pressure points were padded. A roll was placed under the shoulders, and the patient was positioned in a modified beach chair position with the neck extended. The neck, chin, and superior chest were prepped and draped in a sterile fashion.

A/an ___ cm transverse cervical incision was made using a 15-blade scalpel, approximately two fingerbreadths superior to the sternal notch within a skin crease. This was carried down through the skin and subcutaneous tissues with electrocautery. The platysma was encountered and divided with cautery. Musculocutaneous flaps were created superiorly to the thyroid cartilage and inferiorly to the sternal notch using electrocautery. Gentle retractors were placed in the wound to aid in exposure. The strap muscles were divided in the midline with cautery and retracted laterally.

The *right/left* thyroid lobe was mobilized from its areolar attachments using blunt dissection and electrocautery. The thyroid was gently retracted medially, as the strap muscles were separated and retracted laterally. The thyroid gland was then gently retracted inferomedially. The superior pole vessels were identified and sequentially *ligated with __suture/divided energy device* close to the thyroid gland, with careful attention not to injure the external branch of the superior laryngeal nerve.

Using meticulous blunt dissection, and *with the aid of the NIMS monitoring device*, the recurrent laryngeal nerve was identified visually. This was gently pushed away from the thyroid gland. The inferior thyroid vessels were *ligated with ___ suture/ divided with energy device* ties and divided with great care to avoid injury to the recurrent laryngeal nerve. The superior and inferior parathyroid glands were identified and carefully mobilized off of the thyroid gland. The dissection was then continued medially. The trachea was exposed, and the thyroid was dissected medially from its attachments to the trachea up to the ligament of Berry using bipolar cautery. Dissection was extended to the isthmus, which was *suture ligated/divided with energy device.* The specimen was marked with a suture at the superior pole for orientation and handed off to be sent to pathology.

For total thyroidectomy, a similar procedure was carried out on the contralateral lobe. The recurrent laryngeal was identified and protected in a similar fashion. *The parathyroid glands were identified and preserved.* The specimen was marked and passed off the field for pathology.

The wound was copiously irrigated and hemostasis was achieved. *Topical hemostatic agents were applied to aid with hemostasis.* The strap muscles were reapproximated with interrupted *3-0 Vicryl* sutures. The platysma was reapproximated with interrupted *__-0 Vicryl* sutures. *Local anesthetic was injected subcutaneously.* The skin was reapproximated with a running *__-0 Vicryl* subcuticular suture. *Surgical skin adhesive/Steri-Strips* was placed over the incision.

The patient was extubated deep with the vocal cords in view using the C-MAC video laryngoscope. The cords were symmetric on this assessment, with good movement, consistent with intact function of the recurrent nerve. Upon completion of the procedure, a debriefing checklist was completed to share information critical to the postoperative care of the patient. The patient was extubated and taken to recovery in good condition.

95 Open and Percutaneous Dilation Tracheostomy

Joseph R. Esparaz and Charles J. Aprahamian

Indications and Benefits

- Emergency Airway
- A bridge to extubating during prolonged respiratory compromise
- Benefits: Obtaining emergent airway, reducing risk of airway compromise, and creating "secure" airway access

Risks and Alternatives

- Standard risks (bleeding, infection, need for additional procedures, and risks of anesthesia)
- Injury to adjacent structures, such as the innominate artery, the esophagus, strap muscles, and superficial jugular veins
- Post-procedure risk of inadvertent decannulation, loss of airway due to separation of trachea from airway appliance, airway stenosis, and cartilaginous tracheomalacia
- Alternatives: No intervention, open cricothyroidotomy (age appropriate), percutaneous cricothyroidotomy (age appropriate), and endotracheal intubation

J. R. Esparaz (✉)
University of Illinois College of Medicine at Peoria;
OSF Children's Hospital of Illinois, Department of Surgery, Peoria, IL, USA

C. J. Aprahamian
OSF Children's Hospital of Illinois,
Division of Pediatric Surgery, Department of Surgery,
Peoria, IL, USA

Note These Variations

- Open mature stoma tracheostomy
- Percutaneous dilation tracheostomy (age/size appropriate)

Open Tracheostomy

Preoperative Diagnosis Acute respiratory failure

Postoperative Diagnosis Same as preoperative diagnosis

Findings Same as postoperative diagnosis

Procedure(s) Performed Open tracheostomy

Anesthesia *General/regional/procedural sedation*

Specimen None

Drains None

Implants Institution-specific tracheostomy appliances

D. J. Papandria et al. (eds.), *Operative Dictations in Pediatric Surgery*,
https://doi.org/10.1007/978-3-030-24212-1_95

Estimated Blood Loss ___ mL

Indications This is a/an ___*-day/week/month/year*-old *male/female* with *acute respiratory failure* / *(other indication)*. *He/she* was deemed to be a suitable candidate for Open Tracheostomy.

Procedure in Detail Following satisfactory induction of anesthesia, the patient was placed in supine position with a shoulder roll placed to provide neck extension. Extremities were appropriately padded. Timeouts were performed using both preinduction and preincision safety checklists with participation of all present in the operative suite. These confirmed the correct patient, procedure, operative site, and additional critical information prior to the start of the procedure. The neck and chest were then prepped and draped in the usual sterile fashion.

We began by first identifying specific landmarks – cricoid cartilage, thyroid cartilage, and sternal notch. Next, a *vertical/horizontal* incision was made approximately one fingerbreadth cephalad to the sternal notch. Electrocautery dissection was used to help expose the strap muscles, avoiding the external jugular veins. Hemostasis was achieved during dissection. The midline raphe of the strap muscles was incised and continue dissection until trachea was encountered.

Discussion was had with anesthesia team prior to entering trachea, and oxygen was lowered accordingly. Second and third tracheal rings were identified. Monofilament suture was used to secure the tracheal ring medially and laterally and the ring was controlled with a hemostat. An 11-blade scalpel was used to open the trachea, and the endotracheal tube was identified. Anesthesiology team pulled back the endotracheal tube until just out of the field of vision.

[Choose One:]

If open tracheostomy – no formal stoma: The tracheal incision was enlarged by creating an *H-incision/U-incision/cruciate* incision. A tracheal dilator was used for exposure and a ___mm tracheostomy tube was placed into the tracheal defect. The balloon was inflated. The ventilator was connected to the tracheostomy appliance and end-tidal CO_2 was confirmed with anesthesiology team. The appliance was secured to the neck with tracheostomy ties as well as several interrupted ___/0 nylon sutures. Hemostasis was achieved.

If Option B – open mature stoma tracheostomy: The tracheal incision was enlarged into an *I-shaped/trapdoor* incision. Next, the cartilage flaps were sewn to the skin by multiple buried absorbable sutures. A ___mm tracheostomy tube was placed into the tracheal defect. The balloon was inflated. The ventilator was connected to the tracheostomy appliance and end-tidal CO_2 was confirmed with anesthesiology team. The appliance was secured to the neck with tracheostomy ties as well as several interrupted ___/0 nylon sutures. Hemostasis was achieved.

Upon completion of the procedure, a debriefing checklist was completed to share information critical to the postoperative care of the patient. Sponge, needle, and instrument count were performed and correct ×2. The patient tolerated the procedure well, was awakened, and was transported to the post-anesthesia care unit in stable condition thereafter.

Percutaneous Dilation Tracheostomy

Preoperative Diagnosis Acute respiratory failure

Postoperative Diagnosis Same as preoperative diagnosis

Findings Same as postoperative diagnosis

Procedure(s) Performed Percutaneous dilation tracheostomy

Anesthesia *General/regional/procedural sedation*

Specimen None

Drains None

Implants Institution-specific tracheostomy appliances

Estimated Blood Loss ___ mL

Indications This is a/an ___-year-old *male/female* with *acute respiratory failure*/ (*other indication*). *He/she* was deemed to be a suitable candidate for percutaneous dilation tracheostomy.

Procedure in Detail Following satisfactory induction of anesthesia, the patient was placed in supine position with a shoulder roll placed. Extremities were appropriately padded. Timeouts were performed using both preinduction and preincision safety checklists with participation of all present in the operative suite. These confirmed the correct patient, procedure, operative site, and additional critical information prior to the start of the procedure. The neck and chest were then prepped and draped in the usual sterile fashion.

We began by first identifying specific landmarks – cricoid cartilage, thyroid cartilage, and sternal notch. A _______ kit was used. Next, a *vertical/horizontal* incision was made approximately one fingerbreadth cephalad to the sternal notch. The endotracheal tube was pulled back under visualization with direct laryngoscopy until the balloon was seen at the vocal cords. Without additional dissection, the trachea was palpated, and a prefilled needle and syringe were placed inferior to the second tracheal ring in the midline. The needle was advanced while aspirating until air bubbles were identified. The wire was then advanced into the needle. A bronchoscope was inserted into the endotracheal tube identifying the wire was midline in the trachea and traveling caudad. Next, stepwise dilation occurred with the kit-specific dilators. A/an ___-mm tracheostomy tube was then placed over the wire. Both the wire and dilator were then removed. The balloon was inflated and a bronchoscope was inserted via the tracheostomy tube with identification of the carina, confirming placement. The ventilator was connected to the tracheostomy appliance and end-tidal CO_2 was confirmed with anesthesiology team. The appliance was secured to the neck with tracheostomy ties as well as several interrupted nylon sutures. Hemostasis was achieved. Lastly, the endotracheal tube was removed.

Upon completion of the procedure, a debriefing checklist was completed to share information critical to the postoperative care of the patient. The patient tolerated the procedure well, was awakened, and was transported to the post-anesthesia care unit in stable condition thereafter.

96 Cervical Lymph Node Biopsy

Michaela Kollisch-Singule and Jennifer Stanger

Indications and Benefits

- Persistent cervical lymphadenopathy >6 weeks duration
- Cervical lymph node >2 cm or multiples site of adenopathy
- Benefits: Diagnosis of cause of lymphadenopathy (benign, inflammatory/infectious, systemic disease, and malignancy)

Risks and Alternatives

- Standard risks (bleeding, infection, need for additional procedures, and risks of anesthesia)
- Injury to adjacent structures (spinal accessory nerve)
- Head/Neck lymphedema
- Alternatives: Continue observation/medical management, fine needle aspiration

M. Kollisch-Singule (✉)
SUNY Upstate Medical University, Department of General Surgery, Syracuse, NY, USA
e-mail: KolliscM@upstate.edu

J. Stanger
SUNY Upstate Medical University, Department of Pediatric Surgery, Syracuse, NY, USA

Essential Steps

1. Incision over the enlarged lymph node
2. Identify and remove lymph node
3. Ensure hemostasis
4. Close the incision

Note These Variations

- In cases where the lymph node is not palpable, consider the use of ultrasound-guided visualization of the lymph node.

Template Operative Dictation (Open)

Preoperative Diagnosis Enlarged level __ cervical lymph node biopsy

Postoperative Diagnosis Same as preoperative diagnosis

Findings Same as postoperative diagnosis

Procedure(s) Performed Cervical lymph node biopsy

Anesthesia *General and Local*

Specimen Level __ cervical lymph node

D. J. Papandria et al. (eds.), *Operative Dictations in Pediatric Surgery*,
https://doi.org/10.1007/978-3-030-24212-1_96

Drains *None/penrose drain*

Implants None

Estimated Blood Loss ___ mL

Indications This is a/an ___*-day/week/month/year*-old *male/female* who presents with cervical lymph node enlargement first noted __ weeks ago which has not regressed. The node was noted to be *soft/rubbery/firm, tender/nontender*, and *mobile/fixed.* He/she was deemed to be a suitable candidate for cervical lymph node biopsy. The risks and benefits of the procedure were described at length with the patient and guardians and their questions and concerns were addressed; consent was obtained.

Procedure in Detail Following satisfactory induction of anesthesia, the patient was placed in a supine position and appropriately padded. Timeouts were performed using both preinduction and preincision safety checklists with participation of all present in the operative suite. These confirmed the correct patient, procedure, operative site, and additional critical information prior to the start of the procedure. The *right/left* neck was extended and then prepped and draped in the usual sterile fashion.

The level __ lymph node *was/was not* palpable. {An ultrasound was used to help localize the lymph node.} An approximately 2–3-cm incision was made over the lymph node. The dissection was carried down through the deeper tissues with the use of electrocautery. The enlarged lymph node was identified and found to be *soft/firm/mobile/adherent/associated with matted lymph nodes* and approximately __ cm in size. The lymph node was grasped and released from surrounding attachments; lymphatic tributaries were identified and sealed with electrocautery. Care was taken to remove the lymph node in its entirety. The lymph node was subsequently passed off the table and sent *fresh / in formalin / in fetal calf serum / according to institutional protocol for handling lymph nodes* for pathologic analysis.

Hemostasis was achieved with electrocautery. __ mL of local anesthesia was infiltrated into the skin and subcutaneous tissues of the wound bed. {A/an __-inch Penrose drain was placed in the wound and *was/was not* secured at the level of the skin.} The wound was closed with interrupted __ sutures in the deep tissues and dermis. A running __ subcuticular suture was used to reapproximate the skin edges. *Dermabond/Mastisol and Steri-Strips* were placed over the incision.

Upon completion of the procedure, a debriefing checklist was completed to share information critical to the postoperative care of the patient. The patient tolerated the procedure well, *was extubated in the operating room*, and was transported to the post-anesthesia care unit in stable condition thereafter.

Excision of Thyroglossal Duct Cyst 97

Carolyn Gosztyla and Howard I. Pryor II

Indications and Benefits

- Recurrent infections
- Mass effect causing: Pain, globus sensation, dysphagia, or dyspnea
- Current or future malignancy
- Cosmetic deformity
- Benefits: Relief of symptoms related to infection or mass effect, reduction of malignancy risk, resection of malignancy, and improved cosmetic appearance following resection

Risks and Alternatives

- Standard risks include bleeding, infection, need for additional procedures, and risks of anesthesia.
- Hematoma or seroma in the deep spaces of the neck requiring drains or reoperation.
- Injury to the superior laryngeal, lingual, and hypoglossal nerves.
- Recurrence of infected cyst or draining sinus.
- Alternatives: Drainage of an infected thyroglossal duct cyst can temporize or alleviate infectious symptoms, but primary resection, when possible, is recommended to lower the risk of recurrence. Antibiotic treatment should precede surgical intervention.

Essential Steps

Excision of a Thyroglossal Duct Cyst

1. Preoperative confirmation of normal thyroid gland via ultrasound. Occasionally, a lingual thyroid can be mistaken for a thyroglossal duct cyst.
2. A horizontal curvilinear skin incision is made in a skin fold overlying the cyst or a skin ellipse is made containing draining sinus or site of previous drainage.
3. Myocutaneous flaps are raised superiorly and inferiorly in the subplatysmal plane.
4. Careful dissection of the cyst from the adjacent structures is performed to the level of the body of the hyoid bone.
5. Resection of the middle third of the hyoid bone.
6. Continuation of dissection posterosuperiorly to the foramen cecum taking care to leave the mucosa of the tongue intact.
7. Placement of a drain.
8. Multilayer closure with resorbable suture.

C. Gosztyla
Walter Reed National Military Medical Center, Department of General Surgery, Bethesda, MD, USA

H. I. Pryor II (✉)
Division of Pediatric Surgery, Walter Reed National Military Medical Center, Department of Surgery, Bethesda, MD, USA

D. J. Papandria et al. (eds.), *Operative Dictations in Pediatric Surgery*,
https://doi.org/10.1007/978-3-030-24212-1_97

Note These Variations

- Arborization of the cyst tract is common so taking a wider core of tissue surrounding the cyst tract may be necessary.
- The original Sistrunk procedure detailed excision of the foramen cecum along with part of the genioglossus muscle and the raphe of the mylohyoid muscles.

Template Operative Dictation

Preoperative Diagnosis Thyroglossal duct cyst

Postoperative Diagnosis Same as preoperative diagnosis

Findings Same as postoperative diagnosis

Procedure(s) Performed Excision of thyroglossal duct cyst

Anesthesia General

Specimen Thyroglossal duct cyst and tract with mid portion of hyoid bone

Drains __ *Fr Jackson Pratt/Rubber band/ Penrose*

Estimated Blood Loss ___

Indications This is a/an ___-day/-week/-month/-year-old male/female with preoperative diagnosis of thyroglossal duct cyst causing *recurrent infection/globus sensation/dysphagia/dyspnea/malignancy/cosmetic deformity*. He/she was deemed to be a suitable candidate for excision of thyroglossal duct cyst and lingual thyroid was excluded by preoperative imaging.

Procedure in Detail Following satisfactory induction of anesthesia, the patient was placed in *supine/beach chair/flex* position with a bump placed under the shoulders to facilitate extension of the neck. The patient was padded appropriately. Preoperative antibiotics were administered within 30 minutes of skin incision. Timeouts were performed using both preinduction and preincision safety checklists with participation of all present in the operative suite. These confirmed the correct patient, procedure, operative site, and additional critical information prior to the start of the procedure. The neck was then prepped from the lips to just below the clavicles and laterally to the mastoid processes. The patient was draped in the usual sterile fashion.

Local anesthesia consisting of ___*% lidocaine/bupivacaine with/without epinephrine* was injected subcutaneously at the proposed site of skin incision. The weight of the child was ___kg, and a total of ___mL was injected keeping below the maximum recommended dose of local anesthetic for the weight of the child.

A curvilinear skin incision was made horizontally in a skin crease overlying the cyst.

If draining sinus identified or previous drainage performed: *A draining sinus/site of previous drainage procedure* was identified and an ellipse of tissue surrounding the skin opening was excised.

The skin incision was carried through the subcutaneous tissue using electrocautery, and the platysma was transected to enter the subplatysmal plane. Cranial and caudal flaps were raised. The strap muscles were divided vertically through the midline raphe. After careful palpation of the cyst, the adjacent muscle and soft tissue were divided taking care to not enter the cyst cavity. This dissection was continued to the level of the hyoid bone keeping a central cuff of tissue attached to the bone.

The subperiosteal plane was located and a Colorado tip electrocautery needle was used to dissect the soft tissue attachments to skeletonize the middle third of the hyoid bone. The middle third of the hyoid bone was detached from the lateral thirds using *bone cutting forceps/heavy sci ssors/electrocautery*.

Next, an Alice clamp was used to retract the cyst and hyoid bone, and the dissection was continued at a 45-degree angle posterosuperiorly toward the base of the tongue. A cuff of tissue was removed including the raphe of the mylohyoid muscles as well as portions of the genioglossus and hyoglossus muscles immediately adjacent to the foramen cecum. *A gloved hand was inserted into the patient's mouth, and pressure was applied at the base of the tongue overlying the site of the foramen cecum to guide the dissection.*

[Choose One:]

If mucosa not violated: The mucosa was not violated.

If mucosa violated: The mucosa was violated and was repaired using a single 3-0 chromic suture in a figure of eight.

The specimen was removed and was sent as a permanent specimen for pathologic evaluation.

Hemostasis was obtained and the wound was irrigated thoroughly. *The deep musculature of the tongue was approximated using a horizontal mattress stitch of 3-0 Vicryl.* The cut edges of the sternohyoid muscles were reapproximated to the cut edges of the myohyoid muscle. A ___ *Fr Jackson Pratt/Rubber band/Penrose* drain was left in the wound bed and was allowed to course out of the lateral extent of the incision. The strap muscles were reapproximated across the median raphe overlying the drain. The platysma was approximated with resorbable suture. A deep dermal closure was performed using 4-0 Vicryl. The skin was closed with a running subcuticular 5-0 monocryl. The skin was reinforced with *Steri-Strips/Dermabond*. The drain was secured with ___ *Monocryl/nylon*. Kerlix fluffs were fashioned and were secured over the incision with tape.

Upon completion of the procedure, a debriefing checklist was completed to share information critical to the postoperative care of the patient. The patient tolerated the procedure well, was extubated in the operating room, and was transported to the post-anesthesia care unit in stable condition.

Excision of Branchial Cleft Cyst/Sinus

98

Lorraine I. Kelley-Quon

Indications and Benefits

- Persistent branchial cleft cyst/sinus
- Benefits: Removal of nidus for infection

Risks and Alternatives

- Standard risks (bleeding, infection, need for additional procedures, and risks of anesthesia)
- Injury to adjacent structures (glossopharyngeal nerve, vagus nerve, hypoglossal nerve, and carotid sheath)
- Incomplete excision of sinus tract
- Alternatives: None

Essential Steps

1. Cannulation of the sinus
2. Elliptical incision around sinus opening
3. Dissection up the length of the sinus tract
4. Transverse step ladder incision(s) along the length of the sinus tract
5. Suture ligation of the base of the sinus

Template Operative Dictation (Open)

Preoperative Diagnosis Excision of branchial cleft Cyst/sinus

Postoperative Diagnosis Same as preoperative diagnosis

Findings Same as postoperative diagnosis

Procedure(s) Performed Excision of branchial cleft cyst/sinus

Anesthesia General

Specimen Branchial cleft cyst/sinus

Drains None

Implants None

Estimated Blood Loss ___

Indications This is a/an ___*-day/week/month/year*-old *male/female* with a branchial cleft cyst/sinus. He/she was deemed to be a suitable candidate for Excision of branchial cleft cyst/sinus.

L. I. Kelley-Quon (✉)
Children's Hospital Los Angeles, Division of Pediatric Surgery, Department of Surgery, Keck School of Medicine of University of Southern California, Los Angeles, CA, USA
e-mail: lkquon@chla.usc.edu

D. J. Papandria et al. (eds.), *Operative Dictations in Pediatric Surgery*,
https://doi.org/10.1007/978-3-030-24212-1_98

Procedure in Detail Following satisfactory induction of anesthesia, the patient was placed in the supine position and appropriately padded. Timeouts were performed using both preinduction and preincision safety checklists with participation of all present in the operative suite. These confirmed the correct patient, procedure, operative site, and additional critical information prior to the start of the procedure. The bilateral neck was then prepped and draped in the usual sterile fashion.

A lacrimal duct probe was used to cannulate the sinus tract. It was passed superiorly to estimate the length of the sinus. Next, an elliptical incision was made around the sinus opening, and dissection was carried up the length of the sinus tract using sharp dissection to minimize damage to adjacent structures. Traction sutures were placed on the base of the sinus exit site to facilitate dissection. The sinus tract was noted to extend beyond the limits of the initial skin incision so an additional transverse step-ladder incision was made several centimeters superior to the initial incision along the length of the sinus tract. The sinus tract was then passed through the subcutaneous tunnel between the two incisions and exited out the second incision. Dissection continued with traction up to the base of the sinus toward the tonsillar fossa. Suture ligation proximal to the base of the tract was performed using an absorbable suture and the tract was transected and passed off the field as specimen. The incisions were irrigated with warmed saline and hemostasis was checked. The platysma was reapproximated in an interrupted fashion using absorbable suture followed but the subcutaneous and subcuticular layers. A sterile dressing was applied to all incisions.

Upon completion of the procedure, a debriefing checklist was completed to share information critical to the postoperative care of the patient. The patient tolerated the procedure well, *was extubated in the operating room*, and was transported to the post-anesthesia care unit in stable condition thereafter.

Parathyroidectomy

99

Sara A. Mansfield and Jennifer H. Aldrink

Indications and Benefits

- Parathyroid adenoma
- Parathyroid hyperplasia, multiple endocrine neoplasia
- Benefits: Surgical treatment of hypercalcemia

Risks and Alternatives

- Standard risks (bleeding, infection, need for additional procedures, and risks of anesthesia)
- Injury to adjacent structures (recurrent laryngeal nerve, external branch of the superior laryngeal nerve, vascular structures, and trachea)
- Continued/recurrent hyperparathyroidism
- Hypocalcemia (temporary or permanent)
- Hoarseness (temporary or permanent)
- Hematoma with airway compromise

S. A. Mansfield
The Ohio State University Wexner Medical Center, Department of General Surgery, Columbus, OH, USA

J. H. Aldrink (✉)
Nationwide Children's Hospital, The Ohio State University College of Medicine, Division of Pediatric Surgery, Department of Surgery, Columbus, OH, USA
e-mail: Jennifer.Aldrink@nationwidechildrens.org

Essential Steps

1. Preoperative localization of parathyroid adenoma
2. Obtain baseline PTH level
3. Develop subplatysmal flaps and divide strap muscles
4. Expose, identify, and resect abnormal parathyroid gland
5. Draw post-excision PTH and verify adequate drop

Note These Variations

- Four gland exploration with 3½ gland parathyroidectomy or total parathyroidectomy with autoimplantation is indicated for parathyroid hyperplasia.
- Radioisotope-guided parathyroidectomy.
- Minimally invasive parathyroidectomy.
- When multiple adenomas or hyperplastic glands are felt to be the source of hyperparathyroidism then full cervical exploration should be undertaken with excision of any abnormal glands. If all 4 glands are abnormal then either 3.5 glands should be resected or all 4 glands should be resected with autotransplantation of one-half gland into either the chest wall or the brachioradialis muscle of the forearm.

D. J. Papandria et al. (eds.), *Operative Dictations in Pediatric Surgery*,
https://doi.org/10.1007/978-3-030-24212-1_99

- When all 4 glands cannot be identified after full cervical dissection or an abnormal gland cannot be identified in the setting of presumed primary hyperparathyroidism, there are several surgical options. Selective jugular venous sampling for PTH levels may identify the laterality of the offending gland and assist in localization. Intraoperative ultrasonography may identify the gland. A unilateral thyroid lobectomy may be performed on the side of a missing gland to potentially remove an intrathyroidal abnormal parathyroid gland. A transcervical thymectomy may be considered.

Template Operative Dictation (Open)

Preoperative Diagnosis **Diagnosis**

Postoperative Diagnosis Same as preoperative diagnosis

Findings Same as postoperative diagnosis

Procedure(s) Performed Parathyroidectomy

Anesthesia *General*

Specimen Parathyroid gland(s)

Drains {Drains}

Estimated Blood Loss ___

Indications This is a/an ___-*day/week/month/year*-old *male/female* with **Indication**. He/she was deemed to be a suitable candidate for parathyroidectomy.

Procedure in Detail Timeouts were performed using both preinduction and preincision safety checklists to verify correct patient, procedure, site, and additional critical information prior to beginning the procedure. Following induction of general anesthesia *with a NIMS recurrent laryngeal nerve monitoring endotracheal tube*, both arms were tucked at the sides and all pressure points were padded. A roll was placed under the shoulders, and the patient was positioned in a modified beach chair position with the neck extended. The neck, chin, and superior chest were prepped and draped in a sterile fashion.

A/an ___-cm transverse cervical incision was made using a 15-blade scalpel, approximately 2 fingerbreadths superior to the sternal notch within a skin crease. This was carried down through the skin and subcutaneous tissues with electrocautery. The platysma was encountered and divided with cautery. Musculocutaneous flaps were created superiorly to the thyroid cartilage and inferiorly to the sternal notch using electrocautery. Gentle retractors were placed in the wound to aid in exposure. The strap muscles were divided in the midline with cautery and retracted laterally.

The *right/left* thyroid lobe was mobilized from its areolar attachments using blunt dissection and electrocautery. Baseline PTH level was drawn from *an arterial line/peripheral IV*. The thyroid was gently retracted medially, as the strap muscles were separated and retracted laterally. An abnormal appearing right/left superior/inferior parathyroid gland was noted. The gland was gently dissected from the surrounding tissues down to its pedicle. The pedicle of the parathyroid gland was clamped and tied with __/0 suture. The parathyroid was then passed off the field to pathology. A PTH level was drawn at 5 minutes and at 10 minutes post excision from the similar route as previous. Frozen section analysis confirmed abnormal parathyroid tissue. The post-excision 5- and 10-minute PTH returned as ___ and ___which constituted a ___% drop from baseline.

If abnormal parathyroid was not found, or PTH drop inadequate: *Further exploration was continued as the thyroid was retracted medially and explored further superior/inferior to previous. Intraoperative ultrasound was used to identify and abnormal appearing parathyroid (describe location). Selective venous jugular sampling was used to lateralize the side of concern. The tracheoesophageal groove/carotid/jugular sheaths were explored to identify the* *offending gland. An abnormal-appearing right/left superior/inferior parathyroid gland was noted (describe location of the gland). The gland was gently dissected from the surrounding tissues down to its pedicle and excised. Following identification of the abnormal gland, a PTH level was drawn at 5 minutes and at 10 minutes post excision from the similar route as previous.*

The wound was copiously irrigated and hemostasis was achieved. *Topical hemostatic agents were applied to aid with hemostasis.* The strap muscles were reapproximated with interrupted *3/0-vicryl* sutures. The platysma was reapproximated with interrupted __/*0-vicryl* sutures. *Local anesthetic was injected subcutaneously.* The skin was reapproximated with a running __/*0 vicryl* subcuticular suture. *Surgical glue/steri-strips* were placed over the incision.

Upon completion of the procedure, a debriefing checklist was completed to share information critical to the post-operative care of the patient. The patient was extubated and taken to recovery in good condition.

Excision of Benign Soft Tissue Lesions

100

Anthony J. Munaco

Indications and Benefits

- Symptomatic lesions
  - Tenderness
  - Infection
- Changing lesions
- Patient/caregiver anxiety
  - Diagnosis
  - Possibility of malignancy
- Benefits:
  - Alleviation of symptoms
  - Diagnosis

Risks and Alternatives

- Standard risks (bleeding, infection, need for additional procedures, and risks of anesthesia).
  - Injury to adjacent structures (cutaneous nerves)
  - Recurrence
  - Need for reexcision
- Alternatives: Observation, symptom management

A. J. Munaco (✉)
OSF Healthcare Children's Hospital of Illinois, University of Illinois College of Medicine at Peoria, Department of Pediatric Surgery, Peoria, IL, USA
e-mail: amunaco@uic.edu

Essential Steps

1. Determine association of lesion with skin.
2. Complete clinical excision of lesion when feasible.
3. Do not sacrifice critical structures for benign disease

Note These Variations

- Elliptical incision including involved skin
  - Linear incision

Template Operative Dictation (Open)

Preoperative Diagnosis Soft tissue lesion of ___

Postoperative Diagnosis Same as preoperative diagnosis

Findings Same as postoperative diagnosis

Procedure(s) Performed Excision of soft tissue lesion of ___

Anesthesia *General/regional/procedural sedation/local*

D. J. Papandria et al. (eds.), *Operative Dictations in Pediatric Surgery*,
https://doi.org/10.1007/978-3-030-24212-1_100

Specimen ___ cm × ___ cm soft tissue lesion of ___

Drains None

Implants None

Estimated Blood Loss ___

Indications This is a/an ___*-day/week/month/year*-old *male/female* with *symptomatic/changing/concerning* soft tissue lesion of the *right/left* ___. He/she was deemed to be a suitable candidate for excision of soft tissue lesion.

Procedure in Detail Following satisfactory induction of anesthesia, the patient was placed in position to expose the lesion and appropriately padded. Timeouts were performed using both preinduction and preincision safety checklists with participation of all present in the operative suite. These confirmed the correct patient, procedure, operative site, and additional critical information prior to the start of the procedure. The ___ was then prepped and draped in the usual sterile fashion.

The lesion was assessed for association with the skin.

[Choose One:]
If skin involved with lesion: An elliptical incision was made to encompass the skin involvement and deepened into the subcutaneous tissues.

If skin not involved with the lesion: A linear incision was made over the lesion and deepened into the subcutaneous tissues.

The lesion was circumferentially excised. Lesion was *oriented/not oriented* with suture and passed off the table as specimen. Wound was examined and no further palpable lesion was appreciated. *Wound was irrigated.* Hemostasis was achieved. Wound was closed in layers of absorbable suture, and sterile dressing was applied.

Upon completion of the procedure, a debriefing checklist was completed to share information critical to the post-operative care of the patient. The patient tolerated the procedure well, *was extubated in the operating room*, and was transported to the post-anesthesia care unit in stable condition thereafter.

101 Incision and Drainage

Melissa Vanover and Payam Saadai

Indications and Benefits

- Abscess
- Benefits: Control of infection

Risks and Alternatives

- Standard risks (bleeding, infection, need for additional procedures, and risks of anesthesia)
- Injury to adjacent structures (neurovascular)
- Transient bacteremia
- Recurrence
- Scar
- Alternatives: Antibiotics

Essential Steps

1. Localize abscess cavity by *palpation/needle aspiration*
2. *Linear/stab* incision
3. Send fluid sample for culture
4. Break up internal loculations
5. Copious irrigation
6. *Place drain*

Note These Variations

- Localization technique
- Incision
- *Drain/vessel loop/packing* placement

Template Operative Dictation

Preoperative Diagnosis Abscess

Postoperative Diagnosis Abscess

Findings ___mL of pus drained

Procedure(s) Performed Incision and drainage

Anesthesia *General/regional/procedural sedation*

Specimen Fluid for culture

Drains *None/Penrose drain/vessel loop*

Implants None

Estimated Blood Loss ___mL

M. Vanover
University of California, Davis, Department of Pediatric General, Thoracic and Fetal Surgery, Sacramento, CA, USA

P. Saadai (✉)
UC Davis Medical Center/Shriners Hospital for Children, Division of Pediatric Surgery, Sacramento, CA, USA
e-mail: psaadai@ucdavis.edu

D. J. Papandria et al. (eds.), *Operative Dictations in Pediatric Surgery*,
https://doi.org/10.1007/978-3-030-24212-1_101

Indications This is a/an ___-*day/week/month/year*-old *male/female* with abscess(es). He/she was deemed to be a suitable candidate for incision and drainage.

Procedure in Detail Following satisfactory induction of anesthesia, the patient was placed in *supine/prone/lateral decubitus position* and appropriately padded. Timeouts were performed using both preinduction and preincision safety checklists with participation of all present in the operative suite. These confirmed the correct patient, procedure, operative site, and additional critical information prior to the start of the procedure. The ___ was then prepped and draped in the usual sterile fashion. Perioperative antibiotics were *administered/confirmed.*

If no palpable fluctuance*: Needle aspiration was performed to localize the abscess cavity.*

A *linear/stab* incision was made over the *area of maximal fluctuance/abscess cavity* following natural skin lines. *Purulent/serosanguinous/serous* fluid was encountered, and a sample sent for culture. Internal loculations were broken up with a hemostat. The abscess cavity was copiously irrigated with saline.

[Choose One:]

If Penrose drain: *A Penrose drain was placed in the abscess cavity and secured with absorbable sutures.* A dry gauze dressing was placed.

If vessel loop: *A vessel loop was placed in the abscess cavity, brought out through a separate stab incisin, and tied to itself.* A dry gauze dressing was placed.

If packing: *Packing tape/iodoform gauze/betadine-soaked gauze/dry gauze was packed in the abscess cavity.* A dry gauze dressing was placed.

If no indwelling drain or packing: *No drain was left/a second incision was placed to form a cruciate incision, and the corners were excised sharply to promote free drainage of the cavity.*

Upon completion of the procedure, a debriefing checklist was completed to share information critical to the post-operative care of the patient. The patient tolerated the procedure well, *was extubated in the operating room*, and was transported to the post-anesthesia care unit in stable condition thereafter.

Excisional Biopsy of Benign Breast Mass

102

Young Chun and Isam Nasr

Indications and Benefits

- Resection of a benign mass
- Resection of a precancerous but benign mass
- Benefits: Resection of a benign mass and pathologic evaluation of the mass

Risks and Alternatives

- Standard risks (bleeding, infection, need for additional procedures, and risks of anesthesia).
- Injury to adjacent structures ({critical structures}).
- Seroma/hematoma.
- Breast deformity/size mismatch.
- Incomplete excision.
- Alternatives:
  - Continue monitoring without removal of the mass.
  - Medical therapy.

Y. Chun
Johns Hopkins University, Department of Pediatric Surgery, Baltimore, MD, USA

I. Nasr (✉)
Johns Hopkins Hospital, Department of Pediatric Surgery, Johns Hopkins Children's Center, Baltimore, MD, USA
e-mail: inasr1@jhmi.edu

Essential Steps

1. Review of all available images and verification of location and laterality of mass.
2. Locate the mass within the breast.
3. Incision over mass.
4. Hemostatic dissection to and around the breast mass.
5. Remove the mass in its entirety.
6. Mark the mass to allow the pathologist to identify six sides of the mass.
7. The mass is sent to radiology/pathology to verify that either the wire/mass is indeed within the specimen.
8. Carefully inspect the field for hemostasis and control any bleeding appropriately either with cautery or with suture ligation.
9. Close the wound in layers.

Note These Variations

- Preoperative wire localization is often used to help locate the benign breast mass since many are nonpalpable and identifiable only with imaging (i.e., mammogram).
- Intraoperative ultrasound is useful in select cases for the localization of a breast mass. It is

D. J. Papandria et al. (eds.), *Operative Dictations in Pediatric Surgery*,
https://doi.org/10.1007/978-3-030-24212-1_102

especially helpful in identifying smaller masses and surgeons who often use the ultrasound for evaluation of breast masses.
- The technique used to label the margins of the mass differs from surgeon to surgeon. The basic requirement is to ensure that all six sides of the mass are marked. In the event that additional resection of a margin is required, it can be limited to the side in question. Otherwise, all six sides must be reexcised.
- There are different types of skin incisions such as radial incision, curvilinear incision, circumareolar/periareolar incision, and inframammary fold incision. Determination of the skin incision depends on the exact location of the breast mass as well as the shape of the breast itself to give the best cosmetic result.

Template Operative Dictation (Open)

Preoperative Diagnosis Benign breast mass

Postoperative Diagnosis Same as preoperative diagnosis

Findings Same as postoperative diagnosis

Procedure(s) Performed Excisional biopsy of benign breast mass

Anesthesia *General/regional/procedural sedation*

Specimen Breast mass

Drains *JP drain*

Implants None

Estimated Blood Loss __

Indications This is a/an ___*-day/week/month/ year*-old *male/female* with [*right, left*] breast mass. He/she was deemed to be a suitable candidate for an excisional biopsy of a benign breast mass.

Procedure in Detail Following satisfactory induction of anesthesia, the patient was placed in supine position with arms out and appropriately padded. Timeouts were performed using both preinduction and preincision safety checklists with the participation of all present in the operative suite. Those confirmed the correct patient, procedure, operative site, and additional critical information prior to the start of the procedure. The breast was then prepped and draped in the usual sterile fashion.

[Choose One:]

Preoperative wire localization was done to localize the mass: The wire was carefully prepped into the field. A radial incision was made to include the wire, and the dissection plane followed the wire to the mass. The mass was palpated around the tip of the wire. An Allis clamp was placed on the mass to facilitate dissection. The mass was removed with a 1 cm margin. Sutures were placed on the mass to designate six sides of the mass. One silk suture with one tail was placed on the anterior surface, another suture was placed with two tails on the lateral surface of the mass and two sutures were placed on the inferior surface of the mass. The field was examined for hemostasis.

Intraoperative palpation was used to localize the mass: The mass was palpated in the breast. A radial incision was made over the mass with the least distance from the skin. Dissection was carried down to the mass, which was subsequently palpated through the incision. An Allis clamp was placed on the mass to facilitate dissection. The mass was removed with a 1-cm margin. Sutures were placed on three sides of the mass for the pathologist (one suture for the anterior surface, two sutures for the lateral surface, and three sutures for the inferior surface). The field was examined for hemostasis.

Intraoperative ultrasound was used to localize the mass: An ultrasound probe was prepped into the sterile field. The mass was located using the ultrasound probe over the breast tissue. A radial incision was made over the mass with the least distance from the skin. Dissection was carried down to the mass and the was palpated through the incision. An Allis clamp was placed on the mass to facilitate dissection. The mass was removed with a 1-cm margin. Sutures were placed on three sides of the mass for the pathologist (one suture for the anterior surface, two sutures for the lateral surface, and three sutures for the inferior surface). The field was examined for hemostasis.

If there is a large defect after removal of the mass: A Jackson-Pratt drain was left in place.

The incision was closed in layers. Interrupted 3-0 Vicryl stitches were placed to reapproximate the dead space as well as the deep dermal layer. The skin incision was closed using 4-0 Monocryl in a running subcuticular fashion. The incision was dressed using Steristrips, gauze, and Tegaderm.

Upon completion of the procedure, a debriefing checklist was completed to share information critical to the postoperative care of the patient. The patient tolerated the procedure well, *was extubated in the operating room*, and was transported to the postanesthesia care unit in stable condition thereafter.

103 Aspiration/Drainage of Breast Abscess

David Coyle

Indications and Benefits

- Presence of a clinically diagnosed or ultrasound-confirmed breast abscess
- Mastitis failing to respond to antimicrobial therapy complicated by suppuration
- Incision and drainage of a breast abscess is usually only indicated following failure of abscess aspiration with antimicrobial therapy
- Benefits: Sampling of purulent fluid for laboratory analysis may allow optimization of antimicrobial treatment

Risks and Alternatives

- Standard risks (bleeding/hematoma formation, and risks of anesthesia)
- Injury to breast bud, especially in prepubertal girls
- Abscess recurrence
- Long-term cosmetic deformity
- Alternatives: Medical therapy with spontaneous drainage; ultrasound-guided needle aspiration; and incision and drainage

D. Coyle (✉)
Nationwide Children's Hospital, Division of Pediatric Surgery, Columbus, OH, USA
e-mail: David.coyle@nationwidechildrens.org

Essential Steps

Aspiration of Breast Abscess

1. Position the patient supine. ***If the abscess is in the outer quadrants of the breast,*** abduct the upper limb at the shoulder to optimize access.
2. Localization of the abscess cavity: ***If abscess is "pointing" (thinned skin with obvious imminent drainage),*** no further localization is necessary. ***If the abscess location is not immediately obvious***, localization with ultrasound is necessary, which reveals an irregularly shaped cavity with a thickened echogenic wall and a complex hypoechoic center.
3. A wide bore cannula is placed percutaneously into the abscess cavity *with ultrasound guidance/at the point of maximal clinical fluctuance*.
4. A syringe is used to sample pus from the cavity, which is sent for gram staining and culture.
5. A separate syringe is then used to aspirate the cavity empty as fully as possible.
6. The needle is withdrawn, and any remaining pus is manually expressed from the puncture site.
7. A loose gauze-based dressing is placed over the puncture site.

D. J. Papandria et al. (eds.), *Operative Dictations in Pediatric Surgery*,
https://doi.org/10.1007/978-3-030-24212-1_103

Incision and Drainage of Breast Abscess

1. Position the patient supine. ***If the abscess is in the outer quadrants of the breast,*** abduct the upper limb at the shoulder to optimize access.
2. Localization of the abscess cavity: ***If abscess is "pointing" (thinned skin with obvious imminent drainage),*** no further localization is necessary. ***If the abscess location is not immediately obvious***, localization with ultrasound is necessary, which reveals an irregularly shaped cavity with a thickened echogenic wall and a complex hypoechoic center.
3. A circumareolar incision is made as close to the abscess cavity as possible.
4. The abscess cavity is entered sharply or bluntly with a hemostat clip.
5. Pus is sampled from the cavity using a syringe for gram stain and culture.
6. Infected material is evacuated from the abscess cavity.
7. Instrumentation or probing of the cavity is minimized to avoid injuring the breast bud or Cooper's ligaments.
8. The cavity is irrigated with 0.9% saline.
9. The wound is loosely packed with an antimicrobial wick (e.g., povidone iodine soaked gauze wick).
10. A loose gauze dressing is placed over the wound.

Note These Variations

- Where an abscess caused by *Mycobacterium tuberculum* is suspected (i.e., "cold," painless abscess in an at-risk group, e.g., HIV-positive), additional infection control precautions should be utilized in the theatre. Infected fluid should be specifically sent for Ziehl-Nielsen staining and tuberculosis culture.
- In cases of recurrent abscess refractory to medical treatment or with atypical findings such as a painless mass or discharging sinuses, a biopsy from the abscess cavity should be taken for histopathologic assessment, as malignancy or granulomatous changes may occur.
- In neonates, incision and drainage should be avoided where possible, as the risk of subsequent long-term cosmetic deformity is not trivial.

Template Operative Dictation (Aspiration/Incision and Drainage of Breast Abscess)

Preoperative Diagnosis *Right/left*-sided breast abscess

Postoperative Diagnosis Same

Findings Breast abscess at _ o'clock position

Procedure(s) Performed *Aspiration/drainage of breast abscess*

Anesthesia: [Choose One:]
For percutaneous aspiration and if patient will tolerate local anesthesia: *Topical anesthesia with 4% tetracaine* and local infiltration with *2% lidocaine plus epinephrine (1:200,000)*

For all others: *General anesthesia / procedural sedation*

Specimen Pus to Microbiology for gram stain, anaerobic, and aerobic culture

Drains *Antimicrobial wick / packing strip (___ cm)*

Estimated Blood Loss ___ mL

Indications This is a/an _ *-year*-old *female/male* with a right sided breast abscess at the _ o'clock position *confirmed with ultrasound* complicating an episode of non-puerperal mastitis. She was deemed to be a suitable candidate for *Aspiration/Drainage of Breast Abscess*.

Procedure in Detail The patient was placed in supine position and appropriately padded. Timeouts were performed using a preprocedural safety checklist with participation of all present in the operative suite. These confirmed the correct patient, procedure, operative site, and additional critical information prior to the start of the procedure. The *right/left* breast was then prepped and draped in the usual sterile fashion.

[Choose One:]

If Aspiration of Breast Abscess: An ultrasound probe covered with transmission gel was placed in a sterile nonlatex ultrasound probe cover. Using sterile transmission gel, the abscess cavity was localized by ultrasound and a __ gauge cannula was used to access the abscess cavity percutaneously. The cannula needle was removed and pus from the cavity was sampled and sent for microbiology evaluation as described above. The abscess cavity was aspirated under ultrasound guidance until empty and irrigated through the cannula sheath using 0.9% saline. The cannula was removed and a small absorbent dressing was placed over the puncture site.

If Drainage of Breast Abscess: At the site of maximum fluctuance, a circumareolar incision was made, entering the abscess cavity sharply. Pus was expressed from the cavity and sampled for microbiology evaluation as described above. Instrumentation of the abscess cavity to break up septations was minimized. The cavity was irrigated copiously with 0.9% saline. A soft antimicrobial wick was loosely packed into the abscess cavity, and an absorbent gauze pressure dressing was placed over the wound and was secured with medical adhesive tape.

Upon completion of the procedure, a debriefing checklist was completed to share information critical to the postoperative care of the patient. The patient tolerated the procedure well, *was extubated in the operating room*, and was transported to the post-anesthesia care unit in stable condition thereafter.

Excisional Lymph Node Biopsy — 104

Morgan Johnson, Courtney Pisano,
and Gail E. Besner

Indications and Benefits

- Lymphadenopathy
- Concern for malignancy

Risks and Alternatives

- Bleeding
- Infection
- Anesthesia risks
- Injury to nerve or vascular structures near the site of procedure
- Recurrence
- Lymphedema
- Alternatives include observation, complete surgical resection

M. Johnson
The Ohio State University, College of Medicine, Columbus, OH, USA

C. Pisano · G. E. Besner (✉)
Nationwide Children's Hospital, Department of Pediatric Surgery, Columbus, OH, USA
e-mail: gail.besner@nationwidechildrens.org

Essential Steps

Cervical Lymph Node Resection

1. The largest lymph node deemed appropriate should be identified and marked
2. Divide platysma
3. Divide the fascial layers of neck
4. Visualize the lymph node while identifying and avoiding other nearby structures
5. Remove the lymph node while maintaining full integrity of the specimen
6. Check hemostasis
7. Close incision
8. Send specimen fresh to pathology for frozen section

Template Operative Dictation

Preoperative Diagnosis *Enlarged lymph node/concern for malignancy*

Postoperative Diagnosis Same as preoperative diagnosis

Findings *Lymphadenopathy without evidence of infection/other*

D. J. Papandria et al. (eds.), *Operative Dictations in Pediatric Surgery*,
https://doi.org/10.1007/978-3-030-24212-1_104

Procedure(s) Performed Excisional lymph node biopsy

Anesthesia *General/regional/procedural sedation*

Specimen {Specimen}

Drains {Drains}

Implants {Implants}

Estimated Blood Loss ___

Indications This is a/an ___*-day/week/month/year*-old *male/female* presented with *lymphadenopathy/other in L/R neck.* Diagnostic imaging and workup indicated *concern for malignancy/infection/other.* The patient was brought to the operating room for an excisional lymph node biopsy.

Procedure in Detail The patient was brought to the operating room and placed on the operating table in the supine position. Following satisfactory induction of *general/local* anesthesia, a time-out was completed verifying the patient by two identifiers, the procedure to be performed and the operative site. Appropriate perioperative antibiotics were administered, and the *L/R neck* was prepped and draped in the usual sterile fashion.

A horizontal incision was marked directly overlying the palpable enlarged lymph node. *1% lidocaine with 1:100,000 epinephrine was injected.* The incision was made and dissection carried down to the fascia using electrocautery. The fascia was incised and the enlarged lymph node was identified. Lymph node integrity was maintained and removed using sharp dissection. The specimen was sent fresh to pathology for analysis. The area was irrigated with normal saline. Hemostasis was obtained using the electrocautery device. The fascial layers were closed using interrupted 3/0-Vicryl sutures. The subcutaneous fat was closed with 4/0-Vicryl *running/interrupted* sutures followed by a 5/0-Vicryl running subcuticular skin closure. The incision was dressed with *Steri-Strips/topical skin adhesive.*

All sponge, needle, and instrument counts were correct at the end of the procedure. Upon completion of the procedure, a debriefing checklist was completed to share information critical to the postoperative care of the patient. The patient tolerated the procedure well, *was extubated in the operating room*, and was transported to the postanesthesia care unit in stable condition thereafter.

Torticollis

105

Lea Wehrli and Stefan Scholz

Indications

- Persistent contracture of the sternocleidomastoid muscle *with failure of conservative treatment (physical therapy)*
- Progressive hemifacial hypoplasia
- Plagiocephaly
- Compensatory scoliosis
- Diagnosis in children older than one year of age
- Exclusion for other etiologies for torticollis (e.g., ocular, vestibular, bony abnormalities, spasm of other muscle causing torticollis (e.g., trapezius muscle), or inflammatory process of the neck (e.g., retropharyngeal abscess and rheumatoid arthritis)

Benefits

- Resolution of limited range of motion of neck
- Improvement of plagiocephaly, hemifacial hypoplasia

L. Wehrli
Children's Hospital of Pittsburgh of UPMC, Department of Pediatric Surgery, Pittsburgh, PA, USA

S. Scholz (✉)
University of Pittsburgh School of Medicine, Children's Hospital of Pittsburgh, Department of Pediatric Surgery, Pittsburgh, PA, USA
e-mail: stefan.scholz@chp.edu

Risks and Alternatives

- Standard risks (bleeding, infection, need for additional procedures, and risks of anesthesia)
- Most common: Injury to accessory nerve or brachial plexus
- Injury to carotid sheath structures, jugular veins, subclavian vessels, or facial or vagal nerve
- Incomplete tenotomy
- Recurrence
- Esthetically disturbing scar or keloid
- Alternatives: Endoscopic approach though the neck or axilla

Essential Steps

1. Positioning of the patient: Supine position with a small shoulder roll for hyperextension of the neck with minimal reverse Trendelenburg and head rotated toward the nonaffected side.
2. The muscle is best divided at its lower end.
3. A 3–4-cm-long transverse skin incision is made in a skin crease one finger above the sternal and clavicular heads of the affected sternocleidomastoid muscle.
4. The platysma is divided transversely with diathermy and the external jugular vein retracted laterally.

D. J. Papandria et al. (eds.), *Operative Dictations in Pediatric Surgery*,
https://doi.org/10.1007/978-3-030-24212-1_105

5. Identify the converging muscle heads of the sternocleidomastoid muscle and gently dissect the muscle with a right angle off the underlying carotid sheath starting from lateral.
6. Divide the clavicular and sternal portion of the muscle with diathermy in a stepwise fashion.
7. Tightness of the deep cervical fascia between the sternocleidomastoid and the trapezius muscles can usually be palpable once the sternocleidomastoid has been divided. This fascia should also be divided, most importantly, under direct vision to avoid damage to the spinal accessory nerve and the brachial plexus.
8. Confirm complete release of the torticollis with rotation of the head to each side. Any remaining fibrotic muscle bands, which can be palpated during head rotation, should be divided.
9. Hemostasis is confirmed.
10. The platysma is closed with absorbable suture and the skin with absorbable subcuticular suture.
11. The procedure can be performed as a day case and no postoperative restriction of movement is necessary.

Note These Variations

- A Penrose drain can be tunneled under the sternocleidomastoid muscle for retraction to protect underlaying structures prior to division with diathermy.
- Endoscopic transaxillary or lateral cervical subcutaneous approaches are minimally invasive alternatives.

Template Operative Dictation

Preoperative Diagnosis Congenital muscular torticollis

Postoperative Diagnosis Same

Findings Contracted and fibrotic sternocleidomastoid muscle

Procedure Performed Distal tenotomy of the sternocleidomastoid muscle

Anesthesia General

Specimen None

Drains None

Implants None

Estimated Blood Loss Minimal

Indications Persistent torticollis with failure of nonoperative management

Procedure in Detail Following induction of general anesthesia, the patient was placed in a supine position with moderate hyperextension of the neck, reverse Trendelenburg position, and the head rotated toward the nonaffected side. The head was placed on a soft doughnut ring. All exposed bony sites were padded appropriately. Timeouts were performed using both preinduction and preincision safety checklists with participation of all present in the operative suite. These confirmed the correct patient, procedure, operative site, instrumentation, and additional critical information prior to the start of the procedure. The neck was then prepped and draped in the usual sterile fashion. A single-shot antibiotic with skin coverage was given intravenously 30 min prior to the incision.

A 3-cm-long transverse skin incision following a natural skin crease was performed approximately one finger above the clavicle and the well palpable contracted sternocleidomastoid muscle. The platysma was then divided with diathermy along the transverse incision. A Weitlaner wound distractor was placed. The convergence of the sternal and the clavicular portion of the sternocleidomastoid muscle was identified. Starting from lateral, blunt dissection of the muscle was performed with a right-angle instrument. Great care was exercised to avoid injury to underlaying neck structures. Once the muscle was completely mobilized in this area, the right-angle instrument was passed underneath for retraction. The muscle was then completely divided with diathermy in a stepwise manner. Tightness of the deep cervical fascia between the sternocleidomastoid and the trapezius muscles was palpated. The fascia was then separated with scissors under direct vision. Great care was taken to avoid injury to the underlaying carotid sheet, the spinal accessory nerve, and the brachial plexus. Complete release of all fibrotic structures was confirmed with palpation and rotation of the head. Hemostasis was confirmed. The platysma was closed with 4/0 Vicryl interrupted sutures. The skin was closed with a subcuticular running suture with 5/0 Monocryl. Steri-Strips and a sterile dressing are applied to the incision.

Upon completion of the procedure, a debriefing checklist was completed to share information critical to the postoperative care of the patient. The patient tolerated the procedure well, was extubated in the operating room, and was transported to the postanesthesia care unit in a stable condition [1].

Reference

1. Muscular Torticollis. Daentzer D, Stüder D, Wirth CJ. Oper Orthop Traumatol. 2010;22(2):177–87.

Resection of Postaxial Supernumerary Digits

106

Greg Grenier and Julie Balch Samora

Indications and Benefits

- Indication 1: Type A or B postaxial polydactyly
- Benefits: Removal of structure that can affect hand function, creation of an aesthetically pleasing hand (Fig. 106.1)

Risks and Alternatives

- Injury to adjacent structures (Soft tissue structures and neurovascular bundle to the small digit).
- Misclassification of a Type A vs. Type B postaxial polydactylous digit.
- Lack of recognition of an underlying syndrome, particularly in Caucasian patients (Fig. 106.2).
- Suture Ligation of rudimentary digit-loose ligature placed on the digit will occlude venous outflow only, leading to venous congestion and possibly a painful digit. Can prolong complete ischemia time. A ligature placed too far distal on the digit will leave an unsightly stump with the potential for a painful neuroma.
- Staple ligation of rudimentary digit: If the staple is not applied immediately adjacent to the surrounding soft tissue, it will leave an unsightly stump and can possibly cause a painful neuroma.
- Instrumented excision of digit-inappropriate digital block will lead to incomplete anesthesia and a painful procedure for the child if general anesthesia is not utilized. Placing too large of an ellipse can lead to a large wound with the potential need for additional closure methods and/or complications. Incomplete excision of the soft tissue can lead to a residual aesthetically unpleasing stump. Incising the nerve too distally can lead to a symptomatic neuroma. Too much traction on the nerve such that the nerve is cut along with the ulnar digital nerve to the native small digit can lead to decreased sensibility. Inadequate hemostasis of the vessels can lead to prolonged bleeding.
- Alternatives: Observation.

Essential Steps

Suture Ligation of Type B Postaxial Polydactyly

1. Step 1: Recognize that postaxial polydactyly is more common in African American patients and rare in Caucasian patients. If postaxial polydactyly is identified in a Caucasian

G. Grenier (✉)
Ohio University/Doctors Hospital, Department of Orthopedic Surgery, Columbus, OH, USA

J. B. Samora
Nationwide Children's Hospital, Department of Orthopaedics, Columbus, OH, USA

D. J. Papandria et al. (eds.), *Operative Dictations in Pediatric Surgery*,
https://doi.org/10.1007/978-3-030-24212-1_106

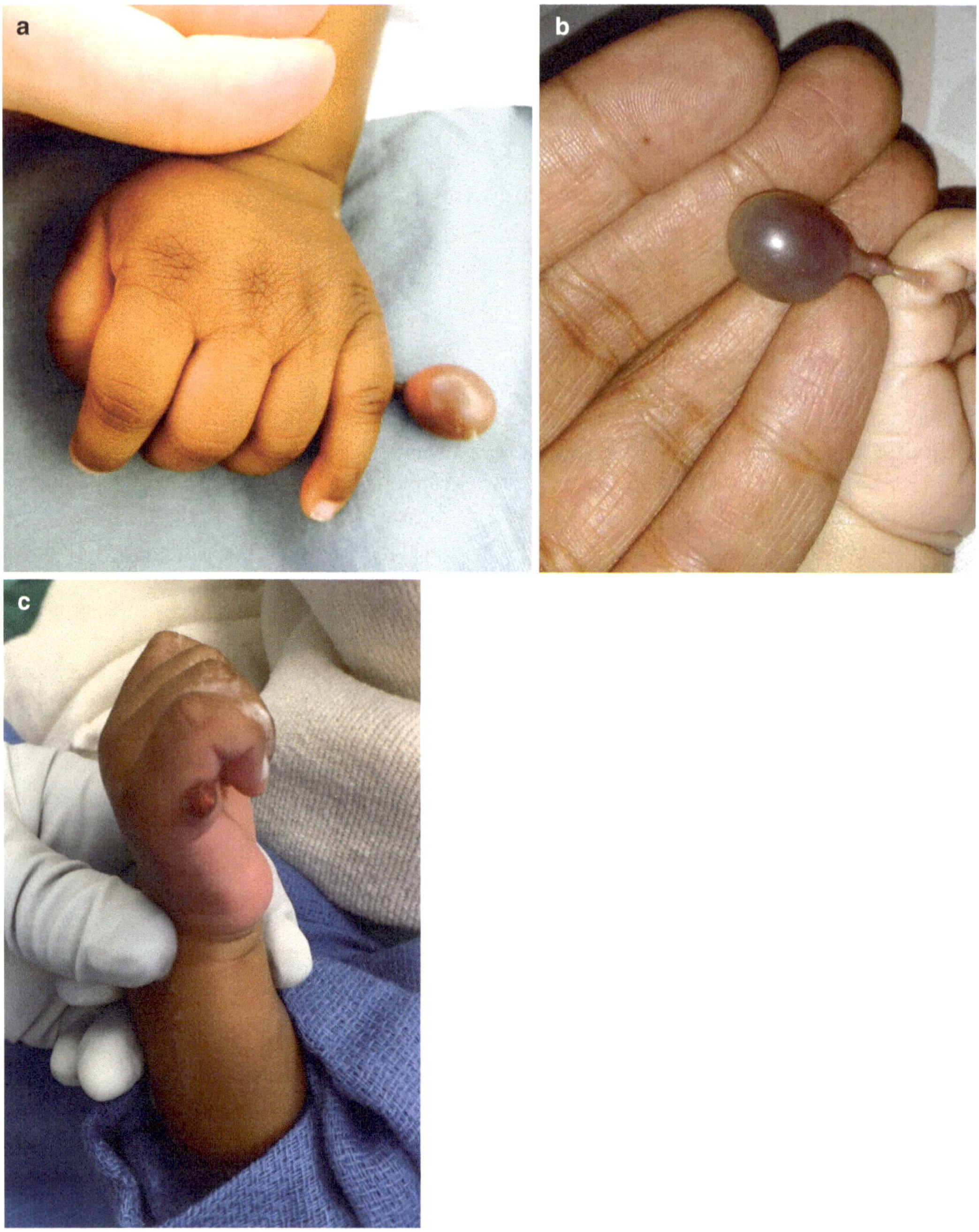

Fig. 106.1 Examples of appearance of a Type A postaxial polydactyly's starting the auto-amputation process, without suture or vascular clip ligation (A, B). When the digits auto-amputate, usually, there is a residual stump that is aesthetically unpleasing and can lead to a painful neuroma (C)

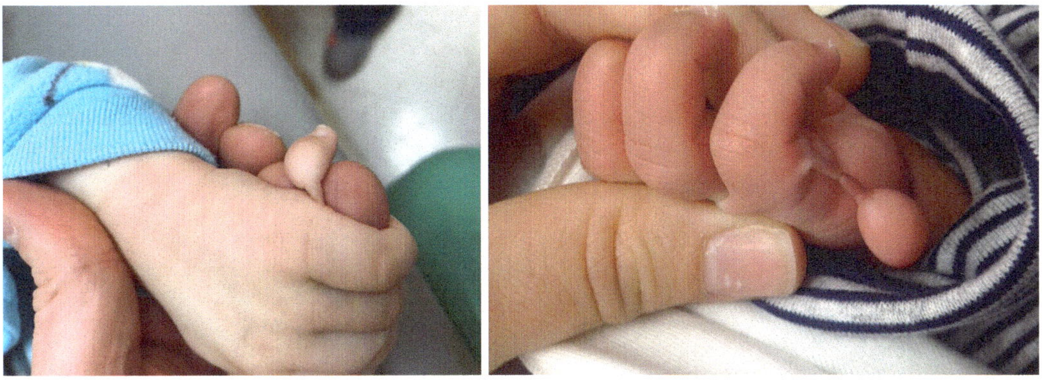

Fig. 106.2 Example of two Caucasian patients with Type A postaxial polydactyly. They were referred to Genetics to evaluate for any associated syndromes

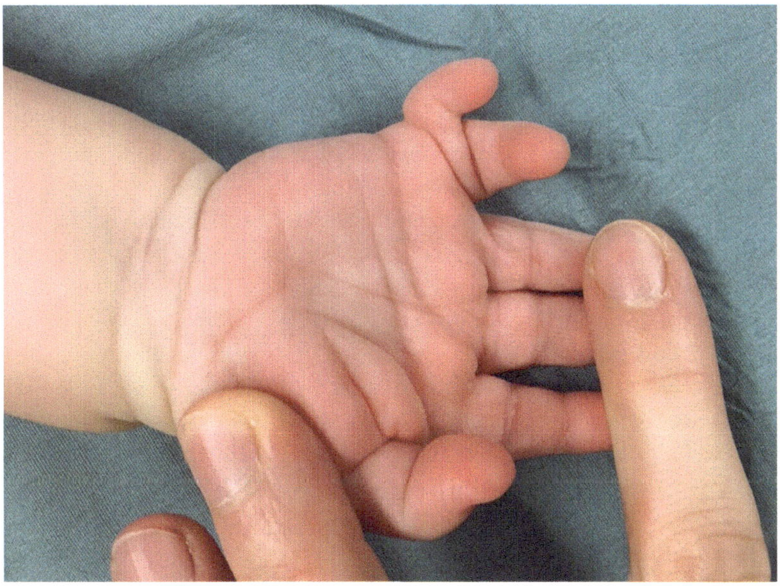

Fig. 106.3 Example of a Type A postaxial polydactyly, which cannot be treated with suture or vascular clip ligation

individual, consider genetic referral for an underlying syndrome (chondroectodermal dysplasia, Ellis-van Creveld syndrome) (Fig. 106.3).

2. Step 2: Identify a true Type B postaxial polydactyly, rudimentary digit attached to the ulnar border of the small digit in a pedunculated fashion.
3. Step 3: The procedure can be completed in the nursery, office, or operating room setting without the need for anesthesia.
4. Step 4: Grasp the pedunculated digit and place on tension to better identify the stalk.
5. Step 5: *Utilizing suture of adequate strength and knot security, tie the suture around the base of the stalk.*
6. Step 6: Evaluate that *suture* is in correct position on the stalk as close to the skin as possible, and is sufficiently tight to occlude blood flow to the digit.
7. Step 7: The digit will become necrotic and fall off, typically within 10 days (reported range of 4–21 days).
8. Step 8: Provide education to families on signs/symptoms of infection which would warrant an expeditious evaluation.

Instrumented Excision of Type B Postaxial Polydactyly

1. Recognize that postaxial polydactyly is more common in African–American patients and rare in Caucasian patients. If postaxial polydactyly is identified in a Caucasian individual, consider genetic referral for an underlying syndrome (chondroectodermal dysplasia, Ellis-van Creveld syndrome).
2. Step 2: Identify a true Type B postaxial polydactyly, rudimentary digit attached to the ulnar border of the small digit in a pedunculated fashion.
3. Step 3: The procedure can be completed in the office under local anesthetic or in the operating room, with or without supplementary anesthetic provision.
4. Step 4: *Patient is placed supine with arm extended on an arm board or hand table.*
5. Step 5: If desired, place a nonsterile tourniquet on the brachium and elevate to 225 mmHg.
6. Step 6: A digital block is performed utilizing either *1% or 2% Lidocaine or 0.25% or 0.5% Bupivacaine.*
7. Step 7: Grasp the pedunculated digit and place on tension to better identify the stalk. A towel clip or point-to-point clamp is a good tool to utilize if no assistance is available.
8. Step 8: Create a longitudinal ellipse, not circular, around the stalk using a small Beaver blade.
9. Step 9: Utilize Littler scissors to dissect the contents of the stalk.
10. Step 10: The vessels are identified, separated from the nerve, and cauterized.
11. Step 11: The nerve to the accessory digit is identified, placed on traction, and cut either with the scissors or the Beaver blade as proximally as possible and allowed to retract. Care is made to protect the native digital nerve.
12. Step 12: If the tourniquet was elevated, it is released and hemostasis is achieved. The digit is assessed for vascularity.
13. Step 13: The wound is closed with horizontal mattress suture using absorbable 5-0 Chromic suture.
14. Step 14: Soft compressive dressings are applied, leaving the fingertip exposed for parents to observe.
15. Step 15: Dressings are removed in 3 days to allow for bathing.

Note These Variations

- Variation 1: Utilization of surgical vascular clip for ligation of rudimentary postaxial digit. All steps are the same as suture ligation.
- Variation 2: In situation where suture is too loose or placed too far distal on stalk, remove and reapply either suture or surgical clip with correct tension and in correct position.
- Variation 3: Type and concentration of local anesthesia utilized is physician-dependent with decision based upon the desired onset time, length of anesthesia, and length of analgesia.

Template Operative Dictation (Open)

Pre-procedure Diagnosis *Right/left/bilateral* Type B postaxial polydactyly

Post-procedure Diagnosis Same as preoperative diagnosis

Findings Same as postoperative diagnosis

Procedure(s) Performed *Right/left/bilateral Type B postaxial polydactyly excision*

Anesthesia *None*

Specimen None

Drains None

Implants None

Estimated Blood Loss Minimal

Indications This is a/an ___-*day/week/month/year*-old *male/female* with Type B postaxial polydactyly. He/she was deemed to be a suitable candidate for *right/left/bilateral Type B postaxial polydactyly excision* via *suture/surgical clip ligation.* Risks, benefits, and alternatives were discussed with the care providers and consent was obtained.

Procedure in Detail In the *office/nursery/operating room,* the patient was *placed in supine, sitting, comfortable position in caregiver's lap, and all bony prominences were appropriately padded.* A timeout was performed with participation of all present. The correct patient, procedure, site, and additional critical information was confirmed prior to the start of the procedure. *The right, left digit(s) was then prepped and draped in the usual sterile fashion.*

The pedunculated digit was grasped with adequate longitudinal tension placed on the digit to better identify the stalk. *A suture of adequate strength and knot security was utilized to tie around the base of the stalk.* Evaluation of the *suture* demonstrated that it was in the correct position on the stalk and tight enough that blood flow to the digit was compromised.

[Choose One:]
If suture ligation: *A suture of adequate strength and knot security was utilized to tie around the base of the stalk.*

If surgical clips: *A surgical clip applicator with an appropriately sized surgical clip was utilized to completely enclose the base of the stalk. The surgical clip was then deployed and visualized to confirm adequate placement and compression on the stalk. A duplicate clip was applied in parallel fashion.*

Upon completion of the procedure, a debriefing checklist was completed to share information critical to the postoperative care of the patient. The patient tolerated the procedure well, and was *handed back to the caregiver, returned to regular room/floor, and transported to the postanesthesia care unit in stable condition.*

Template Operative Dictation (Instrumented Excision)

Preoperative Diagnosis Type B postaxial polydactyly

Postoperative Diagnosis Same as preoperative diagnosis

Findings Same as postoperative diagnosis

Procedure(s) Performed *Right/left/bilateral Type B postaxial polydactyly excision*

Anesthesia General

Specimen Rudimentary digit

Drains None

Implants None

Estimated Blood Loss Minimal

Indications This is a/an ___-*day/week/month/year*-old *male/female* with Type B postaxial polydactyly. He/she was deemed to be a suitable candidate for *Right/left/bilateral Type B Postaxial Polydactyly excision* utilizing surgical instrumentation. Specific risks discussed included, but were not limited to, bleeding, infection, harm to surrounding structures, stiffness, wound healing problems, neuroma formation, numbness, and need for further procedures. After discussion, there was agreement to move forward with operative intervention and informed consent was obtained.

Procedure in Detail The patient was seen in the preoperative area and the appropriate site(s) was/were identified and marked. Following satisfactory induction of anesthesia in the operating room, the patient was placed in *supine position with arm extended on a hand table/arm board* and *all bony prominences were appropriately padded*. Timeouts were performed using preincision safety checklists with participation of all present in the operative suite. The correct patient, procedure, site, and additional critical information were confirmed prior to the start of the procedure. *A nonsterile tourniquet was applied to the right, left upper extremity, which was then prepped and draped in the usual sterile fashion.*

A digital block was performed utilizing *1% or 2% Lidocaine or 0.25% or 0.5% Bupivacaine. The tourniquet was elevated to 225 mmHg.* The postaxial polydactyly was identified and an elliptical incision around the base was created. Adequate tension was applied to the stalk by grasping the digit and applying longitudinal traction, with care to just come through the dermis, so as to protect the neurovascular structures. Longitudinal spreads were made utilizing Littler scissors along the neurovascular structures. The vessels were individually cauterized. The nerve was retracted and cut as proximally as possible, but not harming the native nerve proximal to the bifurcation. *The tourniquet was deflated.* Hemostasis was achieved. The finger was pink and perfused.

The wound was cleaned utilizing sterile saline and 5-0 chromic suture was utilized to close the wound utilizing horizontal mattress sutures. The wound was covered with a 2 × 2, Tegaderm, Kling, and a lightly applied Coban wrap.

All counts were correct ×2 at the end of the case. I was present for the entire procedure. There were no complications.

Upon completion of the procedure, a debriefing checklist was completed to share information critical to the postoperative care of the patient. The patient tolerated the procedure well, *was extubated in the operating room*, and was transported to the postanesthesia care unit in stable condition thereafter.

Template Operative Dictation (Instrumented Excision)

Preoperative Diagnosis Type A postaxial polydactyly

Postoperative Diagnosis Same as preoperative diagnosis

Findings Same as postoperative diagnosis

Procedure(s) Performed Right/left/bilateral Type A postaxial polydactyly excision

Anesthesia General

Specimen Rudimentary digit

Drains None

Implants None

Estimated Blood Loss Minimal

Indications This is a/an ___*-day/week/month/year*-old *male/female* with Type A postaxial polydactyly. He/she was deemed to be a suitable candidate for Right/left/bilateral Type A Postaxial Polydactyly excision utilizing surgical instrumentation. Specific risks discussed included, but were not limited to, bleeding, infection, harm to surrounding structures, stiffness, wound-healing problems, neuroma formation, numbness, and need for further procedures. After discussion, there was agreement to move forward with operative intervention and informed consent was obtained.

Procedure in Detail The patient was seen in the preoperative area and the appropriate site(s) was/were identified and marked. Following satisfactory induction of anesthesia in the operating room, the patient was placed in *supine position with arm extended on a hand table/arm board* and *all bony prominences were appropriately padded*. Timeouts were performed using preincision safety checklists with participation of all present in the operative suite. The correct patient, procedure, site, and additional critical information were confirmed prior to the start of the procedure. *A nonsterile tourniquet was applied to the right, left upper extremity, which was then prepped and draped in the usual sterile fashion.*

A digital block was performed utilizing *1% or 2% Lidocaine or 0.25% or 0.5% Bupivacaine. The tourniquet was elevated to 225 mmHg.* The postaxial polydactyly was identified and an *elliptical incision with proximal extension* or "*racquet- type*" incision was created around the accessory digit. Careful blunt dissection was utilized to identify abductor digiti minimi muscle (ADM). Using a sharp knife, the ADM was subperiosteally detached from its insertion on ulnar border of the base of the proximal phalanx of the accessory digit. The ulnar collateral ligament (UCL) on the ulnar border the metacarpophalangeal joint of the accessory digit was identified. Sharp knife dissection was again utilized to subperiosteally release the UCL distally, making sure to maintain a sleeve of periosteum. *This was then tagged for later identification and reattachment.* The vascular structures to the accessory digit were dissected and ligated. The nerve was cut as proximally as possible, with care not to injure the ulnar digital nerve to the native small finger. Using a combination of blunt and sharp dissection, the remaining tissue, including bone, of the accessory digit was removed. *If bone had to be separated sharply, fluoroscopy was utilized to identify appropriate dissection. Bone wax was applied.* The previously identified and isolated ADM and UCL were mobilized and prepared for reattachment onto the small finger. The UCL was reattached to the base of the ulnar border of the proximal phalanx of the native small finger utilizing *4-0 nonabsorbable Vicryl suture. If an adequate UCL cannot be harvested, a tendon from the type A polydactylous digit can be utilized to create a ligament (Fig.*

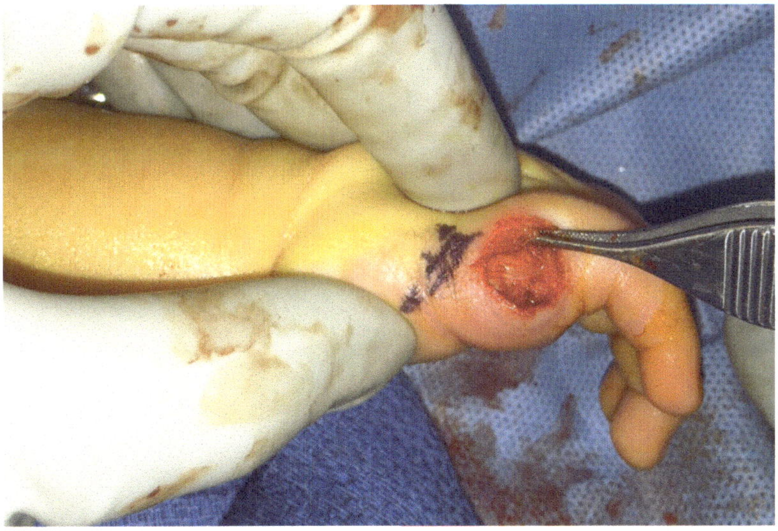

Fig. 106.4 Example of ulnar collateral ligament (UCL) reconstruction using a flexor tendon from the accessory digit, suturing about the metacarpophalangeal joint with 4-0 Vicryl

106.4). The abductor digiti quinti (ADQ) was then reattached onto the ulnar border of the base of the 5th proximal phalanx utilizing *4-0 Vicryl suture*. The metacarpophalangeal joint was evaluated for stability. *The tourniquet was deflated and hemostasis was achieved. 5-0 absorbable Chromic suture* was used to close the skin in horizontal mattress fashion. Sterile soft dressing was applied to the hand, followed by a *cast/splint* for stabilization. Immobilization for 2–4 weeks will be utilized to protect the reconstruction.

All counts were correct ×2 at the end of the case. I was present for the entire procedure. There were no complications.

Upon completion of the procedure, a debriefing checklist was completed to share information critical to the postoperative care of the patient. The patient tolerated the procedure well, *was extubated in the operating room*, and was transported to the postanesthesia care unit in stable condition thereafter (Fig. 106.5).

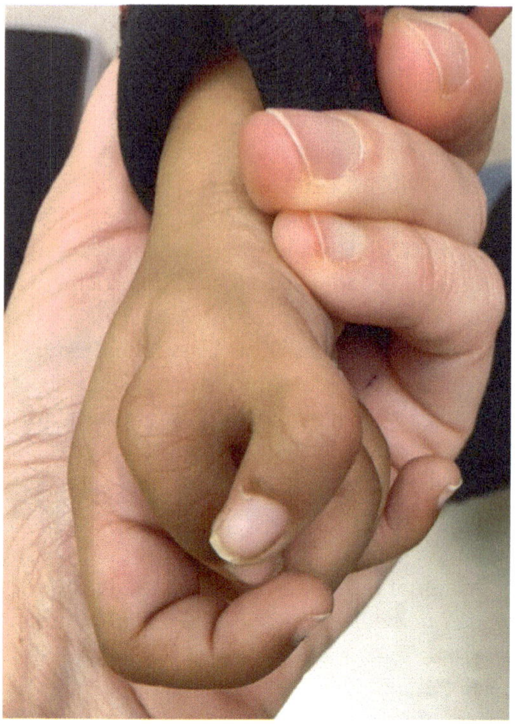

Fig. 106.5 Example of a preaxial polydactyly, which should be referred to a pediatric hand surgeon for management

Two-Incision Four-Compartment Lower Extremity Fasciotomy

107

Carolyn Gosztyla and Eric Jelin

Indications and Benefits

- Lower extremity trauma (crush, blunt, penetrating) with or without long bone fracture and resulting in compartmental hypertension
- Acute vascular injury causing ischemia or impaired venous drainage
- Prolonged extremity immobility (may be related to operative positioning or drug overdose)
- Massive fluid resuscitation in burn or trauma patients
- Benefits: Relief of symptoms related to compartmental hypertension, prevention of muscular necrosis, prevention of myoglobinuria, and renal failure

Risks and Alternatives

- Standard risks (bleeding, infection, need for additional procedures, and risks of anesthesia)
- Injury to adjacent structures including nerve injury and bleeding
- Scarring

C. Gosztyla (✉)
Walter Reed National Military Medical Center, Department of General Surgery, Bethesda, MD, USA

E. Jelin
Johns Hopkins, Department of Surgery, Bloomberg Children's Center, Baltimore, MD, USA

Essential Steps

Lateral Incision with Anterior and Lateral Compartment Fasciotomies

1. Identification of the following landmarks is essential to prevent iatrogenic injury to adjacent structures: fibular head, tibial tuberosity, anterior tibial spine, and lateral malleolus.
2. A longitudinal skin incision is made from the upper calf to the ankle. The optimal location overlies the intramuscular septum which is typically centered between the fibular shaft and the crest of the tibia.
3. A longitudinal incision is made in the fascia of the anterior compartment and the septum is divided to accommodate a second longitudinal H-type incision in the lateral compartment.

Medial Incision with Superficial and Deep Posterior Compartment Fasciotomies

1. A longitudinal incision is made from the upper calf to the ankle in a position 2–3 cm medial to the tibia.
2. The superficial tissue is incised.

D. J. Papandria et al. (eds.), *Operative Dictations in Pediatric Surgery*,
https://doi.org/10.1007/978-3-030-24212-1_107

3. The soleus muscle is released from the tibia longitudinally until the deep posterior compartment is able to be visualized.
4. The deep posterior fascia is incised.

Note These Variations

- Single-incision four-compartment fasciotomy where a single lateral incision is utilized to release all four compartments. In this approach, resection of the fibular head is no longer routinely recommended due to additional risk posed to the peroneal artery and nerve. This approach may be considered in patients with traumatic fibular fracture where the dissection has been partially completed by the traumatic incident.

Template Operative Dictation (Open)

Preoperative Diagnosis *Right/left* lower extremity compartment syndrome resulting from *trauma/vascular repair/fluid resuscitation/prolonged immobility/thrombosis.*

Postoperative Diagnosis Same as preoperative diagnosis

Findings Same as postoperative diagnosis

Procedure(s) Performed Two-incision four-compartment lower extremity fasciotomy

Anesthesia *General/regional/procedural sedation*

Specimen None

Drains *A negative pressure wound dressing was applied/none.*

Implants None

Estimated Blood Loss ___

Indications This ___-*day/week/month/year*-old *male/female* presented with increased pain and swelling of the lower extremity following *trauma/revascularization/fluid resuscitation/prolonged immobility. He/she* was diagnosed with compartment syndrome in the *left/right* lower extremity and deemed to be a suitable candidate for two-incision four-compartment lower extremity fasciotomy. Informed surgical consent was obtained by the *patient/patient's parent/guardian* prior to proceeding to the operating room.

Procedure in Detail Following satisfactory induction of anesthesia, the patient was placed in supine position and appropriately padded. Timeouts were performed using both preinduction and preincision safety checklists with participation of all present in the operative suite. These confirmed the correct patient, procedure, operative site and additional critical information prior to the start of the procedure. *Appropriate antibiotics were administered.* Doppler signals in the foot were obtained prior to starting the procedure. The *right/left* leg was then prepped and draped in the usual sterile fashion.

A longitudinal skin incision was made over lateral aspect of the leg at the midpoint between the fibular shaft and the anterior tibial spine. The incision was deepened through the subcutaneous tissue and skin flaps were raised to expose the muscular fascia. The fascia of the anterior compartment was identified and incised longitudinally, carried along the length of the skin incision. The intramuscular septum was visualized and transected to enter the lateral compartment. The fascia of the lateral compartment was then incised longitudinally and carried to the length of the skin incision creating a "H-type" incision between the anterior and lateral compartments.

Attention was then turned to the medial leg. A longitudinal skin incision was made 2–3 fingerbreadths posterior to the tibial spine. The incision was deepened through the subcutaneous tissue and skin flaps were raised to expose the superficial fascia. The superficial fascia was divided releasing the superficial posterior compartment and providing visualization of the soleus muscle. The soleus muscle attachment to the tibia was released using electrocautery until the deep posterior fascia was visualized. The deep posterior fascia was then incised longitudinally to release the deep posterior compartment. The released muscle was noted to bulge from the opened compartments and was found to be *viable/mottled/ischemic*.

Irrigation of both incisions was performed and hemostasis was confirmed. The wounds were dressed with a negative pressure wound dressing. Doppler signals were confirmed in the foot prior to leaving the operating room.

Upon completion of the procedure, a debriefing checklist was completed to share information critical to the postoperative care of the patient. The patient tolerated the procedure well, was extubated in the operating room, and was transported to the postanesthesia care unit in stable condition.

Splenectomy (Open and MIS Approach)

108

Lorraine I. Kelley-Quon

Indications and Benefits

- Hereditary spherocytosis
- Immune thrombotic purpura
- Sickle cell anemia
- Warm autoimmune hemolytic anemia
- Felty syndrome
- Symptomatic splenic hemangioma
- Traumatic injury
- Benefits: Relief of pain, resolution of hematologic pathologies, and cessation of traumatic blood loss

Risks and Alternatives

- Standard risks (bleeding, infection, need for additional procedures, and risks of anesthesia)
- Injury to adjacent structures (pancreas, small bowel, colon, stomach, and diaphragm)
- Overwhelming postsplenectomy infection
- Alternatives: Medical management of hematologic pathologies, nonoperative management of splenic trauma according to ATLS

L. I. Kelley-Quon (✉)
Children's Hospital Los Angeles, Division of Pediatric Surgery, Department of Surgery, Keck School of Medicine of University of Southern California, Los Angeles, CA, USA
e-mail: lkquon@chla.usc.edu

Essential Steps

1. Upper midline laparotomy incision
2. Mobilize the splenic flexure
3. Enter the lesser sac
4. Ligation of the short gastric vessels
5. Exposure of the hilar vessels
6. Ligation of the hilar vessels
7. Division of the splenodiaphragmatic, splenocolic, and splenorenal attachments
8. Extraction of the spleen

Note These Variations

- Left subcostal incision for open exposure.
- Patient can be placed in lithotomy position with a left lumbar roll for splenectomy, especially if it is to be completed at the same time as a cholecystectomy.

Template Operative Dictation (Open)

Preoperative Diagnosis *Hereditary spherocytosis, immune thrombotic purpura, sickle cell anemia, and Felty syndrome/* ____

Postoperative Diagnosis Same as preoperative diagnosis

D. J. Papandria et al. (eds.), *Operative Dictations in Pediatric Surgery*,
https://doi.org/10.1007/978-3-030-24212-1_108

Findings Same as postoperative diagnosis

Procedure(s) Performed Splenectomy

Anesthesia General

Specimen Spleen

Drains None

Implants None

Estimated Blood Loss ___

Indications This is a/an ___-*day/week/month/year*-old *male/female* with *blunt abdominal trauma/hereditary spherocytosis, immune thrombotic purpura, sickle cell anemia, and Felty syndrome/*____. He/she was deemed to be a suitable candidate for splenectomy.

Procedure in Detail Following satisfactory induction of anesthesia, the patient was placed in the supine position and appropriately padded. Timeouts were performed using both preinduction and preincision safety checklists with participation of all present in the operative suite. These confirmed the correct patient, procedure, operative site, and additional critical information prior to the start of the procedure. The abdomen was then prepped and draped in the usual sterile fashion.

An upper midline incision was made. Electrocautery was used to dissect through the subcutaneous tissue down to the linea alba. The abdomen was entered under direct vision in the midline and the fascial incision was extended superiorly and inferiorly to the edges of the skin incision. A self-retaining retractor was placed to facilitate visualization and the abdomen was inspected for accessory splenic tissue. The stomach was grasped and the lesser sac was entered using a *hand held Ligasure device/clamp-cut-tie technique/electrocautery*. The short gastric vessels were serially ligated along the lesser curvature of the stomach. The splenic artery and vein were visualized at the splenic hilum and circumferentially cleared. Care was taken not to disrupt the pancreatic parenchyma. The splenic artery was ligated using a *handheld Ligasure device/suture ligation/handheld vascular load EndoGIA stapler.* The splenic vein was similarly transected. Attention was turned to lysis of the remaining splenic attachments. The splenodiaphragmatic, splenocolic, and splenorenal attachments were serially divided until the spleen was free. The spleen was then extracted from the abdominal cavity and passed off the field as specimen. The left upper quadrant was copiously irrigated with warmed saline and hemostasis was checked. The laparotomy incision was closed using PDS (polydioxanone suture) in a running fashion. Interrupted Vicryl sutures were used to reapproximate Scarpa's fascia followed by a running subcuticular stitch to close the skin. A sterile dressing was placed.

Upon completion of the procedure, a debriefing checklist was completed to share information critical to the postoperative care of the patient. The patient tolerated the procedure well, *was extubated in the operating room*, and was transported to the postanesthesia care unit in stable condition thereafter.

Template Operative Dictation (Laparoscopic)

Preoperative Diagnosis *Hereditary spherocytosis, immune thrombotic purpura, sickle cell anemia, and Felty syndrome/*____

Postoperative Diagnosis Same as preoperative diagnosis

Findings Same as postoperative diagnosis

Procedure(s) Performed Laparoscopic splenectomy

Anesthesia General

Specimen Spleen

Drains None

Implants None

Estimated Blood Loss ___

Indications This is a/an ___-*day/week/month/year*-old *male/female* with *blunt abdominal trauma/hereditary spherocytosis, immune thrombotic purpura, sickle cell anemia, and Felty syndrome/*____. He/she was deemed to be a suitable candidate for laparoscopic splenectomy (open and minimally invasive surgical (MIS) approach).

Procedure in Detail Following satisfactory induction of anesthesia, the patient was placed in right lateral decubitus position, a break in the operating room (OR) table was positioned to open up the left upper quadrant and the patient was appropriately padded. Timeouts were performed using both preinduction and preincision safety checklists with participation of all present in the operative suite. These confirmed the correct patient, procedure, operative site, and additional critical information prior to the start of the procedure. The abdomen and left chest were then prepped and draped in the usual sterile fashion.

An incision was made at the inferior border of the umbilicus and dissection was carried down to the fascia which was incised with electrocautery. A Veress needle was inserted into the abdomen. Saline was infused and aspirated to confirm intra-abdominal placement. The abdomen was insufflated to 15 mm Hg. A 12-mm trocar was placed transumbilically and a 5-mm 30-degree scope was inserted into the abdomen. No injury upon trocar insertion was appreciated. The abdomen was further inspected and no accessory spleens were identified. Three additional 5-mm trocars were inserted in the left subcostal region. The splenic flexure was mobilized using a 5 mm Ligasure device. The lesser sac was entered and the short gastric vessels were serially ligated to expose the splenic hilum. The hilum was circumferentially cleared. Care was taken to avoid disrupting the pancreatic tail. The camera was then moved to the medial-most subcostal port and a vascular load EndoGIA stapler was inserted into the abdomen via the umbilical trocar. The artery and vein were taken together with a single fire of the stapler. Hemostasis was checked. The splenodiaphragmatic, splenorenal, and splenocolic attachments were serially divided until the spleen was free. The umbilical trocar site was upsized to a 15-mm trocar and a 15-mm Endo Catch bag was inserted into the abdomen. The spleen was placed in the Endo Catch bag which was then closed. Hemostasis was again checked prior to extraction. The bag was then partially drawn out of the umbilical trocar site to expose the splenic parenchyma and the abdomen was desufflated. The spleen was morcellated using ring forceps. The fragments of spleen were passed off the field as specimen. Once the specimen had been sufficiently morcellated, it was extracted through the umbilical trocar site and passed off the field as specimen. The 15-mm trocar was re-inserted into the abdomen, the abdomen re-insufflated, and a final check for hemostasis was performed. The remaining trocars were withdrawn under direct vision followed by the umbilical trocar. The fascia of the umbilical trocar site was closed with polydioxanone suture (PDS) in an interrupted fashion followed by an inverted dermal Vicryl stitch to close the skin. The remaining 5-mm trocar sites were similarly closed using an inverted dermal Vicryl stitch. Local anesthetic was infused into all trocar sites followed by sterile dressings.

Upon completion of the procedure, a debriefing checklist was completed to share information critical to the postoperative care of the patient. The patient tolerated the procedure well, *was extubated in the operating room*, and was transported to the postanesthesia care unit in stable condition thereafter.

109 Splenorrhaphy

Paul K. Waltz and Stefan Scholz

Indications and Benefits

- Splenic trauma requiring operative intervention or inadvertent injury during another procedure
- Benefits: Splenic preservation

Risks and Alternatives

- Standard risks (bleeding, infection, need for additional procedures, and risks of anesthesia).
- Injury to stomach, pancreas, large intestine, and small intestine.
- Continued splenic bleeding.
- Alternatives: Most splenic trauma is successfully managed nonoperatively or with interventional radiology interventions. Unstable trauma patients with multiple injuries and bleeding splenic injury may require total splenectomy. Splenorrhaphy alone or partial splenectomy with splenorrhaphy may be an alternative if the patient's condition allows. Splenorrhaphy may be performed laparoscopically. In case of splenectomy, splenic pieces may be implanted into the omentum for preservation of splenic function.

P. K. Waltz
University of Pittsburgh Medical Center, Department of General Surgery, Pittsburgh, PA, USA

S. Scholz (✉)
University of Pittsburgh School of Medicine, Children's Hospital of Pittsburgh, Department of Pediatric Surgery, Pittsburgh, PA, USA
e-mail: stefan.scholz@chp.edu

Essential Steps

- Midline laparotomy, abdominal exploration, and four-quadrant packing as indicated in case of trauma laparotomy.
- In hemodynamically stable patients, a laparoscopic approach may be a good alternative.
- Retract stomach medially, oral gastric or nasal gastric tube may facilitate exposure.
- Retract colon inferiorly.
- Mobilize the splenic attachments to the colon.
- Mobilize the superior and inferior attachments of the spleen in order to medialize the spleen and elevate it from the retroperitoneum.
- Avoid injury to the pancreatic tail.
- Divide the short gastric vessels.
- Identify the hilum, a vascular clamp can be placed to control the hilum.
- Identify the extent of injury to the spleen.
- *Use monopolar/bipolar/argon beam coagulation, topical hemostatic agents, pledgeted sutures with or without omental packing, absorbable mesh wrapping to control, and repair the injury.*
- Assess for hemostasis.
- Fixate the spleen to adjacent structures to prevent torsion.

D. J. Papandria et al. (eds.), *Operative Dictations in Pediatric Surgery*,
https://doi.org/10.1007/978-3-030-24212-1_109

Note These Variations

- Topical hemostatic agents utilized (i.e., Surgical [Ethicon]).
- Energy sources: argon beam coagulation, bipolar (i.e., Aquamantys [Medtronic]).
- Suture type (typically absorbable on blunt needle), use of pledgets, and type of absorbable mesh.
- Procedure may be performed laparoscopic in selected hemodynamically stable patients with laparoscopic argon beam coagulator and laparoscopic application of hemostatic agents.

Template Operative Dictation

Preoperative Diagnosis Splenic injury

Postoperative Diagnosis Same as preoperative diagnosis

Findings Bleeding injury of the spleen manifested as a *superficial/deep* laceration.

Procedure(s) Performed Splenorrhaphy with *suture/omental patch/mesh wrap.*

Anesthesia *General*

Specimen None

Drains None

Estimated Blood Loss ___

Indications This is a/an ___-day/week/month/year-old male/female with severe blunt trauma and hypotension requiring operative exploration.

Procedure in Detail Following satisfactory induction of anesthesia, the patient was placed in supine position and appropriately padded. Timeouts were performed using both preinduction and preincision safety checklists with participation of all present in the operative suite. These confirmed the correct patient, procedure, operative site, and additional critical information prior to the start of the procedure. The chest, abdomen, and groins were then prepped widely and draped in the usual sterile fashion.

A generous midline laparotomy was deepened through the skin and soft tissue to the linea alba. The peritoneal cavity was entered without injury. Hemoperitoneum was encountered and evacuated. The left upper quadrant was packed with lap sponges to tamponade splenic bleeding. *There were no other sources of bleeding.* The stomach was reflected medially and the splenic flexure of the colon inferiorly. The lap sponges in the left upper quadrant were removed. The spleen was mobilized free of its attachments and reflected medially and superiorly off of the retroperitoneum. Care was taken to avoid injury to the tail of the pancreas. Splenic hemorrhage was controlled with gentle elevation and manual compression. *The splenic hilum was then clamped with a large vascular clamp.* The injury was found to be a *superficial/deep, linea/stellate/complex laceration.*

As the patient was stable, there were no other identified injuries, and the spleen appeared to be salvageable. We elected to proceed with splenorrhaphy. The short gastric vessels were divided. *The upper/lower pole of the spleen was deemed unsalvageable and a partial splenectomy was performed with an energy device.* The injury surface was controlled with *bipolar diathermy/argon beam coagulation, horizontal mattress sutures of chromic on a large blunt needle reinforced with pledgets.* The area was then covered with a hemostatic agent. *Splenorrhaphy was completed with absorbable polyglactin (Vicryl) mesh to tightly wrap and reinforce the spleen.* Following the repair, hemostasis was deemed appropriate. *Topical hemostatic agent was left overlying the repair.* The splenorrhaphy mesh bag was then fixated in place in the upper left quadrant to the diaphragm and the retroperitoneum to prevent postoperative splenic torsion. Thorough exploration of the abdominal cavity revealed no other injury.

The fascia was closed in a *running/interrupted* manner and the skin was closed with fine absorbable sutures in a running fashion. Upon completion of the procedure, a debriefing checklist was completed to share information critical to the postoperative care of the patient. The patient tolerated the procedure well, *was extubated in the operating room*, and was transported to the postanesthesia care unit in stable condition thereafter.

Subtotal Splenectomy or Splenic Cyst Excision

110

Seth Goldstein and Daniel Rhee

Indications and Benefits

- Indication 1: Hematologic disorders including hereditary hemolytic spherocytosis, sickle cell disease (with recurrent or life-threatening splenic sequestration, hypersplenism, and splenic abscess), thalassemia major (with frequent transfusion requirements or massive splenomegaly), and failure of medical management for idiopathic thrombocytopenic purpura.
- Indication 2: Splenic mass, cyst, and abscess.
- Indication 3: Symptomatic splenomegaly or hypersplenism in malignancy.
- Benefits: Treat symptoms of underlying disorder or removal of lesion with preservation of splenic function.

Risks and Alternatives

- Standard risks (bleeding, infection, need for additional procedures, and risks of anesthesia).
- Injury to adjacent structures (stomach, pancreas, and diaphragm).
- Need for total splenectomy: With risk of overwhelming postsplenectomy infection or chronic thromboembolic pulmonary hypertension. If possible, vaccinations of *Streptococcus pneumoniae*, *Neisseria meningitides*, and *Haemophilus influenzae* should be administered before the operation.
- Splenic vein thrombosis, pancreatitis, portal vein thrombosis, and abscess.

Alternatives: Medical management, total splenectomy

Essential Steps: Open

1. Entry into abdomen.
2. Explore the peritoneum.
3. Open the lesser sac through the gastrosplenic ligament and expose the splenic hilum.
4. Divide the lateral splenic attachments, splenocolic, and splenorenal ligaments to fully mobilize the spleen.
5. Identify the major splenic vessels.

Subsection 1: For Partial Splenectomy for Hematologic Disorder or Splenic Mass/Abscess Removal

1. Identify the segmental branches to the upper and lower pole.

S. Goldstein
Ann & Robert H Lurie Children's Hospital of Chicago, Chicago, IL, USA

D. Rhee (✉)
Johns Hopkins School of Medicine, Department of Surgery, Baltimore, MD, USA
e-mail: drhee1@jhmi.edu

D. J. Papandria et al. (eds.), *Operative Dictations in Pediatric Surgery*,
https://doi.org/10.1007/978-3-030-24212-1_110

2. Ligate the blood supply to the area of planned resection (if upper pole, also ligate short gastric arteries).
3. Observe for line of demarcation. If for hemolytic disorder, goal is to leave 10–30% of spleen.
4. Divide parenchyma at the level of the demarcation with sealer/cautery/stapler device.
5. Obtain hemostasis of raw surface with argon beam coagulator, topical agents, suture ligatures, or mattress sutures.
6. Close without drains.

Subsection 2: For Splenic Cyst Excision

1. Drain the splenic cyst.
2. Circumferentially resect the roof of the cyst.
3. Cauterize or coagulate (argon beam coagulator) the base of the cyst.
4. Obtain hemostasis.
5. Close without drains.

Note These Variations

- Variation 1: Open versus laparoscopic access.
- Variation 2: Partial resections for hematologic disease or tumors requires full organ mobilization; cyst excision and fulguration may not demand full dissection depending on location.
- Variation 3: Differences in location and extent of partial resection based on spleen size and indication for operation.
  - For systemic disease such as hereditary spherocytosis, the goal is to near-total debulk, leaving only 10–30% of the spleen.
  - For benign tumors, the goal is to preserve as much parenchyma as possible.
  - Upper pole versus lower pole depending on tumor location or surgeon preference.

Template Operative Dictation

Preoperative Diagnosis *Hereditary hemolytic spherocytosis, sickle cell disease, thalassemia major, immune thrombocytopenic purpura (ITP), splenic mass, or cysts.*

Postoperative Diagnosis Same as preoperative diagnosis

Findings Same as postoperative diagnosis

Procedure(s) Performed Subtotal splenectomy or splenic cyst excision

Anesthesia *General/regional/procedural sedation*

Specimen Spleen, partial

Drains None

Implants None

Estimated Blood Loss ___

Indications This is a/an ___*-day/week/month/year*-old *male/female* presented with *hereditary hemolytic spherocytosis, sickle cell disease, thalassemia major, ITP, splenic tumors or cysts. He/she* was deemed to be a suitable candidate for *subtotal splenectomy or splenic cyst excision*

Procedure in Detail Following satisfactory induction of anesthesia, the patient was placed in supine position *with a bump placed under the left flank* and appropriately padded. Timeouts were performed using both preinduction and preincision safety checklists with participation of all present in the operative suite. These confirmed the correct patient, procedure, operative site, and additional critical information prior to the start of the procedure. *Specific lines/tubes* (i.e., *Foley catheter, OG/NG, SCDs, arterial line) were placed.* Preoperative antibiotics were given. The abdomen was then prepped and draped in the usual sterile fashion.

[Choose One:]
If open for hematologic disease or tumor: A left upper quadrant *transverse/subcostal* incision was made and electrocautery was used to divide the muscles in layers. The posterior sheath and peritoneum were opened sharply to enter the abdominal cavity. *A self-retaining retractor was placed to give adequate exposure and the abdominal cavity was explored.* The spleen was found to be *normal in size/enlarged. (List any other abnormalities found).* The lesser omental sac was opened and the short gastric vessels were divided using *cautery/energy sealing-dividing device.* The main splenic artery and vein with segmental branches were identified as they entered the splenic hilum. The splenocolic, splenorenal, and splenophrenic ligaments were divided by cautery and the spleen was medially rotated and delivered into the wound. *Control of the main splenic vessels was obtained using vessel loops/vascular clamps.* The *upper/lower* pole vessels were individually ligated, taking care to avoid injury to the pancreas. After ligating the segmental vessels supplying the *area/pole*, approximately *10–30%/other %* of perfused spleen volume remained. The spleen was then divided along the line of demarcation, on the devascularized side, using a *cautery/stapler/sealing device.* The specimen was sent off for pathology.

If open for splenic cyst: A left upper quadrant *transverse/subcostal* incision was made and electrocautery was used to divide the muscles in layers. The posterior sheath and peritoneum were opened sharply to enter the abdominal cavity. *A self-retaining retractor was placed to give adequate exposure and the abdominal cavity was explored.* The splenic cyst was identified after *medial/lateral/inferior/superior* manipulation and aspirated, with *clear/cloudy/serous/bloody/other* fluid removed. The roof of the cyst was then excised using *cautery/energy sealing-dividing device,* staying close to the spleen and working circumferentially to remove the outer portion of the cyst, and leaving the base within the spleen. The partial cyst wall was sent for pathology. The bed was *cauterized/coagulated/fulgurated using method of choice.*

If laparoscopic for hematologic disease or tumor: Atraumatic entry into the peritoneum was achieved via *Hasson/Veress technique* and the entire peritoneum was insufflated with CO_2 to a pressure of 12–15 mmHg and visually inspected. Initial impression was [*state findings/spleen appearance*]. UNDER direct visualization, a *3/5/10*-mm port was introduced in the midclavicular line on the left side below the tip of the spleen. Another *3/5/10*-mm port was placed in the midline epigastric area. *An additional port was placed superiorly in the midline subxiphoid area.* The table was placed in reverse Trendelenburg with the left side up. The stomach was grasped and retracted medially to expose the short gastric vessels. These vessels were divided using an *energy sealer-divider device/clips/electrocautery* exposing the splenic hilum. The splenocolic ligaments were then divided using electrocautery allowing retraction of the colon inferiorly and the splenorenal ligaments were then identified and divided. The ligamentous attachments to the upper portion of the spleen were preserved to avoid postoperative volvulus of the remnant spleen.

The main splenic artery and vein were identified *and control was obtained using vessel loops.* The splenic hilum was carefully inspected identifying the segmental branches. The spleen was partially devascularized by ligating the segmental vessels to the *upper/lower* pole using *energy sealer device/ clips/ electrocautery.* The spleen was demarcated and the splenic parenchyma was divided approximately 1 cm away from the line of devascularization using an *energy sealer device/stapler.* Bleeding from the splenic bed was controlled using *argon beam/electrocautery/topical hemostatic agents.* After hemostasis was achieved, the remnant was inspected and estimated that approximately *10–30%/other %* of perfused spleen volume remained. A laparoscopic retrieval bag was then inserted directly into the *umbilical/left lower quadrant* port site and deployed under direct vision. The resected spleen was then placed into the sac and the neck of the sac was exteriorized through the trocar site. *The port site was then enlarged to allow removal/*

morcellation of the spleen was carried out, breaking up with spleen within the bag using suction, finger fracture, and/or forceps. The bag was removed intact from the abdominal cavity and sent off as specimen.

If laparoscopic for cyst: Atraumatic entry into the peritoneum was achieved via *Hasson/Veress technique* and the entire peritoneum was insufflated with CO_2 to a pressure of 12–15 mmHg and visually inspected. Initial impression was [*state findings/spleen appearance*] under direct visualization, a *3/5/10*-mm port was introduced in the midclavicular line on the left side below the tip of the spleen. Another *3/5/10*-mm port was placed in the midline epigastric area. *An additional port was placed superiorly in the midline subxiphoid area.* The table was placed in reverse Trendelenburg with the left side up. The splenic cyst was identified after *medial/lateral/inferior/superior* manipulation and aspirated, with *clear/cloudy/serous/bloody/other* fluid removed. The roof of the cyst was then excised using *cautery/energy sealing-dividing device,* staying close to the spleen and working circumferentially to remove the outer portion of the cyst, and leaving the base within the spleen. The partial cyst wall was sent for pathology. The bed was *cauterized/coagulated/fulgurated using method of choice.*

Bleeding from any raw parenchymal surfaces was controlled using *argon beam coagulator/topic agents/capsular vertical mattress sutures using 2-0 monofilament suture with pledgets/omental buttress/other.* After satisfactory hemostasis, the remaining spleen was inspected and found to be *viable/other.* Abdominal wall fascia was closed with a *running suture using ____/ interrupted ____*. The skin was closed with a *4/0 absorbable Monocryl* suture in a *running* subcuticular technique and was dressed with *surgical skin adhesive.*

Upon completion of the procedure, a debriefing checklist was completed to share information critical to the postoperative care of the patient. The patient tolerated the procedure well, *was extubated in the operating room*, and was transported to the postanesthesia care unit in stable condition thereafter.

Placement of Central Venous Catheter

111

Carolyn Gosztyla and Howard I. Pryor II

Indications and Benefits

- Central intravenous access, short or long term
- Emergency resuscitation
- Central Venous Pressure monitoring
- Infusions of critical or caustic substances (vasoactive medications, chemotherapy, and parenteral nutrition)
- Hemodialysis, plasmapheresis, apheresis
- Pulmonary artery catheterization
- Benefits: Accesses with single or multiple lumen catheter for infusion, dialysis, or hemodynamic monitoring

Risks and Alternatives

- Standard risks include bleeding, infection, need for additional procedures, and risks of anesthesia.
- Early complications: Hematoma, pneumothorax, hemothorax, inadvertent arterial puncture, cardiac arrhythmia, thoracic duct injury, retained guide wire or guide wire embolus, air embolus, hemopericardium, cardiac tamponade, chylothorax, and catheter knots.
- Late: Line infection, catheter fracture, vascular erosion, and vessel stenosis.

Essential Steps

1. Select appropriate catheter type and size based on patient characteristics and indication for insertion.
2. Identify insertion site and appropriate anatomic landmarks. The use of ultrasound for identification of the target vessel is recommended.
3. Position patient in Trendelenburg position (internal jugular or subclavian lines), or reverse Trendelenburg (femoral line).
4. Don hair cover, face mask, sterile gown, and sterile gloves.
5. Prep and drape insertion site, place sterile ultrasound cover if it is used.
6. Prep central line by flushing with sterile saline and ensure that wire threads easily through the catheter.
7. Using anatomic landmarks and/or ultrasound, once again identify target site for insertion.
8. Puncture skin with introducer needle while applying backward pressure on syringe plunger. If using ultrasound, watch for the shadow of the needle appear within the

C. Gosztyla
Walter Reed National Military Medical Center, Department of General Surgery, Bethesda, MD, USA

H. I. Pryor II (✉)
Division of Pediatric Surgery, Walter Reed National Military Medical Center, Department of Surgery, Bethesda, MD, USA

D. J. Papandria et al. (eds.), *Operative Dictations in Pediatric Surgery*,
https://doi.org/10.1007/978-3-030-24212-1_111

lumen and watch for a flash of venous blood in syringe to confirm access.

9. Once access is obtained, place introducer and thread guidewire through the needle. If patient has continuous cardiac monitoring, watch for arrhythmia induced by guidewire
10. Remove needle, leaving guidewire in place. Make small incision adjacent to guidewire to facilitate passage of dilator.
11. Insert dilator over wire, then remove while applying pressure at the insertion site to minimize blood loss.
12. Thread catheter over guide wire taking care to always maintain a grasp on the end of the wire while inserting the catheter to prevent wire embolus.
13. Advance tip of catheter to appropriate position and remove guidewire. Confirm backflow of nonpulsatile bleeding from catheter through all ports, then flush and place hubs or caps.
14. Secure catheter in place, clean site, and apply sterile dressing.

Note These Variations

- If percutaneous access is not available, a venous cut down may be performed to facilitate catheter insertion.
- Tunneled lines are inserted in a similar fashion but the distal end is tunneled away from the venipuncture site under the skin creating an access site at a more functional or sustainable position.
- Vascular access ports are placed in a similar manner to a tunneled central line, but the distal end of the catheter is attached to an access port which is placed in a subcutaneous pocket.

Template Operative Dictation

Preoperative Diagnosis ___ necessitating need for central venous access.

Postoperative Diagnosis Same as preoperative diagnosis

Findings Same as postoperative diagnosis

Procedure(s) Performed Placement of central venous catheter

Anesthesia *General/regional/procedural sedation*

Specimen None

Drains None

Implants __ Fr, *single / dual / triple /* ___ lumen *tunneled* central venous catheter *(Hickman / Broviac / ___).*

Estimated Blood Loss ___

Indications This is a/an ___ *-day/week/month/year*-old *male/female* with a history of ___ and need for durable central venous access. Treatment of this condition necessitated central venous access for *resuscitation/monitoring/infusion/hemodialysis.*

Procedure in Detail:

[Choose One]

Bedside procedure: Informed consent from the patient including a thorough explanation of the risks and benefits of the procedure was obtained. The patient was positioned in Trendelenburg. A procedural time out was performed per institutional policy. This confirmed the correct patient, procedure, operative site, and additional critical information prior to the start of the procedure. The *right/left neck/chest/groin* was then prepped in the usual sterile fashion.

Procedure in the Operating Room: After obtaining informed consent from the patient including a thorough explanation of the risks and benefits of central venous catheter insertion, the patient was taken to the operating room. Following satisfactory induction of anesthesia, the patient was placed in Trendelenburg and appropriately padded. Timeouts were performed using both preinduction and preincision safety checklists with participation of all present in the operative suite. These confirmed the correct patient, procedure, operative site, and additional critical information prior to the start of the procedure. The *right/left neck/chest/groin* was then prepped and draped in the usual sterile fashion.

[Choose One:]

Internal jugular placement: Using ultrasound, the *right/left* internal jugular vein was visualized and an 18 g needle was inserted into the vein and was confirmed with aspiration of blood within the syringe. A guidewire was inserted through the needle using Seldinger technique. The needle was withdrawn. *The wire tip was deemed to be in the appropriate position using surgeon interpreted fluoroscopy/the wire tip was deemed to be in the appropriate position with visualization of ectopy on cardiac monitoring.* A small stab incision was made in the skin adjacent to the wire. A dilator was passed over the guidewire, then removed. The distal tip of the catheter was threaded over the wire while maintaining control of the distal tip of the wire. The guide wire was removed. The catheter was flushed and aspirated without difficulty. *The distal tip was confirmed to be in appropriate position using surgeon-interpreted fluoroscopy.* A *2-0 nylon* suture was used to secure the line to the skin. The site was cleaned and a sterile dressing was placed over the insertion site. The instrument and sponge count was correct at the end of the case. The patient tolerated the procedure *and was transferred to the postoperative recovery area in good condition.*

Subclavian placement: The angle of the clavicle was located *and local anesthetic was injected in the skin and subcutaneous tissue along with the periosteum of the clavicle.* A Cook catheter needle was inserted through the skin and subcutaneous tissue of the *left/right* chest toward the sternal notch. After feeling the clavicle with the needle, the needle was passed under the bone to access the *left/right* subclavian vein. A guidewire was inserted through the needle using Seldinger technique. The needle was withdrawn. *The wire tip was deemed to be in the appropriate position using surgeon interpreted fluoroscopy/the wire tip was deemed to be in the appropriate position with visualization of ectopy on cardiac monitoring.* A small stab incision was made in the skin adjacent to the wire. A dilator was passed over the guidewire, then removed. The distal tip of the catheter was threaded over the wire maintain control of the distal tip of the wire. The guide wire was removed. The catheter was flushed and aspirated without difficulty. *The distal tip was confirmed to be in appropriate position using surgeon-interpreted fluoroscopy.* A *2-0 nylon* suture was used to secure the line to the skin. The site was cleaned and a sterile dressing was placed over the insertion site. The instrument and sponge count was correct at the end of the case. The patient tolerated the procedure *and was transferred to the postoperative recovery area in good condition.*

Femoral placement: Using ultrasound, the *right/left* femoral vein was visualized and a Cook catheter needle was inserted into the vein and was confirmed with aspiration of blood within the syringe. A guidewire was inserted through the needle using Seldinger technique. The needle was withdrawn. A small stab incision was made in the skin adjacent to the wire. A dilator was passed over the guidewire, then removed. The distal tip of the catheter was threaded over the wire maintain control of the distal tip of the wire. The guide wire was removed. The catheter was flushed and aspirated without difficulty. A *2-0 nylon* suture was used to secure the line to the skin. The site was cleaned and a sterile dressing was placed over the insertion site. The instrument and sponge count was correct at the end of the case. The patient tolerated the procedure *and was transferred to the postoperative recovery area in good condition.*

***Tunneled internal jugular/subclavian catheter placement*:** Using ultrasound guidance, an introducer needle was used to locate the *right/left internal jugular/subclavian* vein. After aspiration of venous blood, a guidewire was inserted through the needle using Seldinger technique. The needle was withdrawn. The distal tip of the wire was confirmed to be in the appropriate position using surgeon-interpreted fluoroscopy. A small stab incision was made adjacent to the wire. Next a separate incision was made in the *right/left* chest. A subcutaneous tunnel was created and the distal tip of the catheter was pulled through the tunnel to the level of the cuff. The catheter was cut to appropriate length. A dilator was threaded over the wire followed by introduction of the introducer sheath. The wire was removed and the distal tip of the catheter was threaded through the introducer sheath which was simultaneously withdrawn. The catheter was flushed and aspirated without difficulty. *The distal tip was confirmed to be in appropriate position using surgeon-interpreted fluoroscopy.* A *2-0 nylon* suture was used to secure the line to the skin. The stab incision at the neck was closed with a *4-0 monocryl* suture. The catheter site was cleaned and a sterile dressing was placed over the insertion site. The catheter was flushed with an appropriate volume of heparinized saline. The instrument and sponge count were correct at the end of the case. The patient tolerated the procedure *and was transferred to the postoperative recovery area in good condition.*

A postprocedure chest X-ray was reviewed to verify position of the catheter and to assess for procedure-related complications.

112 Placement of Catheters for Hemodialysis/Pheresis (HD) Utilizing Ultrasound (US) and Fluoroscopy

Rebecca M. Rentea and Richard J. Hendrickson

Indications and Benefits

- Continuous Veno-Venous Hemofiltration (CVVH)
- Plasmapheresis
- Hemodialysis
- Continuous renal replacement therapy (CRRT)

Risks and Alternatives

- Standard risks (bleeding, infection, need for additional procedures, and risks of anesthesia)
- Injury to adjacent structures (Internal jugular vein, carotid artery, and lung parenchyma)
- Benefits: Provides suitable access for dialysis

Essential Steps

Insert Subsection Titles in Bold Italic as Needed (or Omit for Simple Procedures)

1. Surgical timeout confirming: review anatomy, history, and relevant labs.
2. Review local protocols regarding HD catheter insertion.
3. Obtain standard card/tray.
4. Place ultrasound machine opposite side of planned insertion.
5. Patient supine in slight Trendelenburg with head turned to the side opposite from planned insertion site.
6. Stand at head of the bed.
7. Use ultrasound probe to confirm the vein is in expected location and is patent and compressible with nonpulsatile venous flow.
8. Prep and drape the patient.
9. Cover ultrasound probe.
10. Anesthetize overlying skin and soft tissue.
11. Ultrasound probe should be centered over the vein in cross-sectional view. The needle tip should be centered with the probe. While holding the ultrasound probe in the nondominant hand, insert 16-gauge needle at a 45 degree angle to the skin about 1–2 cm cephalad to the ultrasound probe, in the same plane. A micropuncture needle (20 gauge) and guidewire 0.018 may be used initially. Once guidewire confirmed, then dilation may be done with a larger dilator to accommodate a 0.35 guidewire and then proceed as follows.
12. Apply negative pressure to the syringe as the needle is slowly advanced. When blood returns, ensure it is dark brown and nonpulsatile. Then advance the guidewire using the Seldinger technique. The guidewire should be seen in the

R. M. Rentea (✉) · R. J. Hendrickson
Children's Mercy, University of Missouri -Kansas City, Department of Pediatric Surgery, Kansas City, MO, USA
e-mail: rrentea@cmh.edu

D. J. Papandria et al. (eds.), *Operative Dictations in Pediatric Surgery*,
https://doi.org/10.1007/978-3-030-24212-1_112

vein. Observe for cardiac ectopy on the electrocardiogram (EKG) monitor which confirms the wire within the heart. Obtain a fluoroscopic image to confirm satisfactory placement of the wire. Best to have the wire directed down in the Inferior Vena Cava (IVC).

13. Pass of the ultrasound probe and finish the procedure.
14. Use fluoroscopically periodically to ensure proper wire placement. Best to be directed down the IVC. When using dilators, use *live* fluoroscopy to ensure safe travel over the wire of the catheter. When placing catheter through peel away sheath, use spot fluoroscopy as sheath is removed a few times to ensure that catheter tip is at the right atrial/superior vena cava Right atrial/Superior Vena Cava (RA/SVC) junction and has not flipped to another location.
15. Test each lumen with injectable saline to ensure brisk flow with aspiration and injection.
16. Optional use of contrast to confirm catheter placement.
17. Check fluoroscopic image once catheter in place to ensure smooth course of catheter from exit site to internal jugular, and tip is at or beyond the RA/SVC junction.
18. Pack the catheter with heparin according to hospital policy for catheter size and/or patient age/weight.

Note These Variations

- Kits vary.
- Ultrasounds vary.
- Can utilize small "finder needles" and exchange over larger wires first.
- Some catheters are tunneled, cuffed, or have a port attached.

Template Operative Dictation

Preoperative Diagnosis __ with need for central venous access for *hemodialysis/plasmapheresis*

Postoperative Diagnosis Same as preoperative diagnosis

Findings Same as postoperative diagnosis

Procedure(s) Performed Placement of catheters for hemodialysis/pheresis (HD) utilizing ultrasound (US) and fluoroscopy

Anesthesia *General/regional/procedural sedation*

Indications This is a/an ___-*day/week/month/year*-old *male/female* with ___. He/she was deemed to be a suitable candidate for placement of catheters for hemodialysis/pheresis (HD) utilizing ultrasound (US) and fluoroscopy.

Procedure in Detail Following satisfactory induction of anesthesia, the patient was placed in supine position and appropriately padded. Timeouts were performed using both preinduction and preincision safety checklists with participation of all present in the operative suite. These confirmed the correct patient, procedure, operative site, and additional critical information prior to the start of the procedure. The neck (site) was then prepped and draped in the usual sterile fashion.

Patient was placed supine, in slight Trendelenburg, with the neck turned to the contralateral side. The right/left neck was chest was prepped widely draped. A _____ brand ultrasound machine with ____MHz probe was used to confirm the internal jugular vein was in its usual anastomotic position and was patent and pliable and had nonpulsatile venous blood flow. A ___ brand pheresis catheter kit was utilized. All parts were flushed and tested prior to use. The skin and subcutaneous tissues were anesthetized with ___ ml of __ 0.25% bupivacaine (1 mg/kg).

The _ internal jugular vein was identified using ultrasound guidance and was percutaneously accessed on the first stick utilizing a 16-gauge needle. Obvious venous blood was returned. The guidewire was visualized in the vein. The guidewire was then placed under fluoroscopic guidance into appropriate position. We observed for any cardiac ectopy on the EKG monitor. A small incision was made at the guidewire exit site.

For a tunneled or cuffed catheter: An incision was placed on the anterior chest wall for the tunneled catheter to exit site and a *tunneler/hemostat* was used to dissect a curved path to the site of internal jugular venotomy. We made sure that the entrance into internal jugular vein was off center to allow a smooth contour, from exit site into internal jugular vein, and avoided a kink of the internal jugular vein when it is punctured at 90 degrees. The catheter was brought through the tunnel *and the cuff positioned __ cm deep to the skin edge.*

Utilizing Seldinger technique, a dilator was passed over the wire to dilate the subcutaneous tissue. The introducer sheath was placed over the wire and the catheter was positioned through the introducer sheath using fluoroscopic guidance. The dilator was exchanged for the catheter and the catheter smoothly advanced.

The guidewire was removed without difficulty, and the catheter ports were aspirated, flushed with saline, and capped without complication. Fluoroscopy [with/without contrast injection] was utilized to confirm the tip of the catheter to be at the SVC/RA junction. The catheter was secured with ___ at the desired depth and a dressing applied. A sterile dressing was applied _ and the catheter was left accessed.

Upon completion of the procedure, a debriefing checklist was completed to share information critical to the postoperative care of the patient. The patient tolerated the procedure well, *was extubated in the operating room*, and was transported to the postanesthesia care unit in stable condition thereafter.

Extracorporeal Membrane Oxygenation (Venovenous) Cannulation

113

Laura A. Galganski and Payam Saadai

Indications and Benefits

- Potentially reversible respiratory failure with severe hypoxia or hypercarbia
- Secondary cardiac failure from hypoxia, sepsis or metabolic derangement
- Benefits: Allows time for correction of severe cardiopulmonary dysfunction or diagnosis of irreversible cause of dysfunction. Greater simplicity in placement compared to arteriovenous extracorporeal membrane oxygenation (ECMO)

Risks and Alternatives

- Standard risks (bleeding, infection, need for additional procedures, risks of anesthesia).
- Injury to adjacent structures (right common carotid artery, right vagus nerve)
- Intracranial hemorrhage
- Blood stream infection
- Alternatives: Venoarterial extracorporeal membrane oxygenation, adjunctive ventilation with inhaled nitric oxide, high-frequency jet or oscillatory ventilation

Essential Steps

1. Choose appropriately sized cannulas
2. Position patient with head turned to left; use a shoulder roll for gentle neck hyperextension
3. Administer intravenous heparin (100 units/kg)

For Open Placement

1. Create a transverse right cervical incision and split sternocleidomastoid muscle bluntly to expose carotid sheath.
2. Open carotid sheath and identify right common carotid artery (RCCA) and right internal jugular vein (RIJV).
3. Obtain proximal and distal control of RIJV and ligate the RIJV cranially.
4. Three minutes after heparin injection, perform venotomy, place clamped venous cannula, and advance until the tip is halfway between the sternal notch and xiphoid.

L. A. Galganski
University of California, Davis, Department of Pediatric General, Thoracic and Fetal Surgery, Sacramento, CA, USA

P. Saadai (✉)
UC Davis Medical Center/Shriners Hospital for Children, Division of Pediatric Surgery, Sacramento, CA, USA
e-mail: psaadai@ucdavis.edu

D. J. Papandria et al. (eds.), *Operative Dictations in Pediatric Surgery*,
https://doi.org/10.1007/978-3-030-24212-1_113

For Percutaneous Placement

1. Using ultrasound guidance, access the RIJV with a needle, and advance a guide wire in to the vein.
2. Advance serial dilators over the guide wire followed by the cannula.

If Second Venous Drainage Catheter Is Needed

1. Using ultrasound guidance, access the femoral vein with a needle, and advance a guide wire in to the vein.
2. Advance serial dilators over the guide wire followed by the cannula.
3. Release the clamp, allowing it to completely fill, reclamp, and secure the cannula.
4. Connect to the ECLS circuit using addition of saline at connection to avoid air in circuit.
5. Confirm position of cannula with fluoroscopy or echocardiography.
6. *If open technique*, obtain hemostasis and partially close incision.

Note These Variations

- A semi-percutaneous technique can be used with open dissection to identify the right internal jugular vein followed by percutaneous access of the vein.
- Second venous drainage catheter can be placed via open cut down technique.

Template Operative Dictation

Preoperative Diagnosis *Respiratory/cardiac failure*

Postoperative Diagnosis *Respiratory/cardiac failure*

Findings Same as postoperative diagnosis

Procedure(s) Performed Extracorporeal membrane oxygenation (venovenous) cannulation

Anesthesia *General/regional/procedural sedation*

Implants ___ Fr venous cannula

Estimated Blood Loss ___ mL

Indications This is a/an ___*-day/week/month/year*-old *male/female* with *respiratory/cardiac failure*. He/she was deemed to be a suitable candidate for extracorporeal membrane oxygenation (venovenous) cannulation.

Procedure in Detail Following induction of anesthesia, the patient was placed in supine position with the head turned to the left and a shoulder roll in place for extension of the neck. Timeout confirmation was performed using both preinduction and preincision safety checklists with participation of all present. These confirmed the correct patient, procedure, operative site, and additional critical information prior to the start of the procedure. The right neck and chest were then prepped and draped in the usual sterile fashion.

[Choose One:]
If Open: A right transverse cervical incision was made over the sternocleidomastoid muscle and blunt dissection was used to divide the muscle, exposing the carotid sheath. The carotid sheath was opened and both right common carotid artery and right internal jugular vein were identified. *The right common carotid artery was encircled with a Silastic loop in the event that future conversion to arteriovenous cannulation is required.* The right internal jugular vein was ligated proximally with __*silk* and controlled distally *with a vessel loop.* Intravenous injection 100 units/kg of heparin was administered and allowed to circulate for 3 minutes. A venotomy was then created in the right internal jugular vein *using an 11 blade*. A ___ Fr double-lumen venovenous cannula was directed into the vessel lumen and advanced until the tip was half of the distance

from the sternal notch to the xiphoid process. The clamp on the cannula was released, allowing it to fill with blood and remove any air before it was reclamped. The cannula was then secured in place using two ___*-0 silk ties over a Silastic bolster*. The sterile circuit was then connected with careful addition of saline at the juncture to prevent air. Following initiation of the circuit, cannula placement was confirmed with *fluoroscopy/echocardiography*. The cannula was secured to the patient's neck with additional nonabsorbable sutures. Hemostasis was achieved and the skin incision was closed in a *running/interrupted* fashion with nonabsorbable monofilament suture.

If Percutaneous: The right internal jugular vein was accessed under ultrasound guidance using a ___ gauge needle and a guidewire was advanced. Position in the right internal jugular vein was confirmed with ultrasound. Dilators were sequentially advanced over the wire and a ___Fr double-lumen venovenous cannula was then placed over the wire using the Seldinger technique. The wire was removed and blood was allowed to fill the cannula and remove any air before it was reclamped. The sterile circuit was then connected to the cannula with careful addition of saline at the juncture to prevent the addition of air. Following initiation of the circuit, cannula placement was confirmed with *fluoroscopy/echocardiography*. The cannulae were secured to the patient's neck with additional nonabsorbable sutures.

Upon completion of the procedure, a debriefing checklist was completed to share information critical to the postoperative care of the patient. The patient tolerated the procedure and remains in critical condition.

114 Extracorporeal Membrane Oxygenation (Arteriovenous) Cannulation

Payam Saadai and Laura A. Galganski

Indications and Benefits

- Primary cardiac failure
- Severe congenital diaphragmatic hernia (CDH) with severe pulmonary hypertension
- Neonates and infants whose size precludes use of venovenous extracorporeal membrane oxygenation (ECMO)
- Benefits: Allows time for correction of severe cardiopulmonary dysfunction or diagnosis of irreversible cause of dysfunction

Risks and Alternatives

- Standard risks (bleeding, infection, need for additional procedures, risks of anesthesia).
- Injury to adjacent structures (right common carotid artery, right internal jugular vein, right atrium)
- Intracranial hemorrhage or ischemia
- Arterial embolization
- Blood stream infection
- Alternatives: Venovenous extracorporeal membrane oxygenation, adjunctive ventilation with inhaled nitric oxide, high-frequency jet, or oscillatory ventilation

Essential Steps

1. Choose appropriately sized cannulas.
2. Position patient with head turned to left; use a shoulder roll for gentle neck hyperextension.
3. Create a transverse right cervical incision and split sternocleidomastoid muscle bluntly to expose carotid sheath.
4. Open carotid sheath and identify right common carotid artery (RCCA) and right internal jugular vein (RIJV).
5. Obtain proximal and distal control of RCCA and RIJV.
6. Administer intravenous heparin (100 units/kg).
7. Three minutes after heparin injection, ligate the artery distally (cranially), perform arteriotomy, and dilate the artery.
8. Place the clamped arterial cannula and advance until tip is one-third of the distance between sternal notch and xiphoid.
9. Release the clamp to allow it to completely fill, reclamp, and secure the cannula.
10. Ligate the vein distally (cranially), perform venotomy, and place clamped venous

P. Saadai (✉)
UC Davis Medical Center/Shriners Hospital for Children, Division of Pediatric Surgery, Sacramento, CA, USA
e-mail: psaadai@ucdavis.edu

L. A. Galganski
University of California, Davis, Department of Pediatric General, Thoracic and Fetal Surgery, Sacramento, CA, USA

D. J. Papandria et al. (eds.), *Operative Dictations in Pediatric Surgery*,
https://doi.org/10.1007/978-3-030-24212-1_114

cannula and advance until the tip is halfway between the sternal notch and xiphoid.

11. Release the clamp, allowing it to completely fill, reclamp, and secure the cannula.
12. Connect to the ECLS circuit using addition of saline at connection to avoid air in circuit.
13. Confirm position of cannula with fluoroscopy or echocardiography.
14. Obtain hemostasis and close incision.

Note These Variations

- Intravenous heparin may be given prior to incision.
- Catheters may be lubricated with mineral oil prior to intravenous placement.
- A second cephalad venous catheter or a femoral vein catheter can be placed to aid in venous drainage.
- Femoral artery cannulation can be used instead of the right common carotid artery; however, this will require a distal reperfusion catheter into the posterior tibial or superficial femoral artery to provide blood flow to the limb.

Template Operative Dictation

Preoperative Diagnosis *Cardiopulmonary failure*

Postoperative Diagnosis *Cardiopulmonary failure*

Findings Same as postoperative diagnosis

Procedure(s) Performed Extracorporeal membrane oxygenation (arteriovenous) cannulation

Anesthesia General anesthesia

Implants ___ Fr arterial cannula, ___ Fr venous cannula

Estimated Blood Loss ___ ml

Indications This is a/an ___*-day/week/month/year*-old *male/female* with *respiratory/cardiac failure*. He/she was deemed to be a suitable candidate for Extracorporeal Membrane Oxygenation (Arteriovenous) Cannulation.

Procedure in Detail Following induction of anesthesia, the patient was placed in supine position with the head turned to the left and a shoulder roll in place for extension of the neck. Timeout confirmation was performed using both preinduction and preincision safety checklists with participation of all present. These confirmed the correct patient, procedure, operative site, and additional critical information prior to the start of the procedure. The right neck and chest were then prepped and draped in the usual sterile fashion.

A right transverse cervical incision approximately 2–3 cm in length was made one finger's breath above the clavicle over the inferior right sternocleidomastoid muscle. Blunt dissection was used to divide the muscle, exposing the carotid sheath. The carotid sheath was opened and both right common carotid artery and right internal jugular vein were isolated and controlled proximally and distally *with vessel loops*. Intravenous injection 100 units/kg of heparin was administered and allowed to circulate for 3 minutes. A venotomy was created in the right internal jugular vein *using an 11 blade*. The ___ Fr cannula was placed until the tip was half of the distance from the sternal notch to the xiphoid process. The clamp was released, allowing it to fill with blood and remove air before it was reclamped. The cannula was then secured in place using *two 2-0 silk ties over a silastic bolster*.

An arteriotomy was created in the right common carotid artery *using an 11 blade*. The artery was dilated and the ___ Fr clamped cannula was placed until the tip was one-third of the distance from the sternal notch to the xiphoid process. The clamp was released, allowing it to fill with blood and remove all air before it was reclamped. The cannula was then secured in place using *two 2-0 silk tie over a silastic bolster.*

The sterile circuit was then connected to the appropriate cannulae with careful addition of saline at their junctures to prevent air. Following initiation of the circuit, cannula placement was confirmed with *fluoroscopy/echocardiography*. The cannulae were secured to the patient's neck with additional nonabsorbable sutures. Hemostasis was achieved and the skin incision was closed in a *running/interrupted* fashion with nonabsorbable monofilament suture.

Upon completion of the procedure, a debriefing checklist was completed to share information critical to the postoperative care of the patient. The patient tolerated the procedure and remains in critical condition.

Extracorporeal Membrane Oxygenation Decannulation

115

Payam Saadai and Laura A. Galganski

Indications and Benefits

- Improvement in respiratory or cardiac failure no longer requiring extracorporeal membrane oxygenation
- Benefits: Removes need for anticoagulation, circuit contamination

Risks and Alternatives

- Standard risks (bleeding, infection, need for additional procedures, risks of anesthesia).
- Injury to adjacent structures (right common carotid artery, vagus nerve, internal jugular vein)
- Intracranial ischemia
- Alternatives: Ongoing extracorporeal life support

P. Saadai (✉)
UC Davis Medical Center/Shriners Hospital for Children, Division of Pediatric Surgery, Sacramento, CA, USA
e-mail: psaadai@ucdavis.edu

L. A. Galganski
University of California, Davis, Department of Pediatric General, Thoracic and Fetal Surgery, Sacramento, CA, USA

Essential Steps

1. Position patient with head turned to left; use a shoulder roll for neck hyperextension.
2. Reverse anticoagulation.
3. Clamp cannulae and disconnect from circuit.

For Open Decannulation

1. Open incision to expose right internal jugular vein *and right common carotid artery if arteriovenous ECMO.*
2. Obtain control of vessels.
3. Remove cannulas and ligate vessels.
4. Obtain hemostasis and close incision.

For Percutaneous Decannulation

1. Divide sutures securing cannula in place.
2. During inspiratory hold, remove the cannula and hold direct pressure over the venotomy.

If a Second Venous Drainage Cannula Was Utilized

1. Follow as above depending on open or percutaneous placement.

D. J. Papandria et al. (eds.), *Operative Dictations in Pediatric Surgery*,
https://doi.org/10.1007/978-3-030-24212-1_115

Note These Variations

- Repair of artery and vein can be considered if the cannulation duration was short and is most successful in pediatric or adolescent patients.

Template Operative Dictation

Preoperative Diagnosis Resolved *respiratory/cardiac failure*

Postoperative Diagnosis Resolved *respiratory/cardiac failure*

Findings Successful decannulation from extracorporeal membrane oxygenation

Procedure(s) Performed Extracorporeal membrane oxygenation decannulation

Anesthesia *General/regional/procedural sedation*

Estimated Blood Loss ___

Indications This is a/an ___*-day/week/month/year*-old *male/female* with resolved *respiratory/cardiac failure.* He/she was deemed to be a suitable candidate for extracorporeal membrane oxygenation decannulation.

Procedure in Detail Following induction of anesthesia, the patient was placed in position with the head turned to the left and a shoulder roll in place for extension of the neck. Timeouts were performed using both preinduction and preincision safety checklists with participation of all present. These confirmed the correct patient, procedure, operative site, and additional critical information prior to the start of the procedure. The right neck and chest were then prepped and draped in the usual sterile fashion. Anticoagulation was reversed and cannulae were clamped

[Choose One:]
If Open: The incision was reopened and the vessels were exposed. Proximal and distal control was obtained. Sutures securing the cannulae were divided and the cannulae and silastic bolsters were removed. The distal vessels were ligated. Hemostasis was achieved and the incision was closed.

If Percutaneous: The sutures securing the cannula were divided. The cannula was removed and direct pressure was applied over the venotomy site until hemostasis was achieved. *A pressure dressing was applied.*

Upon completion of the procedure, a debriefing checklist was completed to share information critical to the postoperative care of the patient. The patient tolerated the procedure well and remains in critical condition.

Creation of Distal Splenorenal Shunt

116

Jamie R. Robinson, James A. O'Neill, and Harold N. Lovvorn III

Indications and Benefits

- Liver cirrhosis when transplantation is not an option, extrahepatic portal hypertension when other measures fail, and gastroesophageal variceal bleeding with failure of pharmacological treatment and sclerotherapy in a patient without severe ascites [1]
- Recurrent gastroesophageal variceal bleeding after appropriately placed TIPS in a patient without severe ascites
- Benefits:
  - Decompresses esophageal and gastric varices
  - Maintains prograde portal flow into the liver
  - Avoids extensive hepatic hilar mobilization that could complicate future liver transplantation
  - Decreased incidence of encephalopathy compared to nonselective portosystemic shunts

Risks and Alternatives

- Standard risks (bleeding, infection, need for additional procedures, risks of anesthesia)
- Injury to adjacent structures (gastric veins, spleen, pancreas, duodenum, stomach, kidney)
- Postoperative ascites
- Recurrent bleeding from varices
- Portal venous thrombosis
- Encephalopathy
- Adhesions
- Alternatives:
  - TIPS
  - Nonselective portocaval shunting

Essential Steps

Entrance to the Abdomen

1. *Long left subcostal incision with an extension across the right rectus muscle or long midline incision from xiphoid to below navel.*
2. Limited abdominal exploration with avoidance of vascular adhesions.
3. Liver examination *and biopsy.*

J. R. Robinson (✉)
Vanderbilt University Medical Center, Department of General Surgery, Nashville, TN, USA
e-mail: jamie.r.robinson@vumc.org

J. A. O'Neill
Vanderbilt University Medical Center, Department of Pediatric Surgery, Vanderbilt Children's Hospital, Nashville, TN, USA

H. N. Lovvorn III
Monroe Carell Jr. Children's Hospital at Vanderbilt, Department of Pediatric Surgery, Nashville, TN, USA

D. J. Papandria et al. (eds.), *Operative Dictations in Pediatric Surgery*, https://doi.org/10.1007/978-3-030-24212-1_116

4. Ligate and divide the umbilical vein.
5. *Measure pre-shunt pressures* via *catheterization of a large central omental vein.*

Identification and Mobilization of the Splenic Vein

6. Open the lesser sac via division of the gastrocolic omentum.
7. Divide the right gastroepiploic vein and any collaterals.
8. Preserve the direct venous connections between the spleen and stomach (short gastric veins and the left gastroepiploic vein).
9. Use palpation to identify the inferior border of the pancreas.
10. Mobilize the pancreas anteriorly and cephalad.
11. Ligate and divide any lymphatic channels to limit chylous ascites.
12. Identify the splenic vein posterior to the pancreas.
13. Dissect the inferior and posterior aspect of the splenic vein.
14. Dissect the splenic vein from its pancreatic branches by ligating both sides and dividing the small vessels.
15. Ligate the inferior mesenteric vein.
16. Mobilize the splenic vein circumferentially to its confluence with the superior mesenteric vein and laterally to a point that allows the vein to be brought down to the renal vein without kinking or tension, *often 6–7 cm.*
17. Divide any large, communicating venous channels, including the coronary vein, at its junction with the splenic or portal vein.

Identification and Mobilization of the Left Renal Vein

18. Elevate the transverse mesocolon *and reflect the splenic flexure of the colon medially* to expose the left renal vein.
19. Mobilize circumferentially the left renal vein for approximately 6 cm.
20. *Often it is helpful for mobilization to ligate the adrenal and gonadal veins.*
21. Ligate adjacent lymphatics to prevent chylous ascites.

Splenorenal Anastomosis

22. *Mark the superior and inferior ends of the splenic vein with traction sutures.*
23. Apply a small bulldog vascular clamp to splenic vein 3 cm proximal to confluence with the superior mesenteric vein to prevent bleeding upon division.
24. Divide the splenic vein close to its junction with the superior mesenteric vein to reduce venous thrombosis.
25. Close the mesenteric end with *continuous 5-0 polypropylene suture, tie, large clip, or vascular stapler.*
26. Release the cephalad retraction of the pancreas to ensure length of splenic vein is adequate but not too long to prevent kinking.
27. *Create an oblique orifice in the splenic vein or slit the vein to allow for a long anastomosis.*
28. Apply small vascular clamp or vessel loop to occlude renal vein proximal and distal to site of anastomosis.
29. Remove a 1.5–2.0-cm long, narrow ellipse of renal vein on its superior border.
30. Anastomose the distal end of the splenic vein to the side of the left renal vein.
31. For the anastomosis, create a continuous posterior row of 5-0 polypropylene suture and interrupted anterior row of 5-0 sutures.
32. Release the splenic vein clamp prior to tying of the final anterior suture to remove air and flush out any blood clots from the anastomosis.

Measure Shunt Pressures and Closure

33. *Measure blood flow through the shunt using a vascular line transducer.*
34. Ensure adequate hemostasis throughout the abdomen.

35. Close the wound in layers for a water tight closure, *retention sutures may be used.*

Note These Variations

- The inferior mesenteric vein may join the superior mesenteric vein. In this situation, it is important not to mistake the superior mesenteric vein for the splenic vein.
- It may be helpful to divide the splenic vein at its junction with the superior mesenteric vein and then perform the dissection of the splenic vein off of the pancreas. However, if this approach is chosen, the renal vein should be dissected first in order to reduce the time of increased pressure in collaterals of the splenic vein.
- A modified technique to selective distal splenorenal shunting is complete division of the left renal vein near the renal hilum and anastomosis of its distal portion to the side of the splenic vein near the confluence with superior mesenteric vein. In this variation, suture ligation of the splenic vein is performed between the anastomosis and the superior mesenteric vein. Care must be taken not to disrupt lumbar venous collaterals on the proximal renal vein so that blood egress from the left kidney may continue.
- Placement of retention sutures to ensure a water tight closure may be useful.
- The body and tail of the pancreas can be mobilized off the splenic vein to the splenic hilum to attempt to reduce the development of vascular collaterals between the mesenteric venous system and the splenorenal shunt.
- Pre- and post-shunt pressures may be measured.

Template Operative Dictation

Preoperative Diagnosis Recurrent esophagogastric variceal bleeding

Postoperative Diagnosis Recurrent esophagogastric variceal bleeding

Findings Large esophagogastric varices

Procedure(s) Performed Creation of a distal splenorenal shunt

Anesthesia *General*

Specimen *Liver biopsy*

Drains None

Implants None

Estimated Blood Loss ___

Indications This patient is a/an ___-*day/week/month/year*-old *male/female* with portal hypertension and recurrent gastroesophageal variceal bleeding following failure of *pharmacological and sclerotherapy/TIPS*. S/he was deemed to be a suitable candidate for Creation of a Distal Splenorenal Shunt.

Procedure in Detail Following satisfactory induction of general anesthesia, the patient was placed in *supine position with elevation of the left side to a 15/30-degree angle*. Pressure points were appropriately padded. Timeout was performed using both preinduction and preincision safety checklists with participation of all present in the operative suite to confirm the correct patient, procedure, operative site, and additional critical information preceding the start of the operation. *Specific lines/tubes (Foley catheter, nasogastric tube, sequential compressions devices, arterial line, central venous catheter)* were placed. The lower chest and abdomen were then prepped and draped in the usual sterile fashion.

Starting at the mid-rectus on the right side, a subcostal incision was made crossing the midline and extended well onto the left flank/A large midline incision starting at the xyphoid was made. Routine exploration of the abdominal cavity was performed. The liver was examined *and biopsied.* The umbilical vein was ligated and divided. *Catheterization of a large central omental vein was performed to measure pre-shunt pressures.*

The lesser sac was entered via the division of the gastrocolic omentum. Proper luminal position of the nasogastric tube was confirmed. The right gastroepiploic vein was divided and the opening of the lesser sac was extended toward the spleen. The short gastric veins and left gastroepiploic vein were intentionally left intact. The inferior border of the pancreas was identified and mobilized anteriorly and cephalad. Any lymphatic channels were doubly ligated and divided. The splenic vein was identified posterior to the pancreas and mobilized circumferentially to its confluence with the superior mesenteric vein and laterally for *6–7 cm*. The inferior mesenteric vein and pancreatic branches to the splenic vein were ligated and divided. The coronary vein was ligated and divided at its junction with the *splenic/portal* vein.

The splenic flexure of the colon was mobilized medially to expose the left renal vein circumferentially for *6 cm. The adrenal and gonadal veins were ligated and divided.* All adjacent lymphatics were doubly ligated and divided. A small vascular clamp was placed on the splenic vein proximal to its confluence with the superior mesenteric vein and point of division. Next, the splenic vein was divided adjacent to its junction with the superior mesenteric vein. The mesenteric end was closed with a *continuous 5-0 suture/tie and large clip*. The length of the splenic vein was measured to ensure adequate length to the left renal vein to prevent twisting or kinking. An *oblique orifice/slit* was made in the vein to allow for a long anastomosis. A 1.5–2.0-cm long, narrow ellipse of renal vein was removed on its superior border. The splenic vein was anastomosed to the left renal vein with a continuous posterior 5-0 suture and interrupted anterior 5-0 sutures. The noncrushing vascular clamp on the splenic vein was released prior to tying of the final anterior suture to remove air and flush out any blood clots. *The blood flow through the shunt was measured using a vascular line transducer.* Adequate hemostasis throughout the abdomen was confirmed and the fascia was closed with a *running suture of ___/interrupted suture of ___*. Wound was closed in a water tight closure *and retention sutures were placed.*

Upon completion of the procedure, a debriefing checklist was completed to share information critical to the postoperative care of the patient. The patient tolerated the procedure well, *was extubated in the operating room,* and was transported to the postanesthesia care unit in stable condition thereafter.

Reference

1. Warren WD, Salam AA, Hutson D, Zeppa R. Selective distal splenorenal shunt. Technique and results of operation. Arch Surg. 1974;108(3):306–14.

Temporal Artery Biopsy

117

Justin A. Sobrino and Jason D. Fraser

Indications and Benefits

- Suspected giant cell arteritis or other systemic vasculitis affecting the temporal artery
- Benefits: Diagnostic certainty of a treatable disease process [1]

Risks and Alternatives

- Standard risks (bleeding, infection, need for additional procedures, risks of anesthesia)
- Injury to temporal branches of the facial nerve resulting in ipsilateral brow droop
- Negative biopsy
- Inadequate biopsy (short length, skip lesions missed, venous specimen) with a possibility of second, contralateral biopsy needed
- Alternatives: Empiric steroid therapy, imaging (color duplex ultrasonography, high-resolution MRI) [1–3]

Essential Steps

1. Identify and mark the temporal artery with palpation or ultrasound as needed.
2. Select the temporal or preauricular approach and make the corresponding incision.
3. Dissection to expose the artery with flaps as needed.
4. Ligation of arterial branches and terminal segments of the specimen.
5. Excise several centimeters of the temporal artery. The length may be limited to 1–2 cm for palpable disease, however, in asymptomatic disease, longer specimens are preferred as skip lesions are common [2, 3].
6. Confirm that the specimen is sent in formalin for permanent pathology. In cases of uncertainty, sending the specimen fresh for confirmation that the artery has been biopsied is reasonable.

Note These Variations

- Biopsies are ideally obtained prior to initiation of steroid therapy, though biopsies may be obtained after up to 2 weeks of therapy without negatively impacting histopathologic analysis [1].
- Some advocate biopsy of the temporal artery trunk through a preauricular incision given the consistency of the location [3].

J. A. Sobrino · J. D. Fraser (✉)
Department of Surgery, Children's Mercy Hospital and Clinics/University of Missouri - Kansas City, Kansas City, MO, USA
e-mail: jdfraser@cmh.edu

D. J. Papandria et al. (eds.), *Operative Dictations in Pediatric Surgery*,
https://doi.org/10.1007/978-3-030-24212-1_117

- Most will advocate unilateral biopsy initially, particularly for localizing symptoms, with subsequent contralateral biopsy reserved for nondiagnostic initial pathology. Others advocate initial bilateral biopsy [2].

Template Operative Dictation (Open)

Preoperative Diagnosis Suspected vasculitis involving the temporary artery

Postoperative Diagnosis Same as preoperative diagnosis

Findings Same as postoperative diagnosis

Procedure(s) Performed Temporal artery biopsy

Anesthesia *General/regional/procedural sedation*

Specimen Segment of the *left/right* temporal artery

Drains None

Implants None

Estimated Blood Loss ___

Indications This is a/an ___-*day/week/month/year*-old *male/female* with a suspected vasculitis involving the temporal artery. *He/she* was deemed to be a suitable candidate for Temporal Artery Biopsy. The risks, benefits, and alternatives to the procedure were discussed in detail with the *patient/guardian* and they have agreed to proceed.

Procedure in Detail Following satisfactory induction of anesthesia, the patient was placed in supine position and appropriately padded. Timeouts were performed using both preinduction and preincision safety checklists with participation of all present in the operative suite. These confirmed the correct patient, procedure, operative site, and additional critical information prior to the start of the procedure. The scalp and face were then prepared and draped in the usual sterile fashion.

Local anesthetic was injected over the selected area. A skin incision was made and blunt dissection was performed to expose the temporal artery and its branches. Arterial branches were ligated. Once an adequate length was exposed on the artery, the proximal and distal portions were ligated. The specimen was extracted and passed off of the table for pathology. The field was irrigated and made hemostatic. The wound was closed in layers. Sterile dressings were applied.

Upon completion of the procedure, a debriefing checklist was completed to share information critical to the postoperative care of the patient. The patient tolerated the procedure well, *was extubated in the operating room*, and was transported to the postanesthesia care unit in stable condition thereafter.

References

1. Hellmann DB. Giant cell arteritis, polymyalgia rheumatica, and Takayasu's arteritis. In: Firestein GS, Budd RC, Gabriel SE, McInnes IB, O'Dell JR, editors. Kelley and Firestein's textbook of rheumatology. 10th ed. Philadelphia, PA: Elsevier. p. 1520–40.
2. Warrington KJ, Cooper LT. Vasculitis and other uncommon Arteriopathies. In: Cronenwett JL, Jonston KW, editors. Rutherford's vascular surgery. 8th ed. Philadelphia, PA. p. 1154–66.
3. Meyers AD, Said S. Temporal artery biopsy: concise guidelines for otolaryngologists. Laryngoscope. 2004;114(11):2056–9.

118 Supraclavicular Right/Left First Rib Resection

Justin A. Sobrino, Pablo Aguayo, and David Juang

Indications and Benefits

- Neurogenic pain
- Axillary vein compression
- Axillary artery compression

Risks and Alternatives

- Alternatives: Physical therapy
- Injury to axillary vein or artery
- Nerve injury: Brachial plexus, intercostal brachial nerve, long thoracic nerve
- Recurrent symptoms
- Pneumothorax

Essential Steps

1. The patient is positioned in a supine position with the head turned away from the operative side.
2. The head of the table should be elevated slightly to reduce venous pressure and expose the operative field.
3. The clavicular head of the sternocleidomastoid mastoid muscle is divided to enhance exposure.
4. The phrenic nerve is identified near the medial border on the anterior surface of the anterior scalene muscle. The nerve is carefully freed and protected to prevent diaphragmatic palsy.
5. The anterior scalene muscle is divided at its insertion near the first rib taking care to avoid injury to the overlying subclavian vein. The muscle is further divided as close to its transverse process origins as possible to complete the resection.
6. The subclavian artery is identified in the inferior portion of the wound and can be easily isolated, should associated arterial pathology warrant surgical correction.
7. The middle scalene muscle is identified posterior and lateral to the root of the brachial plexus.
8. The subclavian artery passes along the medial border of the middle scalene muscle as it courses over the first rib.
9. The long thoracic nerve marks the lateral boundary of the middle scalene muscle division.
10. Cervical ribs are usually embedded within the fibers of the middle scalene muscle and are easily resected at the time of the middle scalenectomy.

J. A. Sobrino · P. Aguayo · D. Juang (✉)
Department of Surgery, Children's Mercy Hospital and Clinics/University of Missouri - Kansas City, Kansas City, MO, USA

D. J. Papandria et al. (eds.), *Operative Dictations in Pediatric Surgery*,
https://doi.org/10.1007/978-3-030-24212-1_118

11. The first rib is circumferentially freed from any muscular attachments, including the intercostal muscles and the subclavian artery.
12. The first rib is transected anteriorly and posteriorly. The remaining remnants are removed with a rongeur.
13. The wound is irrigated and the patient is checked for a pneumothorax.
14. The wound is closed in anatomic layers with absorbable sutures.

Note These Variations

- First rib resections can be performed through a supra and infraclavicular incisions or through a transaxillary approach.

Template Operative Dictation (Open)

Preoperative Diagnosis *Right/left* thoracic outlet syndrome

Postoperative Diagnosis Same as preoperative diagnosis

Findings Same as postoperative diagnosis

Procedure(s) Performed Supraclavicular right/left first rib resection

Anesthesia *General*

Indications This is a/an ___*-day/week/month/year*-old *male/female* with symptoms of thoracic outlet syndrome with *neurogenic/venous arterial compression. He/she* was deemed to be a suitable candidate for a supraclavicular right/left first rib resection. The risks and benefits of the first rib resection were discussed with the patient and *he/she* has elected to undergo surgical intervention.

Procedure in Detail Following satisfactory induction of anesthesia, the patient was placed in a supine position and appropriately padded. The head was turned away from the operative side. Timeouts were performed using both preinduction and preincision safety checklists with participation of all present in the operative suite. These confirmed the correct patient, procedure, operative site, and additional critical information prior to the start of the procedure. The head of the table was then elevated slightly. The neck, shoulder, and upper chest were then prepped and draped in the usual sterile fashion.

A transverse incision was made 1–2 cm cephalad and parallel to the clavicle, beginning at the clavicular head and extending approximately 8 cm laterally. The incision was deepened with electrocautery through the subcutaneous tissue and the platysma muscle. Subplatysmal flaps were developed to the level of the cricoid cartilage and to the clavicle. The external jugular vein and omohyoid muscles were divided in the midwound. The clavicular head of the sternocleidomastoid mastoid muscle was divided to enhance medial exposure. Just deep to the sternocleidomastoid muscular fibers, the internal jugular vein was dissected on its lateral border and carefully retracted medially. The underlying scalene fat pad was mobilized along its medial, superior, and inferior borders and then reflected on a pedicle laterally. [On the left side, the thoracic duct should be identified and carefully ligated as it arches through the anterior inferior medial corner of the scalene fat pad.] The anterior scalene muscle was then identified directly beneath this fat pad. The phrenic nerve was identified on the anterior surface of this muscle near its medial border. The nerve was carefully freed and protected. The anterior scalene muscle was divided at its insertion near the first rib taking care to avoid injury to the overlying subclavian vein. The muscle was then further divided as close to its transverse process origins as possible to complete the resection. The subclavian artery was identified in the inferior portion of the wound.

Attention was then turned to resection of the middle scalene muscle. It was identified posterior and lateral to the root of the brachial plexus. The C5 and C6 nerve trunk were mobilized along its lateral border and gently retracted caudally. The subclavian artery was carefully dissected from the medial border of the muscle as it courses over the first rib. The long thoracic nerve was identified and protected along the muscles' anterolateral surface. The middle scalene fibers were divided along the first rib attachments. The long thoracic nerve marked the lateral boundary of the muscle division. The operative field was then palpated to detect the presence of other fibrous constrictions. Any associated fibromuscular bands in the exposed area of the brachial plexus including those associated with the C7 vertebral and Sibson's fascia were excised.

If Cervical Rib Found: A cervical rib was identified within the fibers of the middle scalene muscle numbers was resected.

The first rib was then freed with blunt finger dissection along the inferior rib surface to detach the intercostal muscle fibers. Laterally, the brachial plexus was displaced and the body of the first rib was divided cleanly just distal to the tubercle. The posterior rib remnant was removed with a rongeur as close to the transverse processes as possible. The subclavian artery was carefully separated from the top of the first rib, and the intercostal muscles and pleura were separated from the underside of the ribs. The first rib was then grasped with a clamp and used as a lever to assist with its anterior division. The anterior division of the first rib was then completed just past the anterior scalene tubercle close to the costochondral junction. The remaining anterior rib remnants were removed with a rongeur.

Once the major portions of the rib had been removed, the remaining stumps are palpated and shortened using a rongeur. The wound was thoroughly irrigated. There was no evidence of any defects in the pleura. The wound was then closed with absorbable suture and sterile dressings applied. Sponge and needle counts were completed.

Upon completion of the procedure, a debriefing checklist was completed to share information critical to the postoperative care of the patient. The patient tolerated the procedure well, *was extubated in the operating room*, and was transported to the postanesthesia care unit in stable condition thereafter.

Debridement of Burn Wounds 119

Rita D. Shelby and Renata B. Fabia

Indications and Benefits

- Shallow burns that are expected to heal without the need for skin grafting.
- Initial procedure for staged wound excision for large, deep burns with sloughing epithelium and debris.
- Benefits: The procedure cleans the wound and allows it to heal more rapidly with reduced risk of infection.

Risks and Alternatives

- Extensive bleeding, infection, need for additional procedures, risk related to anesthesia.
- Pain, hypothermia
- Inadvertent excision and injury of healthy tissue with mechanical debridement
- Alternatives: Enzymatic debridement

Essential Steps

Burn Wound

1. Appropriate wound exposure and cleansing
2. Wound curetting, scraping, roughening or cutting/VersaJet
3. Obtain adequate hemostasis
4. Burn dressing
5. Splinting as necessary to preserve extremity function

Note These Variations

- In contrast to burn wound excision, the surface of debrided wounds is not ready to support immediate placement of permanent wound cover including skin grafts, and other wound covers.
- Enzymatic debridement is an effective alternative for the removal of eschar from burn wounds when conservative mechanical wound debridement is not feasible due to bleeding disorders or other considerations. It is typically reserved for chronic and nonhealing wounds.

R. D. Shelby
Nationwide Children's Hospital, Ohio State University Wexner Medical Center, Department of Pediatric Surgery, Columbus, OH, USA

R. B. Fabia (✉)
Nationwide Children's Hospital, Pediatric General Surgery, Columbus, OH, USA
e-mail: Renata.Fabia@nationwidechildrens.org

D. J. Papandria et al. (eds.), *Operative Dictations in Pediatric Surgery*,
https://doi.org/10.1007/978-3-030-24212-1_119

Template Operative Dictation

Preoperative Diagnosis *Burn wound infection/ partial-thickness/full-thickness contact/flame/ scald/grease/steam/___* burn, *__%* TBSA, involving the __.

Postoperative Diagnosis Same as preoperative diagnosis

Findings Same as postoperative diagnosis

Procedure(s) Performed Debridement of Burn Wounds of the __

Anesthesia *General/procedural sedation*

Drains *None/catheter dressing drains for irrigation of silver sustained-release dressing*

Estimated Blood Loss ___

Indications This is a/an *___-day/week/ month/year-*old *male/female* with __ % TBSA *partial-thickness/full-thickness burn/burn wound infection* of the *location. He/she* was deemed to be a suitable candidate for Debridement of Burn Wounds in order to allow *proper healing/preparation for skin grafting.*

Procedure in Detail Following satisfactory induction of anesthesia, the patient was placed in *supine/prone* and appropriately padded. Timeouts were performed using both pre-induction and preincision safety checklists with participation of all present in the operative suite. These confirmed the correct patient, procedure, operative site, and additional critical information prior to the start of the procedure. Precaution was taken to assure preservation of body temperature including warming of the operating suite, use of heat lamps, and warm irrigation solution. The preexisting *dressing/wound cover* was removed. Appropriate sites for placing monitoring devices were chosen and monitoring devices were secured. The *chosen area of body* was then prepped and draped in the usual sterile fashion.

[Choose One:]

For Large Deep Burns: Using a *curette/forceps/ scissors/scratch pad/saline-soaked laparotomy gauze/hydrosurgical debridement device, foreign bodies/sloughing epithelium/devitalized tissue* was debrided from *the* ___ until a grossly clean tissue level was achieved.

For Superficial Partial-thickness Burns: Using a *curette/forceps/scissors/scratch pad/ saline-soaked laparotomy gauze/hydrosurgical debridement device, foreign bodies/sloughing epithelium/devitalized tissue* was debrided from *the* ___ until healthy, well-perfused tissue level was achieved.

Adequate hemostasis was achieved with application of *direct pressure with saline/ epinephrine-soaked sponges/Thrombin spray/ and/or electrocautery*. After achieving satisfactory debridement and hemostasis, the wound was dressed by application of *burn dressing/ dermal substrate/xenograft/allograft/adherent dressing* which was secured to the wound with *interrupted absorbable __-0 sutures/skin staples/steri-strips/ glue* and was covered by *Kerlix gauze/topical antibiotic ointment and nonadherent dressing/Mepilex/silver impregnated dressing* and wrapped in *Kerlix roll/ACE wrap. A splint was then applied by Occupational Therapy to immobilize the affected extremity in a position of function.*

Upon completion of the procedure, a debriefing checklist was completed to share information critical to the postoperative care of the patient. The patient tolerated the procedure well, *was extubated in the operating room/remained intubated*, and was transported to the *postanesthesia care unit/intensive care unit* in stable condition thereafter.

120 Thoracic and Abdominal Escharotomy

Rita D. Shelby and Renata B. Fabia

Indications and Benefits

- Full-thickness circumferential or near circumferential burns of the thorax preventing adequate chest wall excursion with impending or established respiratory compromise
- Full-thickness circumferential or near circumferential burns of the abdomen with impending or established abdominal compartment syndrome
- Benefits: Prevention or relief of burn-induced respiratory failure and/or abdominal compartment syndrome

Risks and Alternatives

- Extensive bleeding, infection, need for additional procedures

R. D. Shelby
Nationwide Children's Hospital, Ohio State University Wexner Medical Center Department of Pediatric Surgery, Columbus, OH, USA

R. B. Fabia (✉)
Nationwide Children's Hospital, Pediatric General Surgery, Columbus, OH, USA
e-mail: Renata.Fabia@nationwidechildrens.org

Essential Steps

Thoracic

1. A longitudinal incision is made on both sides of the chest along the anterior axillary line, extending to the costal margin.
2. A proximal transverse incision below the clavicles across the upper chest is made and connects the longitudinal incisions; attention should be made to spare the nipples.
3. A distal transverse incision across the upper abdomen connecting the distal aspect of the longitudinal incisions.
4. Incisions should be made with electrocautery or scalpel completely through the full-thickness eschar until subcutaneous tissue is visualized and audible or visual release of pressure is confirmed.
5. Ensure all firm attachments are sufficiently released by running fingers or a small clamp through the incisions into deeper tissues.

Abdomen

1. Mark the incision along the anterior axillary line from the subcostal region to the mid-abdomen; mark transverse incision across supra-umbilical abdomen.

D. J. Papandria et al. (eds.), *Operative Dictations in Pediatric Surgery*,
https://doi.org/10.1007/978-3-030-24212-1_120

2. Lateral incisions should extend from the bilateral subcostal regions extending distally to mid-abdomen.
3. Transverse incision should extend across the supra-umbilical abdominal region connecting the two lateral longitudinal incisions.
4. Incisions should be made with electrocautery or scalpel completely through the full-thickness eschar until the subcutaneous tissue is visualized and audible or visual release of pressure is confirmed.
5. Ensure all firm attachments are sufficiently released by running fingers or a small clamp through the incisions into deeper tissues.

Note These Variations

- Severe abdominal burns not responding to escharotomy with worsening abdominal compartment syndrome will require escalation to decompressive laparotomy.

Template Operative Dictation

Preoperative Diagnosis Full-thickness circumferential or near circumferential burn with eschar

Postoperative Diagnosis Same as preoperative diagnosis

Findings Same as postoperative diagnosis

Procedure(s) Performed Thoracic and abdominal escharotomy

Anesthesia *General/procedural sedation*

Estimated Blood Loss ___

Indications This is a/an ___*-day/week/month/year*-old *male/female* with full-thickness *circumferential/near circumferential* burns of the *chest and/or abdomen*. Rising compartment pressures were resulting in *impending respiratory/multi-organ failure*. He/she was deemed to be a suitable candidate for thoracic and abdominal escharotomy.

Procedure in Detail Following satisfactory induction of anesthesia, the patient was placed in supine position and was appropriately padded. Time outs were performed using both preinduction and preincision safety checklists with participation of all those present in the operative suite. These confirmed the correct patient, procedure, operative site, and additional critical information prior to the start of the procedure. The *chest and abdomen* were prepped and draped in the standard sterile fashion.

Marking of planned incisions was completed. Eschar edges were infiltrated with 1% lidocaine plus 1:100,000 epinephrine. Using *a scalpel/electrocautery*, the thoracic eschar was incised along the anterior axillary line on bilateral sides of the chest, extending to the *costal margin/upper abdomen/mid-abdomen*. Following, this a proximal transverse incision was made below the clavicles across the upper chest, and another incision was made across the upper abdomen, *in the supra-umbilical region*. Both transverse incisions were extended laterally, connecting with the longitudinal incisions. The incisions were carried down to the subcutaneous tissue and immediate release of tissue pressure was *observed/audible*. Adequate release was confirmed with appropriate respiratory and circulatory function which was confirmed by the anesthesiology team. Hemostasis was then obtained using electrocautery and all wounds were thoroughly irrigated. The wounds were then dressed with *Silvadene/antibacterial dressing/silver impregnated* along with an absorbent outer dressing.

Upon completion of the procedure, a debriefing checklist was completed to share information critical to the postoperative care of the patient. The patient tolerated the procedure well, *was extubated in the operating room*, and was transported to the postanesthesia care unit in stable condition thereafter.

Upper Extremity Escharotomy and Fasciotomy

121

Rita D. Shelby, Rajan K. Thakkar, and Kim A. Bjorklund

Indications and Benefits

- Full-thickness circumferential or near circumferential burns of the upper extremities with impending or established vascular compromise
- Traumatic injuries of the upper extremities with impending or established vascular compromise
- Benefits: Prevention or relief of burn/trauma induced compartment syndrome, restoration of tissue perfusion to prevent loss of function or loss of limb

Risks and Alternatives

- Extensive bleeding, infection, need for additional procedures.
- Nerve injury.
- Exposure of vital structures.
- Alternatives: Close monitoring for signs of vascular compromise, fasciotomy may be indicated if there is no improvement of perfusion following escharotomy.

Essential Steps

Upper Extremity Escharotomy, Including Hand

1. With the patient positioned supine, mark medial and lateral incisions in the longitudinal mid-axial line between the extensor and flexor surfaces.
2. The medial incision should extend from axilla to the base of the small finger, anterior to the medial epicondyle to avoid ulnar nerve injury.
3. The lateral incision should extend from just distal to the proximal humeral head to 1–2 cm past the area of the burn or to the proximal phalanx of the thumb if the burn extends to the hand.
4. At the level of the wrist, observe for the superficial branch of radial nerve .
5. Digital incisions should be performed along the mid-axial line between the neurovascular bundle and the extensor mechanism; the thumb incision should be on the radial side, with all other digital incisions on the ulnar side to avoid future problems with pinch.

R. D. Shelby
Nationwide Children's Hospital, Ohio State University Wexner Medical Center, Department of Pediatric Surgery, Columbus, OH, USA

R. K. Thakkar (✉)
Nationwide Children's Hospital, Pediatric General Surgery, Columbus, OH, USA
e-mail: Rajan.Thakkar@nationwidechildrens.org

K. A. Bjorklund
Nationwide Children's Hospital, Department of Plastic, Reconstructive and Hand Surgery, Columbus, OH, USA

D. J. Papandria et al. (eds.), *Operative Dictations in Pediatric Surgery*,
https://doi.org/10.1007/978-3-030-24212-1_121

6. Two longitudinal incisions should be placed on the dorsal hand along the index and ring metacarpal bones.
7. Incisions should be made with electrocautery or scalpel completely through the full-thickness eschar until subcutaneous tissue is visualized and audible or visual release of pressure is confirmed.
8. Ensure all firm attachments are sufficiently released by running fingers or a small clamp through the incisions into deeper tissues.

Upper Extremity Fasciotomy, Including Hand

1. May be performed by extending medial escharotomy incisions.
2. Carpal tunnel decompression is performed by releasing the transverse carpal ligament through a palmar crease incision between the thenar and hypothenar eminence.
3. For the brachial compartments, a lateral incision from the deltoid insertion distally to the lateral epicondyle, sparing any large cutaneous nerves.
4. At the fascial level, the intermuscular septum between the anterior compartment (containing the biceps and brachialis) and the posterior compartment (triceps) is identified and released via longitudinal incisions.
5. Take care to preserve the radial nerve as it passes through the septum from the posterior to anterior compartment.
6. For antebrachial compartments, two longitudinal incisions are required on the dorsal (extensor) and volar (flexor) surfaces.
7. For the dorsal compartment, a straight line incision extending through the fascia is made from just distal to the elbow down to the proximal wrist.
8. For the volar compartments, the S-shaped incision extends transversely across the wrist flexion crease to the ulnar side, curves gently across the mid-forearm and back to the ulnar side at the elbow.
9. At the elbow, the volar incision is curved lateral to the medial epicondyle, then, the deep fascia is released.
10. Careful dissection is warranted at the antecubital fossa, to avoid injury to the brachial artery and median nerve.
11. Hand fasciotomy consists of 4 incisions to ensure that all 10 compartments of the hand are adequately released.
12. A longitudinal incision along the radial aspect of the thumb metacarpal releases the thenar compartment.
13. Dorsal longitudinal incision along the index finger metacarpal releases the 1st and 2nd dorsal interossei and volar interossei, as well as adductor pollicis.
14. Dorsal longitudinal incision over the ring finger metacarpal releases the 3rd and 4th dorsal and volar interossei.
15. A longitudinal incision along the ulnar aspect of the small digit releases the hypothenar muscles.
16. Take care to make incisions away from any neurovascular bundles.

Note These Variations

- Severely burned extremities may require performance of fasciotomy concurrently with escharotomies.
- Digital escharotomies remain controversial.

Template Operative Dictation

Preoperative Diagnosis Full-thickness circumferential or near circumferential upper extremity burn with eschar, *with presence of elevated compartment pressures.*

Postoperative Diagnosis Same as preoperative diagnosis

Findings Same as postoperative diagnosis

Procedure(s) Performed Upper extremity escharotomy and fasciotomy

Anesthesia *General/procedural sedation*

Estimated Blood Loss ___

Indications This is a/an ___*-day/-week-/month/-year*-old *male/female* with full-thickness *circumferential/ near circumferential* burns of the *right/left/forearm/arm/hand.* Rising compartment pressures were resulting in concern for impending *neurovascular compromise.* He/she was deemed to be a suitable candidate for Upper Extremity Escharotomy and Fasciotomy.

Procedure in Detail Following satisfactory induction of anesthesia, the patient was placed in supine position, with *the upper extremities in neutral position,* and was appropriately padded. Timeouts were performed using both preinduction and preincision safety checklists with participation of all those present in the operative suite. These confirmed the correct patient, procedure, operative site, and additional critical information prior to the start of the procedure. The *right/left upper extremity and/or right/left hand* was then prepped and draped in the standard sterile fashion.

Marking of planned incisions was completed. Eschar edges were infiltrated with 1% lidocaine. Using *a scalpel/electrocautery,*

[Choose One:]

If upper extremity escharotomy: The eschar was incised medially, extending from the axilla distally to the base of the small digit. The incision was carried down to the subcutaneous tissue and anterior to the medial epicondyle. An immediate release of tissue pressure was observed. Attention was turned laterally; this incision was carried distally from just distal to the proximal humeral head to the proximal phalanx of the thumb. Again, immediate release of tissue pressure was observed. Hemostasis was obtained using electrocautery and all wounds were thoroughly irrigated. Adequate circulation was confirmed with palpation of pulses and compartments were noted to be soft. The wounds were then dressed with *Silvadene/Antibacterial/silver impregnated dressing* along with an absorbent outer dressing.

If hand escharotomy: The digital eschar of the *right/left* hand was incised on the ulnar aspect of the index through the small digits, and the radial aspect of the thumb. There was no obvious injury to the neurovascular bundles. Then two longitudinal incisions were performed on the dorsal surface of the hand along the index and ring metacarpal bones. Hemostasis was obtained using electrocautery and all wounds were thoroughly irrigated. Adequate circulation to each digit was confirmed and compartments were noted to be soft. The wounds were then dressed with *Silvadene/Antibacterial/silver impregnated dressing* along with an absorbent outer dressing. The hand was dressed and splinted in a position of function to minimize contracture.

If {upper extremity fasciotomy}: A lateral skin incision from the deltoid insertion to the lateral epicondyle was made, sparing large cutaneous nerves. The incision was extended through the fascial level. The intermuscular septum between the anterior and posterior compartments was then identified, and the fascia overlying each compartment was released in a longitudinal manner. Care was taken to avoid injury of the radial nerve as it passes through the intermuscular septum. Then our attention was turned to the forearm compartments. A longitudinal incision was made on the dorsal surface of the forearm from just distal to the lateral epicondyle extending down to the midline proximal wrist, ensuring the incision extended through the fascia. The forearm was rotated, exposing the volar surface. A palmar incision was made between the thenar and hypothenar muscles releasing the carpal tunnel. The incision was then extended transversely across the wrist flexion crease to the ulnar side of the wrist, arched across the volar forearm in a curvilinear fashion, and back to the ulnar side of the elbow. At the elbow, just radial to the medial epicondyle the incision was extended across the elbow joint. The deep fascia was then released using longitudinal incisions. The fascial attachments at the antecubital fossa were released utilizing clamps with careful dissection, protecting the brachial artery and median nerve from injury. This completed the procedure. Hemostasis was ensured using electrocautery and all wounds were thoroughly irrigated. Sterile moist dressings were placed in skin incisions and long-arm splints ensuring minimal flexion of the elbow were applied.

If hand fasciotomy: A longitudinal incision on the radial aspect of the thumb was made to release the thenar compartment. Then an incision on the dorsal surface of the index metacarpal was made, releasing the first and second dorsal and volar interossei. Another dorsal incision over the ring metacarpal was made to release the third and fourth dorsal and volar interossei. Finally, an incision along the ulnar aspect of the small finger was made to release the hypothenar muscles. Adequate circulation to each digit was confirmed and compartments were noted to be soft. *Sterile moist dressings* were placed within the incisions along with an outer absorbent dressing. Skin incisions were left open. All digits were dressed and the hand splinted in a position of function to minimize contracture.

Upon completion of the procedure, a debriefing checklist was completed to share information critical to the postoperative care of the patient. The patient tolerated the procedure well, *was extubated in the operating room*, and was transported to the postanesthesia care unit in stable condition thereafter.

122 Lower Extremity Escharotomy and Fasciotomy

Rita D. Shelby and Rajan K. Thakkar

Indications and Benefits

- Full-thickness circumferential or near circumferential burns of the lower extremities with impending or established vascular compromise
- Traumatic injuries of the lower extremities with impending or established vascular compromise
- Benefits: Prevention or relief of burn/trauma induced compartment syndrome

Risks and Alternatives

- Extensive bleeding, infection, and need for additional procedures.
- Nerve injury.
- Exposure of vital structures.
- Alternatives: Close monitoring for signs of vascular compromise, fasciotomy may be performed if there is no improvement in perfusion following escharotomy.

Essential Steps

Lower Extremity Escharotomy

1. With the patient positioned supine, mark the medial and lateral incision in the longitudinal mid-axial line between the extensor and flexor surfaces.
2. Medial incision should extend from proximal adductor muscles, extending posterior to the medial malleolus to avoid injury to the long saphenous vein and saphenous nerve, distally to the great toe.
3. Lateral incision should extend from the hip, extending distally through the mid-lateral line to avoid the common peroneal nerve, and continue to travel laterally, posterior to the lateral malleolus while continuing to the lateral surface of the fifth toe.
4. Incisions should be made with electrocautery or scalpel completely through the full-thickness eschar until subcutaneous tissue is visualized and audible or visual release of pressure is confirmed.
5. Ensure all firm attachments are sufficiently released by running fingers or a small clamp through the incisions into deeper tissues.

R. D. Shelby
Nationwide Children's Hospital, Ohio State University Wexner Medical Center, Department of Pediatric Surgery, Columbus, OH, USA

R. K. Thakkar (✉)
Nationwide Children's Hospital, Pediatric General Surgery, Columbus, OH, USA
e-mail: Rajan.Thakkar@nationwidechildrens.org

D. J. Papandria et al. (eds.), *Operative Dictations in Pediatric Surgery*,
https://doi.org/10.1007/978-3-030-24212-1_122

Lower Extremity Fasciotomy

1. Two longitudinal incisions from the distal thigh/upper leg to the ankle, 3 cm lateral to the tibia, one of which will be anterolateral while the second is posteromedial.
2. The incisions should extend the entire length of the calf to allow release of all respective compartments.
3. The anterolateral incision is made through the fascia to release the anterior and lateral compartments.
4. The second incision is the posteromedial incision which is made from the distal thigh/upper leg to the ankle, 3 cm medial to the tibia.
5. The longitudinal incision through the soleus muscle exposes the posterior fascia, releasing the superficial posterior and deep posterior compartments.
6. Take care to make incisions away from any neurovascular bundles.

Note These Variations

- Severely burned extremities may require performance of fasciotomy concurrently with escharotomies.
- This is a two-incision approach to the four-quadrant lower leg fasciotomy. This can also be accomplished via a single incision which requires an excision of a large segment of the fibula. This approach is rarely performed in the pediatric patient due to the significant deformity that results.

Template Operative Dictation

Preoperative Diagnosis Full-thickness circumferential or near circumferential lower extremity burn with eschar, *with presence of elevated compartment pressures*

Postoperative Diagnosis Same as preoperative diagnosis

Findings Same as postoperative diagnosis

Procedure(s) Performed Lower extremity escharotomy and fasciotomy

Anesthesia *General/procedural sedation*

Estimated Blood Loss ___

Indications This is a/an ___*-day/week/month/year*-old *male/female* with full-thickness *circumferential/ near circumferential* burns of the *lower extremities/elevated compartment pressures of the lower extremity.* Rising compartment pressures were resulting in *neurovascular compromise.* He/she was deemed a suitable candidate for Lower Extremity Escharotomy and Fasciotomy.

Procedure in Detail Following satisfactory induction of anesthesia, the patient was placed in supine position, with *the lower extremities in neutral position,* and was appropriately padded. Timeouts were performed using both preinduction and preincision safety checklists with participation of all those present in the operative suite. These confirmed the correct patient, procedure, operative site, and additional critical information prior to the start of the procedure. The *right/left lower extremity,* was then prepped and draped in the standard sterile fashion. Marking of planned incisions was completed. Eschar edges were infiltrated with 1% lidocaine plus 1:100,000 epinephrine. Using *a scalpel/electrocautery,*

[Choose One:]
If lower extremity escharotomy: The eschar was incised medially, extending proximally from the adductor muscles, posterior to the medial malleolus, distally to the lateral aspect of the great toe. The incision was carried down to the subcutaneous tissue and immediate release of tissue pressure was observed. Attention was turned laterally, and this incision was carried distally from the hip, extending through the mid-lateral line, avoiding the common peroneal nerve, posterior to the lateral malleolus extending to the lateral surface of the fifth toe. Again, immediate release of tissue pressure was observed. Hemostasis was obtained using electrocautery and all wounds

were thoroughly irrigated. Adequate circulation was confirmed with palpation of pulses and compartments were noted to be soft. The wounds were then dressed with *Silvadene/antibacterial dressing/silver impregnated* along with an absorbent outer dressing.

If lower extremity fasciotomy: A longitudinal incision lateral and parallel to the tibia extending from the proximal leg to the ankle was performed. The incision was extended through the subcutaneous tissue until the fascia was identified while sparing large cutaneous nerves. Skin flaps on either side of the incision were elevated to expose the anterior and lateral compartments of the leg. The fascia overlying the anterior compartment was then incised longitudinally. The same was performed of the fascia overlying the lateral compartment. The underlying muscles were noted to bulge through the fascial incisions, signifying release. Our attention was then turned to the medial aspect. A longitudinal incision medial and parallel to the tibia was made extending from the proximal leg, a few centimeters below the knee, to a 3 cm above the medial malleolus. The incision was extended down to the subcutaneous tissue, until fascia was encountered. The superficial posterior fascia was incised in a longitudinal manner, releasing the superficial posterior compartment. The soleus muscle was then identified and incised until the deep posterior fascia was identified. The deep posterior fascia was then incised, again in a longitudinal manner along the length of the incision, releasing the deep posterior compartment. Adequate circulation was confirmed with palpation of pulses and compartments were noted to be soft. Hemostasis was then obtained using electrocautery. All wounds were thoroughly irrigated. *Sterile moist dressings* were placed within the incisions along with an outer absorbent dressing.

Upon completion of the procedure, a debriefing checklist was completed to share information critical to the postoperative care of the patient. The patient tolerated the procedure well, *was extubated in the operating room*, and was transported to the postanesthesia care unit in stable condition thereafter.

Excision and Autografting of Burn Wound

123

Rita D. Shelby and Renata B. Fabia

Indications and Benefits

- Full-thickness burn wounds
- Deep, nonhealing partial-thickness wounds
- Benefits: Acceleration of wound healing, decreased risk of infection of burn wounds

Risks and Alternatives

- Extensive bleeding, infection, need for additional procedures, and risks of anesthesia.
- Pain, hypothermia.
- Delayed healing.
- Removal of healthy tissue with mechanical debridement.
- Graft loss.
- Alternatives: VersaJet water dissector debridement and enzymatic debridement are effective alternatives for the removal of eschar from burn wounds when conservative mechanical wound debridement is not feasible due to bleeding disorders or other considerations. Of note, enzymatic debridement is typically reserved for chronic and nonhealing wounds.

Essential Steps

1. Adequate wound exposure and cleansing
2. Adequate excision of all devitalized tissue
3. Hemostasis
4. Harvesting of sufficient split-thickness skin graft from appropriate donor area
5. Application of graft tissue to wound bed
6. Application of appropriate burn dressing to grafted area and donor site

Note These Variations

- None

Template Operative Dictation

Preoperative Diagnosis *Deep partial-thickness/ full-thickness* burn, *burn wound infection*, %TBSA, size, location

Postoperative Diagnosis Same as preoperative diagnosis

R. D. Shelby
Nationwide Children's Hospital, Ohio State University Wexner Medical Center, Department of Pediatric Surgery, Columbus, OH, USA

R. B. Fabia (✉)
Nationwide Children's Hospital, Pediatric General Surgery, Columbus, OH, USA
e-mail: Renata.Fabia@nationwidechildrens.org

D. J. Papandria et al. (eds.), *Operative Dictations in Pediatric Surgery*,
https://doi.org/10.1007/978-3-030-24212-1_123

Findings *Deep partial-thickness/full-thickness* burn to (area of body)

Procedure(s) Performed Excision of burn tissue from {area of the body} and split-thickness skin graft from {area of the body} to {area of the body in % TBSA for children <10 years old, and in cm^2 for children >10 years old)

Anesthesia *General/regional*

Drains *None/dressing drains for irrigation of silver sustained-release dressing*

Estimated Blood Loss ___

Indications This is a/an ___-day/week/month/year-old male/female with *deep partial-thickness/full-thickness* burn to *body area*. He/she was deemed to be a suitable candidate for Excision and Autografting of Burn Wound.

Procedure in Detail Following satisfactory induction of anesthesia, the patient was placed in *supine/prone position* and appropriately padded. Timeouts were performed using both preinduction and preincision safety checklists with participation of all present in the operative suite. These confirmed the correct patient, procedure, operative site, and additional critical information prior to the start of the procedure. Precaution was taken to assure preservation of body temperature including warming of the operating suite, use of heat lamps, and warm irrigation solution. The preexisting wound dressing was removed in stages to ensure temperature preservation, and appropriate monitoring devices were secured. The *site of burn and site of donor tissue* were then prepped and draped in the usual sterile fashion.

A *Weck Goulian/Watson knife/Rosenberg knife/sharp scissors/dermatome/VersaJet* was used to excise *necrotic/devitalized* from the *body areas* extending to the *deep dermis/subcutaneous tissue/fascia* until well perfused, viable tissue was encountered. This was performed sequentially with intervals to assure appropriate hemostasis with *topical hemostatic product/application of direct pressure/epinephrine-soaked sponges/Thrombin spray and/or electrocautery.* After achieving satisfactory excision and hemostasis, the wound was covered with sterile moist sponges, to avoid drying of tissue.

Attention was turned to the donor site. The *body area* was exposed, *hair removed/not removed,* and mineral oil was applied to *body area*, ensuring to adequately cover entire donor site. The *Zimmer/De Soutter/etc.* dermatome set at *thickness* was utilized to harvest a *size in cm* split-thickness skin graft. The harvested skin was then placed in normal saline to preserve moisture. Hemostasis to the donor site was obtained using *topical hemostatic product/application of direct pressure/epinephrine-soaked sponges/Thrombin spray and/or electrocautery.*

The harvested skin graft sheets were then meshed *in number-ratio* using *Zimmer/Brennen/etc.* skin graft mesher. Once adequate mesh was obtained, skin graft was placed on prepared burn wound bed, trimming and adding subsequent sheets to adequately fit the size and shape of the wound. The graft was secured to the wound by *silk/nylon/etc. sutures/ skin staples/ fibrin glue/gauze dressing/ and/or non-adherent dressing.*

The grafts were covered with *name of dressing, followed by burn fluffs and wrapped with name of wrapping product or wound Vacuum-Assisted Closure (VAC) closure device with continuous negative pressure set at (mmHg) and the presence of no air leak was confirmed.* Splints were applied over dressing to keep *name joints* in functional position and were then secured with conform wrap. Donor sites were dressed with *Xeroform gauze/Telfa nonadherent gauze/Vaseline gauze/etc.*

Upon completion of the procedure, a debriefing checklist was completed to share information critical to the postoperative care of the patient. The patient tolerated the procedure well, *was extubated in the operating room*, and was transported to the *postanesthesia care unit/Intensive care unit* in stable condition thereafter.

Burn Contracture Release

124

Rita D. Shelby and Renata B. Fabia

Indications and Benefits

- Hypertrophic scar causing limitation of function of affected body part
- Hypertrophic scarring resulting in contracture of surrounding structures and associated pain
- Benefits: Release of skin tension, relief of pain associated with hypertrophic scarring, and improved joint range of motion

Risks and Alternatives

- Extensive bleeding, infection, need for additional procedures, and risks of anesthesia.
- Wound dehiscence.
- Scar widening.
- Further hypertrophy of scars.
- Hyperpigmentation.
- Keloid formation.
- Alternatives: Serial casting or prolonged splinting, as well as new techniques including autologous fat grafting, gene therapy, laser contracture release, and local injection of substances that inhibit scar formation. Use of tissue expander, free flaps, and other surgical techniques exists in the treatment of burn contracture release, but are beyond the scope of this chapter.

Essential Steps

Contracture Release, Scar Lengthening, Placement of Skin Substrate

1. Adequate contracture site exposure and cleansing
2. Marking of sites of excision
3. Excision and incision of contracted tissue, development of flaps
4. Z-plasty, V-Y plasty or other lengthening procedure, and preparation of wound bed for placement of skin substrate
5. Placement of skin substrate (Matrix, Integra, etc.)
6. Application of dressing

Placement of Skin Graft

1. Adequate contracture site exposure and cleansing
2. Marking of sites of excision

R. D. Shelby
Nationwide Children's Hospital, Ohio State University Wexner Medical Center, Department of Pediatric Surgery, Columbus, OH, USA

R. B. Fabia (✉)
Nationwide Children's Hospital, Pediatric General Surgery, Columbus, OH, USA
e-mail: Renata.Fabia@nationwidechildrens.org

D. J. Papandria et al. (eds.), *Operative Dictations in Pediatric Surgery*,
https://doi.org/10.1007/978-3-030-24212-1_124

3. Excision and incision of contracted tissue, development of flaps
4. Preparation of wound bed for placement of skin graft
5. Harvesting full-thickness skin graft from appropriate donor site
6. Processing and placement of skin graft
7. Closure of donor site and application of dressings

Note These Variations

- None

Template Operative Dictation

Preoperative Diagnosis Burn contracture to (area of body)

Postoperative Diagnosis Same as preoperative diagnosis

Findings Same as postoperative diagnosis

Procedure(s) Performed Burn contracture release (area of the body) with *Z-plasty/V-Y-plasty/other lengthening procedure/ and/or placement of named skin substrate/or full-thickness skin graft* from (area of the body).

Anesthesia *General/regional*

Drains None

Estimated Blood Loss ___

Indications This is a/an ___-day/week/month/year-old male/female with *hypertrophic scar of (body part) causing limitation of function of (body part)/hypertrophic scarring of (body part) leading to pulling of surrounding structures and associated pain*. He/she was deemed to be a suitable candidate for burn contracture release.

Procedure in Detail Following satisfactory induction of anesthesia, the patient was placed in *supine/prone position* and appropriately padded. Timeouts were performed using both preinduction and preincision safety checklists with participation of all present in the operative suite. These confirmed the correct patient, procedure, operative site, and additional critical information prior to the start of the procedure. The *site of contracture and site of donor tissue* were then prepped and draped in the usual sterile fashion, and abduction of *extremity* was performed to fully expose contracture.

A marking pen and ruler was utilized to plan the incisions, as well as the *skin flap advancement/or donor* burn contracture release: template operative dictation: *site area*. A *scalpel/electrocautery* was used to incise the scar in a series of *Z/V-Y/linear fashion along the length of the contracted scar for total length of incision/elliptical excision extending to the subcutaneous area ensuring good blood supply*. Flaps were raised, appropriately undermined and scar tissue carefully excised. Hemostasis was achieved using electrocautery. After ensuring satisfactory release of the tension on *skin/tendons/subcutaneous tissue* and desired range of motion of the *joint/commissure/anatomic area*, the wound was reassessed for appropriate closure.

If Lengthening Procedure: *Z-plasty/V-Y/other plasty* total length *in cm* technique was performed and followed with laying the flaps in appropriate order to lengthen the scar. The flaps were then sutured in place using *named suture* in an *interrupted/continuous* fashion.

[Choose One:]

If Skin Substrate: The created *size in cm* wound was covered with skin substrate of *meshed or non-meshed Integra/wound Matrix/other product* and secured in place using *named suture/skin staples*.

If Skin Graft: Our attention was turned to harvesting a full-thickness skin graft from *body area*. After infiltrating skin with saline and 1:200000 epinephrine, an elliptical incision in the direction of natural skin creases was made. A segment of full-thickness skin measuring *size in* *cm* was excised using *a scalpel/electrocautery*. All attachments to subcutaneous tissue were removed sharply using dissecting scissors. The graft tissue was placed in sterile saline to keep moist. Then, primary closure of the donor site was performed using named *suture* in a layered fashion *after undermining the wound edges*. The graft was then positioned dermis down and trimmed to fit wound bed. It was then secured to the wound edges using *named sutures,* followed by a series of "pie-crust" incisions on the surface of the graft to ensure drainage of any potential collection of fluid. The wound was dressed with *bolster dressing/gauze fluffs/*etc. and the donor site was dressed with *gauze fluffs/Kerlix roll/*etc. The area was wrapped with *Ace bandage/ coban/*etc. and the *splint/cast* was applied with the *body part* in functional position to prevent contracture.

Upon completion of the procedure, a debriefing checklist was completed to share information critical to the postoperative care of the patient. The patient tolerated the procedure well, *was extubated in the operating room*, and was transported to the *post anesthesia care unit/Intensive care unit* in stable condition thereafter.

125 Placement of Peritoneal Dialysis Catheters

Rebecca M. Rentea and Richard J. Hendrickson

Indications

- Access for peritoneal dialysis

Risks and Alternatives

- Standard risks (bleeding, infection, need for additional procedures, and risks of anesthesia)
- Injury to adjacent structures
- Bacterial or fungal peritonitis
- Bowel perforation
- Catheter site infection
- Catheter migration
- Catheter obstruction

Essential Steps

1. Access the peritoneal cavity via the umbilicus.
2. Insert the catheter (Pediatric Swan Neck Curl Cath Catheter into the peritoneal cavity).
3. Place the proximal cuff in the preperitoneal space.
4. Create a tunnel from the catheter entrance to exit site.
5. Place the distal cuff in the subcutaneous tissue at least 2 cm from the exit site and no sutures at exit site.
6. Exit site should be lateral and downward facing.
7. Flush the catheter several times to ensure satisfactory function and flow of the catheter once completely inserted and after abdominal closure.

Note These Variations

- Laparoscopic versus open
- Type and size of catheter
- Positioning of exit site

Template Operative Dictation

Preoperative Diagnosis *Renal failure/acute kidney injury*

Postoperative Diagnosis Same as preoperative diagnosis

Findings Same as postoperative diagnosis

Procedure(s) Performed *Open/Laparoscopic* placement of peritoneal dialysis catheter

R. M. Rentea (✉) · R. J. Hendrickson
Children's Mercy, University of Missouri -Kansas City, Department of Pediatric Surgery, Kansas City, MO, USA
e-mail: rrentea@cmh.edu; rjhendrickson@cmh.edu

D. J. Papandria et al. (eds.), *Operative Dictations in Pediatric Surgery*,
https://doi.org/10.1007/978-3-030-24212-1_125

Anesthesia *General*

Specimen Omentum

Implants __ Fr, __ cm peritoneal dialysis catheter

Indications This is a/an ___-year-old male/female with renal insufficiency requiring dialysis. *He/she* was deemed to be a suitable candidate for placement of a peritoneal dialysis catheter.

Procedure in Detail Following satisfactory induction of anesthesia, the patient was placed in supine and appropriately padded. Timeouts were performed using both preinduction and preincision safety checklists with participation of all present in the operative suite. These confirmed the correct patient, procedure, operative site, and additional critical information prior to the start of the procedure. The abdomen was then prepped and draped in the usual sterile fashion. A catheter was chosen based on size by measuring the distance between the umbilicus and the symphysis pubic. The location of the exit site of the catheter was marked on the patient's right side halfway between the mid-clavicular and anterior axillary lines, and out lateral and inferior to the initial incision located just lateral to the umbilicus.

[Choose One:]

If Open: A 2-cm vertical incision was made in the anterior rectus sheath approximately 2–3 cm below the umbilicus. The incision was deepened through the subcutaneous tissues. Hemostasis was assured. The anterior rectus sheath was opened and the muscle fibers bluntly dissected. The posterior rectus sheath was sharply incised and the abdominal cavity entered. A partial omentectomy was performed. Adequate area for peritoneal dialysis was visualized within the abdominal cavity. The patient was placed in the Trendelenburg position, and the catheter was placed over a stylet and advanced into the peritoneal cavity. The intraperitoneal segment was advanced into the peritoneal cavity and the cuff into the preperitoneal space. The peritoneum and rectus sheaths were closed with __ *absorbable suture* ensuring that the catheter was not caught in the suture line. A tunnel was created to the exit site *lateral/caudal* to the entrance site. The distal cuff was placed subcutaneously 3–4 cm from the exit site. The wound was copiously irrigated. Scarpa's fascia was closed with *3*-0 Vicryl.

If Laparoscopic: Access is gained to the peritoneum via the umbilicus with a 5 mm trocar and establish a pneumoperitoneum of 12–15 mm Hg with carbon dioxide. Laparoscopy allows for complete inspection of the peritoneal cavity for any pathology and to also identify patent internal inguinal rings. If patent internal rings are identified, then either laparoscopic or open inguinal hernia repairs are performed. *An additional 5-mm assist port was placed in the left upper quadrant to help facilitate visualization and to permit deployment of a grasper to manipulate the catheter.*

If Omentectomy Performed: Next, we performed an omentectomy. The available omentum was retrieved via the umbilicus and sequentially ligated with the LigaSure vessel sealer/Vicryl ties and electrocautery. The omentum was then *retrieved in an EndoCatch bag/passed off the field* and discarded.

The appropriate length Swan dual cuff curl catheter based upon the patient's size is chosen. After marking out the anticipated catheter track on the skin of the abdomen, an incision was made in the skin to the right of midline and the dissection is carried down to the anterior fascia of the rectus muscle where a transverse incision is made. A purse-string monofilament suture was placed in the anterior fascia. Next, a STEP access needle and sheath were inserted through this opening and carefully advanced to the preperitoneal space with laparoscopic guidance. The sheath was tilted and carefully advanced in the preperitoneal space downward toward the pelvis where it was allowed to enter the peritoneum just above the dome of the bladder. Once fully deployed within the peritoneal cavity, the needle was removed, and the sheath left in place.

A Peel-Away Introducer Sheath Set was inserted, starting with placing the included guidewire through the STEP sheath and advancing it into the pelvis under direct visualization. The STEP sheath was removed and the dilator and sheath was advanced over the guidewire down into the pelvis. The guidewire and dilator were removed leaving the 20-French sheath down in the pelvis.

Next, the dialysis catheter was inserted and advanced through the Peel-Away sheath. The Peel-Away sheath was then removed while holding the cuff with a pair of forceps below the level of the anterior rectus sheath. Once the sheath was removed, the cuff remained below the rectus muscle.

A 5 mm grasper was deployed per the assist port to direct the catheter into an optimal position. Laparoscopy was used to confirm that the radio-opaque stripe was not twisted and that the inner cuff has not migrated into the peritoneum. Next, a second incision was made out lateral and inferior to the initial incision so that the second cuff was positioned within the tunnel about 2 cm from the exit site, and the catheter was facing in a downward position. The catheter was then tunneled from the first or medial incision downwards and laterally.

Once flow into the catheter and drainage out of it was documented, the anterior fascia purse-string suture was tied around the catheter to help anchor the cuff under the anterior rectus sheath to prevent leakage. The subcutaneous tissue was closed in layers followed by skin closure. The fascia was then closed with *3*-0 Vicryl.

Incisions were then closed using *5*-0 Vicryl in subcuticular fashion and a sterile dressing was applied. No sutures were placed at the catheter exit site. The catheter was instilled with saline and was allowed to drain and showed no evidence of hemoperitoneum or fecal contamination. A sterile dressing was then applied at the catheter site *with the assistance of the dialysis team.*

Upon completion of the procedure, a debriefing checklist was completed to share information critical to the postoperative care of the patient. The patient tolerated the procedure well, *was extubated in the operating room*, and was transported to the postanesthesia care unit in stable condition thereafter.

Index

D. J. Papandria et al. (eds.), *Operative Dictations in Pediatric Surgery*,
https://doi.org/10.1007/978-3-030-24212-1

The manufacturer's authorised representative in the EU is Springer
Nature Customer Service Centre GmbH, Europaplatz 3, 69115 Heidelberg,
Germany. If you have any concerns regarding our products, please
contact ProductSafety@springernature.com

Printed and bound by CPI Group (UK) Ltd, Croydon, CR0 4YY
05/10/2026
02228132-0012